P9-AOJ-770

More Anti-Inflammation Diet Tips and Recipes

Protect Yourself from Heart Disease, Arthritis,
Diabetes, Allergies, Fatigue and Pain

Jessica K. Black, ND

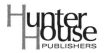
Hunter House PUBLISHERS

Copyright © 2013 by Jessica K. Black, ND

All rights reserved. No part of this publication may be reproduced or transmitted in any form or by any means, electronic or mechanical, including photocopying and recording, or introduced into any information storage and retrieval system without the written permission of the copyright owner and the publisher of this book. Brief quotations may be used in reviews prepared for inclusion in a magazine, newspaper, or for broadcast. For further information please contact:

Hunter House Inc., Publishers
PO Box 2914
Alameda CA 94501-0914

Library of Congress Cataloging-in-Publication Data
Black, Jessica.
More anti-inflammation diet tips and recipes : protect yourself from heart disease, arthritis, diabetes, allergies, fatigue, and pain / Jessica K. Black, ND.
pages cm
Includes bibliographical references and index.
ISBN 978-0-89793-621-7 (pbk.) — ISBN 978-0-89793-622-4 (spiral)
1. Inflammation—Diet therapy—Recipes. I. Title.
RB131.B584 2012
641.5'6318—dc23   2012030028

Project Credits

Cover Design: Brian Dittmar Design, Inc.

Book Production: John McKercher

Dev. Editor: Mary Claire Blakeman

Copy Editor: Kelley Blewster

Proofreader: Lori Cavanaugh

Indexer: Nancy D. Peterson

Managing Editor: Alexandra Mummery

Acquisitions Assistant: Susan McCombs

Editorial Intern: Tu-Anh Dang-Tran

Special Sales Manager: Judy Hardin

Rights Coordinator: Candace Groskreutz

Customer Service Manager:
Christina Sverdrup

Order Fulfillment: Washul Lakdhon

Administrator: Theresa Nelson

Computer Support: Peter Eichelberger

Publisher: Kiran S. Rana

Printed and bound by Sheridan Books, Ann Arbor, Michigan
Manufactured in the United States of America

9 8 7 6 5 4 3 2 1   First Edition   12 13 14 15 16

DETROIT PUBLIC LIBRARY

3 5674 05507793 8

More Anti-Inflammation Diet Tips and Recipes

"Modern medicine does not always have answers for the prevention and healing of inflammatory syndromes. This book should provide a comprehensive guide for both patients and clinicians who treat these conditions. Dr. Black's experience and insight is encyclopediac, and she brings this to the table with finesse."

— Navnit Kaur, MD
Board Certified Anesthesiologist, Portland, Oregon

"*More Anti-Inflammation Diet Tips and Recipes* by Jessica Black, ND, is a superb book that I will be frequently recommending to my patients. Dr. Black's original book made a profound impact on both my personal and professional lives, and I have had many patients incorporate her ideas and recipes with great improvements in their health. Thank you, Dr. Black, for providing such a great resource!"

— Sarah Vlach, MD
Physiatrist, Idaho Falls, Idaho

CHASE BRANCH LIBRARY
17731 W. SEVEN MILE RD.
DETROIT, MI 48235
578-8002

"I was a big fan of Dr. Black's first book about the anti-inflammatory diet. I used it to train my staff and to educate my patients, and I am very grateful to her for providing such a resource to me. So needless to say, I was excited to read her follow-up to that book. My particular therapeutic approach is to decrease inflammation and increase micronutrient health for my patients, so it's no surprise that this book is very useful to me professionally.... The recipes themselves are wonderful! Easy-to-follow, with 'healthy tidbit' points of education and nutritional analyses, the recipes are edifying and satisfying! I highly recommend this book to any health-care practitioner or any patient. It is essential to the integrative approach to healing!"

— Dushyant Viswanathan, MD, Integrative Internist,
Medical Director of The Columbia Center
for Integrative Medicine, Elkridge, Maryland

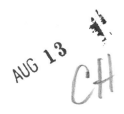
AUG 13
CH

✖

DEDICATION

This book is dedicated to my wonderful family:
my two beautiful daughters and my spirited husband.

Other Books by Jessica K. Black
The Anti-Inflammation Diet and Recipe Book
*Living with Crohn's and Colitis: A Comprehensive Naturopathic Guide
for Complete Digestive Wellness*

Ordering
Trade bookstores in the U.S. and Canada please contact:

Publishers Group West
1700 Fourth Street, Berkeley CA 94710
Phone: (800) 788-3123   Fax: (800) 351-5073

For bulk orders please contact:
Special Sales
Hunter House Inc., PO Box 2914, Alameda CA 94501-0914
Phone: (510) 899-5041   Fax: (510) 865-4295
E-mail: sales@hunterhouse.com

Individuals can order our books by calling (**800**) **266-5592**
or from our website at **www.hunterhouse.com**

Contents

* Detailed recipe listings for each section are given on these pages.

Important Note

The material in this book is intended to provide a review of information regarding an anti-inflammation diet. Every effort has been made to provide accurate and dependable information. The contents of this book have been compiled through professional research and in consultation with medical professionals. However, health-care professionals have differing opinions, and advances in medical and scientific research are made very quickly, so some of the information may become outdated.

Therefore, the publisher, authors, and editors, as well as the professionals quoted in the book, cannot be held responsible for any error, omission, or dated material. The authors and publisher assume no responsibility for any outcome of applying the information in this book in a program of self-care or under the care of a licensed practitioner. If you have questions concerning your nutrition or diet, or about the application of the information described in this book, consult a qualified health-care professional.

Introduction

I have found that the best way to combat chronic inflammation is to incorporate anti-inflammatory foods into one's daily diet. That is why I am sharing new recipes with you in this book, which complements my previous book *The Anti-Inflammation Diet and Recipe Book*.

Chronic inflammation is directly connected to many chronic health problems, ranging from arthritis and Alzheimer's to diabetes and heart disease. No matter your age or health status, an anti-inflammation diet will provide some benefit to you. In my experience working with thousands of patients, those who've adopted some or all aspects of this diet have enjoyed significant improvements in health, including but not limited to weight loss, improved lipid profiles, decreased pain, improved energy, improved mood, and reduced allergies and asthma symptoms.

This book can be used as a guide for you to follow to improve your dietary and lifestyle habits and reduce your risk for chronic disease. Besides new recipes, it offers more thorough and updated research on the effects of inflammation. And it is full of personally tested tips and tricks for adopting and maintaining an anti-inflammatory lifestyle for the long term. As a busy mom of two who also writes books and maintains two offices for my practice as a naturopathic physician, I understand the need for healthy food options that are also convenient. I will help you take those difficult first steps toward change by including meal-planning ideas throughout the book and by including a special tidbit of information with each recipe — sometimes pertaining to a spice used, and sometimes suggesting a simple lifestyle change for reducing stress, improving digestion, or preventing illness. I believe it is part of my duty as a naturopathic physician to educate as many people as possible about how to survive longer with better health. Surviving longer in poor health is not the goal here, which brings up the important topic of how we address illness and health in general.

Health Paradigm: Treat Symptoms or Treat People?

Broadly speaking, the paradigm followed by most practitioners of conventional medicine today is "diagnose and treat disease" or "diagnose and treat symptoms." Unfortunately, this model too often fails to actually get to the bottom of patients' ailments, even with a full battery of pharmaceuticals available to address the symptoms. Sometimes the symptoms are controlled and sometimes they are not, but nothing in the patient's internal environment changes. Nothing happens to improve the health of the patient and the course of his or her illness. The disease process remains intact and can even worsen under medicated symptom management. I like to describe this sort of symptom management as akin to a mechanic's clipping the wire to the "check engine" light. That light comes on for a reason, and if we simply prevent it from coming on without fixing the root cause, the problem will continue and possibly worsen. For example, elevated blood pressure is due to a malfunction of the heart, kidneys, or emotions. If it is treated only with blood pressure medication the underlying problem or problems will still exist, untreated. Over time, either a larger dose of medication will be required to eliminate the symptom or the patient will be switched to a different or stronger med. The scenario of a patient taking multiple and stronger forms of medication over the course of years to manage new or worsening symptoms is all too common.

In the last few decades, patients have come to understand the shortfalls of symptom-management medicine, and many are demanding something different. Consider how many individuals now consult with alternative practitioners compared to decades ago, and how many use natural products of all sorts, ranging from supplements to cosmetics to foods. The Centers for Disease Control and Prevention issued a National Health Statistics Report in 2007 that stated that almost 4 out of 10 adults (and 1 out of 10 children) use a form of complementary and alternative medicine (CAM).[1] Of the reasons provided in the report by people who use CAM, one of them was that mainstream medicine couldn't help them. Alternative-medicine practitioners multiply in number each year—and demand for our services continues to increase—because of the failure of symptom-management medicine to treat the root causes of illness. I have met many medical doctors at conferences who are eager to learn CAM therapies. Because patients are demanding a change, the physician who is willing to change and learn will be able to help more patients.

What Is Naturopathic Medicine?

A licensed naturopathic physician (ND) attends a four-year, graduate-level naturopathic medical school. The coursework includes all of the same basic science courses as conventional medical school. In addition, it emphasizes holistic and nontoxic approaches to therapy, with a strong emphasis on disease prevention and optimizing whole-body wellness. The naturopathic curriculum also includes training in clinical nutrition, homeopathic medicine, botanical medicine, naturopathic manipulation technique, and counseling. Naturopathic physicians take professional board exams in order to be licensed by a state or other jurisdiction as a primary care, general practice physician.

Naturopathic doctors rely on strict regimens of natural medicines to treat illness. Rather than trying to attack specific diseases, naturopathic physicians focus on cleansing and strengthening the body as a whole. Using the naturopathic approach to improving one's diet parallels a naturopathic approach to disease: Take away the causative factor. That's the main message of this book: Removing inflammation-causing foods results in less inflammation in the body and thus less of the damage and symptoms that are caused by inflammation.

Disease or illness ensues when the body loses track of how to maintain important daily rhythms that are vital to its survival. Sometimes disease comes on quickly, with symptoms that are visible or readily apparent. But sometimes disease is slow to form and keeps its indicators hidden deep within the body, where they must be discovered by blood tests or by symptoms that manifest subtly and gradually. This slow process is what occurs during chronic inflammation.

We now know more than ever the importance of reducing inflammation to maintain good health. Because chronic inflammation is linked to most of the fatal diseases affecting people in developed countries worldwide, if you want to enjoy good health it is important to assess your diet and lifestyle and make improvements where necessary. We cannot continue to ignore the fact that our current dietary practices have resulted in significant illness and obesity at epidemic levels. Comfort foods, fried goodies, too few vegetables, sweet drinks, and overprocessed foods are the major culprits.

Please know that it is possible to turn things around when it comes to your health, and it is never too late to make changes. Reducing inflammation will prolong your life and improve your health. In the chapters that follow I'll talk more about inflammation and its detrimental effects, and I will offer concrete actions that you can take to minimize inflammation and counteract its harmful effects. My intention in describing the pervasive problem of inflammation isn't to frighten you. Knowledge is power, as the saying goes, and my hope is that having this knowledge will inspire and empower you to create positive changes in your life and your health.

PART I

Inflammation and Wellness

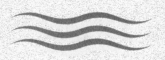

CHAPTER 1

What Is Inflammation and Why Do You Need to Reduce It?

Inflammation has become a hot topic in the last decade. Current research has helped us to understand that chronic inflammation is related to a host of illnesses, including some of the most deadly conditions worldwide. In this chapter I want to help you understand inflammation. Why does it matter? How do we know that chronic inflammation is harmful? What is the difference between "good" and "bad" inflammation?

Inflammation: An Overview

Inflammation plays an important role in our health. It is part of the intricate immune system, our body's first line of defense against bacteria, viruses, and other foreign invaders. Too much of a good thing, though, can be counterproductive and in some cases may prove deadly. Although the job of the immune system is to protect the body, when faced with long-term exposure to modern irritants like smoking, lack of exercise, and a diet of high-fat, high-calorie, and highly processed foods, the inflammation process goes into overdrive. These are the circumstances under which inflammation causes harm to bodily tissues.

The long list of irritants that may trigger a chronic (long-term) inflammatory response includes substances that were never meant to be ingested or absorbed by our bodies. We have created a toxic environment that can cause illness after long-term exposure, especially if those effects are not counteracted with positive lifestyle measures. Just a few of these offending substances are:

- air pollutants
- alcohol

- chemicals added to cosmetics, lotions, and other body-care products
- food additives/food dyes (e.g., MSG)
- harsh cleaning chemicals
- heavy metals
- hormones, such as the synthetic chemicals added to animal feed to encourage growth
- nicotine and chemicals added to cigarettes
- over-the-counter drugs
- pesticides
- pharmaceutical/prescription drugs
- preservatives
- radon
- street drugs

All of these dangerous substances, and many more that aren't listed here, pose potential threats to the body. When exposed to such toxins the body responds naturally by starting to attack. The attack may be so small in scale that you can't feel it or sense it. Often, the response may fail to show up on a blood test until a person is well into an illness.

How does inflammation help to guard a healthy body? It is a response from the immune system that serves to protect and heal tissue. Inflammation helps to heal injuries, prevent bacteria in a wound from becoming dangerous, repair tissue damage, and remove debris from the body. When the body is subjected to any sort of harm—from, for example, an insect bite, a viral or bacterial infection, an injury resulting in a cut or scrape, a joint sprain, a food allergy, or repetitive use of weight-bearing joints—the immune system initiates the inflammation process as a signal that cell repair and protection are needed.

In the case of viral or bacterial invasion, immune cells directed at defeating the offending organism are sent to the area to act as the first line of defense in an effort to decrease the foreign invader's ability to spread throughout the body.

In the case of a joint sprain, swelling, heat, and redness are the result of a direct and immediate inflammatory response whereby immune cells are delivered to the area to help rebuild and repair tissue. Inflammation also serves to immobilize the joint to prevent further injury.

In the case of the gastrointestinal system, inflammation plays a role in managing the impressive regulatory border.

A regulatory border within the body functions to allow access to important substances and to deny access to unwanted ones. It does so by using chemical messengers and hormones as "keys." The gastrointestinal tract is one of our most important regulatory borders. It permits healthful nutrients and beneficial bacteria into the body, and it keeps out unwanted microorganisms and potentially harmful larger food particles.

Inflammation at the Cellular Level
(A Discussion for the Science Buff)

A number of cells are important in the inflammatory cascade. The process of inflammation begins when the immune system triggers certain cells in the body to release cytokines, or proteins that send signals to other cells. Cytokines may be inflammation-promoting or inflammation-inhibiting. Cytokines that promote inflammation stimulate the release of immune cells locally (to one area of the body) or systemically (throughout the whole body).

The cells that release cytokines are known as leukocytes, or white blood cells; we generally think of them as our immune cells. In fact, there are several types of leukocytes, and all of them play a different role in the inflammatory process. To name just a few, monocytes are cells that engulf foreign invaders or material. T lymphocytes, or T cells, help to initiate and direct the immune response and form memory responses for future infections. B lymphocytes help to make antibodies needed for bacterial resistance. Lymphocytes are the cells that are often out of balance in inflammatory diseases.

These all-important leukocytes are produced and stored within the complex matrix of lymphatic tissue. The lymphatic system is comprised of the thymus gland, the spleen, the lymph nodes (located throughout the whole body), and the lymphatic tissue that lines the small intestine (called Peyer's patches, or aggregated lymphatic follicles). Lymphatic tissue and lymph nodes line every nerve and blood vessel in the body and function as a "highway" for immune cells and waste products. Immune cells use the lymphatic system to travel, repair, and fight. Wastes are constantly transported along the lymphatic system on their way to being exported through our main elimination organs: the kidney, liver, gastrointestinal tract, and skin.

Making sure the lymphatic system is working properly is important in the treatment of all diseases—especially inflammatory bowel disease—because as we eliminate waste, it reduces stress on the elimination organs like the bowel, thereby supporting improved function. Accumulation of toxins in the bowel can confuse the immune response in inflammatory bowel disease patients.

Another important leukocyte is the mast cell. The cytokines released by mast cells recruit all of the other types of immune cells to the site where the body is being attacked. The result is an immediate and robust inflammatory response. In the case of an injured ankle, for example, it is the mast cells that release the cytokines that cause the ankle to swell in as little as a minute after injury occurs. Mast cells appear to be the primary inflammatory mediator.

In addition to releasing cytokines, mast cells also secrete histamine, which is important in initiating local immune responses. Histamine is responsible for the irritation and redness you notice around a swollen bug bite. It stimulates blood vessels to allow larger quantities of white blood cells and proteins to pass through to an affected area to facilitate a successful attack on foreign invaders or to stimulate the healing response during an injury.

Histamine is good at stimulating the body to react, but it is sometimes responsible for heightening the response to an exaggerated or pathological degree. When histamine plays a part in a hyperreaction, it is referred to as an allergic reaction. Allergic reactions can vary in severity from mild to lethal. This is why medicines known as antihistamines can sometimes reduce inflammatory bowel disease symptoms; they reduce the body's allergic response as well as the inflammation caused by reactions to food or other chemicals. Histamines are also important in regulating function within the gastrointestinal tract.

Why Do You Need to Reduce Inflammation?

Now let's consider how inflammation can harm the body. When too much inflammation is present, it causes damage to tissues such as blood vessels and joints. In response, the body may create more inflammation in an attempt to fix the problem. This leads to a vicious cycle that is hard to break without drastically changing dietary and lifestyle habits.

Chronic inflammation (inflammation that is present for the long term) in an area of the body can cause a shift in the type of inflammatory cell found in the area, which can lead to destructive and healing responses taking place simultaneously. The body will maintain this balance as long as it can, but if the inflammation is present for long enough the harmful processes will start to win out, potentially leading to illness.

We now understand, much more clearly than we did even a decade ago, that inflammation plays a role in most chronic illnesses. In part this is because inflammation is such a widespread phenomenon within the body. Because inflammatory messengers ride along the highway of blood and lymph vessels, inflammatory processes can occur in the body's every nook and cranny.

Here is a list of some—but not all—of the diseases associated with inflammation:

Diseases Associated with Chronic Inflammation

- Alzheimer's disease, memory loss, and other forms of dementia[1]
- cardiovascular diseases[2] such as atherosclerosis, clotting, heart attack
- stroke
- diseases that end in the suffix "-itis" (e.g., arthritis, sinusitis, bursitis)
- periodontal disease[3]
- cystic fibrosis
- COPD (chronic obstructive pulmonary disease)[4]
- insulin resistance, diabetes[5]
- IBD (inflammatory bowel disease), Crohn's disease, ulcerative colitis
- celiac disease
- cancer[6]

Now let's take a look at a list of the top-ten health threats in the United States:

Top-Ten Health Threats in the United States According to the CDC, 2009[7]

- heart disease: 598,607 people affected
- cancer: 568,607 people affected
- COPD (emphysema, chronic bronchitis): 137,082 people affected
- stroke (cerebrovascular diseases): 128,603 people affected
- accidents (unintentional injuries): 117,176 people affected

- Alzheimer's disease: 78,889 people affected
- diabetes: 68,504 people affected
- influenza and pneumonia: 53,582 people affected
- kidney disease (nephritis, nephrotic syndrome, nephrosis): 48,714 people affected
- intentional self-harm (suicide and attempted suicide): 36,547

Placing this list side by side with the preceding one plainly answers the question of why you need to reduce inflammation: almost all of the top-ten health threats are directly related to inflammation. We all have a high likelihood of developing one of these health problems, each of which can lead to death. Of course, death is inevitable, but it's how we live until that moment that is important to me. We needn't live our lives resigned to the prospect of growing sicker and more disabled as we age. In a perfect world, one would be at one's healthiest for the longest time possible, then become ill and quickly perish without much suffering. It is my hope that individuals who care for themselves and their bodies attain this goal. It is not too late to take accountability for your habits and change them to enhance your future. You can also inspire your friends and associates to adopt healthier lifestyles by setting an example, and you can certainly influence your children's lifelong habits by introducing good practices into your home starting today.

Finally, I was shocked to see that the tenth leading health threat was suicide/attempted suicide. (This differed from 2007's statistics, which listed septicemia, or blood poisoning, as the tenth.) It's important to address your mental and emotional well-being as part of a holistic approach to health. Suicide is often preceded by depression, anxiety, or bipolar tendencies. If you feel your emotions are out of control, please seek help to obtain the balance you need.

Are You at Risk for Chronic Inflammation?

Sometimes it is clear from a person's genetic history that he or she is at risk for developing an illness that is related to inflammation. Obesity, heart disease, diabetes, and many other inflammation-related conditions run in families. Take a good look at your elders' and siblings' health history and decide for yourself if you may be at risk. I would say that most individuals are at risk for inheriting some form of inflammatory condition. Sometimes we inherit the probability through genetics, but we can also inherit it through learned behaviors around food, exercise, and our reaction to stress. Growing up in a household with family members who are sedentary and who frequently indulge in fast food almost guarantees that you'll need to apply yourself to adopt new habits.

Table 1. Inflammation Risk Factors

Risk Factors for Elevated Inflammation	Changes to Make to Alter the Risks
Diabetes, especially if poorly controlled	Eliminate all sugar and sugar substitutes
Family history of heart disease	Exercise, anti-inflammation diet (AI diet)
Gum disease	AI diet, visit a dentist, brush and floss often, don't allow mercury-amalgam fillings
Heart disease	Exercise, AI diet
Long-term, untreated infections	AI diet, take herbs to boost immune system and decrease inflammation
Obesity or excess weight	Lose weight, exercise
Poor diet	AI diet
Sedentary lifestyle, lack of regular exercise	Exercise
Smoking	Stop smoking
Stress	Exercise, meditation, deep breathing

Testing for Inflammation

Blood tests can help to determine a patient's level of inflammation. Here are a few of the more common ones.

Erythrocyte Sedimentation Rate (ESR) Test

Sed rate, or erythrocyte sedimentation rate (ESR), can be tested at a doctor's office to determine how much inflammation is present in one's system. This figure is not a stand-alone diagnostic tool but along with other blood work and a complete history and physical can be extremely helpful in diagnosing and treating a patient. When a patient's blood is placed in a tall, thin tube, red blood cells (erythrocytes) gradually settle to the bottom. Inflammation can cause the cells to clump together. Because clumps of cells are denser than individual cells, they settle to the bottom more quickly. The sed rate test measures the distance red blood cells fall in a test tube in one hour. The farther the red blood cells have descended, the greater the inflammatory response of the patient's immune system. ESR is often elevated in individuals suffering from arthritis or an autoimmune disease. ESR may be more helpful in monitoring a patient's response to treatment than in determining a diagnosis.

C-Reactive Protein Test

Often, ESR is coupled with other tests. CRP, or C-reactive protein, is another major test that reveals chronic inflammation. The level of CRP, a protein found in the blood, rises in response to inflammation. It's important to note that levels of CRP increase and decrease slowly; therefore, low-grade inflammation can be present without the elevation of CRP or ESR.

Blood Tests for Heart Disease

Other blood tests are specific for heart disease risk. It is no longer enough to simply measure your total cholesterol and your blood pressure. When getting blood work done, other tests should be included, such as CRP, a full lipid panel including triglycerides and types of cholesterol, apolipoprotein B, homocysteine, fibrinogen, lipoprotein A, and brain natriuretic peptide, also called B-type natriuretic peptide (BNP).

BNP, a protein produced by the heart and blood vessels, helps the body eliminate fluids, relaxes blood vessels, and funnels sodium into the urine. It may be present in high levels if the heart is under stress or damaged. Apolipoprotein B is a component of LDL, the "bad cholesterol" that helps facilitate the movement of cholesterol into the cells. Testing for levels of apolipoprotein B may reveal more about cardiac health than simply measuring LDL. Homocysteine is used by the body for repair; it helps to build and maintain tissue and is important in the manufacture of proteins. Elevated levels may mean your body is having to do repair work. Fibrinogen is a clotting protein. Excess fibrinogen can help gauge elevated clotting risk, plaquing risk, and risk of stroke.

As you can see, many of these markers tell us when there are deeper issues going on. This goes back to the unique ability of the body to do what is needed to survive. The body doesn't increase a substance like homocysteine to kill you. It does so because a repair job is needed somewhere.

Red Flags

Think of these cardiovascular markers in your blood work as red flags. "Oops, my cholesterol is up; I had better change something to improve it." Or, "Looks like my homocysteine is elevated; that means my body must be working on something. I should do all that I can to remove excess stress on the body to allow it to heal, and I should take action to support the cardiovascular system in general."

Pharmaceutical medications aimed at lowering cholesterol do only that: lower cholesterol. Yes, they may reduce the risk of heart attack, but they are not changing the picture or working to reverse the disease process that is occurring. In fact, they may be taking cholesterol away from important places that need it, like the brain. Cholesterol is a good transporter; therefore, if the body has high toxicity or inflammation, often cholesterol levels will increase. The solution to pollution is dilution. Cholesterol is a waxy, fatlike substance that tends to cause a diluting effect by swallowing the "bad" chemicals in the body. If the body is increasing cholesterol to act as protection, then it will be unlikely to give that cholesterol up. A cholesterol-lowering drug targets not only the cholesterol in the bloodstream but may also target the cholesterol that is used for other mechanisms such as hormone manufacture or nervous system support. Your body will be much more willing to let these mechanisms go because it will always prioritize survival. We know this by reviewing what occurs under stress. During an extremely stressful situation, the body will completely shut off digestion and healing, because it is more concerned about immediate survival. Let me repeat this: the body will do anything to survive. All symptoms we see are the result of the body's attempt to stay alive.

Let's face it. Inflammation, when uncontrolled, causes damage. It serves a purpose for healing from sickness or acute injury, but when left to linger in the body it harms healthy tissue. Inflammation has been associated with many illnesses that are extremely prevalent in our society; no one is immune from its effects. That means it's important to be proactive now about reducing inflammation by making good choices. Do it for your health. We can't eliminate all of the daily assaults on our bodies, so let's influence the factors we can. Paying attention to your diet is the easiest way to reduce the effects of inflammation. That's the topic of the next chapter.

CHAPTER 2

Addressing the Dietary Triggers of Inflammation

The important triggers of inflammation are diet, other lifestyle habits, injury, stress, and environment. Diet is probably the most significant of these. That should come as no surprise. After all, it is fairly common knowledge that poor diet has been directly linked to many illnesses, such as diabetes, heart disease (including atherosclerosis), dementia, stroke, obesity, some types of cancer, and kidney disease—all of which we identified in the first chapter as being related to inflammation.

My understanding of inflammation has blossomed in the past few years as I have done more research on immune system balance and how food choices can affect inflammation.

Foods that cause inflammation are foods that are high in toxins, poor fats, artificial ingredients, unhealthy chemicals, and unwanted sugars. They are foods that aren't nutrient dense, are too easy to digest, and are too high in calories. The first half of this chapter examines the impact that a diet containing too many of these sorts of undesirable foods can have on inflammation levels. The second half describes the dietary changes you can make to reduce inflammation and improve your health.

Glycemic Index

Glycemic index measures a food's impact on blood sugar (glucose) levels. The higher a food's GI, the more elevated your blood sugar will become as a result of consuming that food. High-GI foods tend to be foods that are high in carbohydrates without the benefit of also being high in bulk, fiber, or nutrients. They are typically packed with sugar and calories. Regularly consuming such foods will result in abnormally elevated glucose levels, which can lead to metabolic issues, weight gain, and type-2 diabetes. The body is not meant to withstand a continued elevation in glucose.[1] Over time, consistently elevated glucose negatively impacts lipid levels, triglyceride levels, and inflammation levels. It leads to insulin resistance, weight gain, elevated blood pressure, poor mood, and disrupted sleep. For a table listing the glycemic index for many common foods, please visit www.glycemicindex.com.

The general rule for good dietary practice is to avoid all high-GI foods, considered to be anything with a rating of 70 or over. Consume only in moderation foods with a medium glycemic index, from 56 to 69. Eat generously all low-GI foods (55 or below). Low-GI foods control appetite better, facilitate weight loss, and reduce inflammation by reducing blood glucose levels.

Know that paying attention to the GI of the foods you eat is only one aspect of the anti-inflammation diet (AI diet). Just because linguini, for example, fits the bill by being low on the GI chart doesn't mean that you should indulge in endless servings of linguini. In fact, as you will learn later in the chapter, the AI diet encourages you to avoid eating gluten (a protein found in wheat and certain other grains) due to its inflammatory propensity.

Healthy and Unhealthy Fats

Unhealthy fats were discussed in depth in my first book, *The Anti-Inflammation Diet and Recipe Book*. What I will repeat here is that we should avoid *all* fried foods and fast foods. Certain frying practices can change the chemical structure of even a healthy cooking oil to produce what is known as a "trans fat." Other names for trans fat are "partially hydrogenated oil" or "partially hydrogenated fat." These unhealthy fats have a direct connection to inflammation, heart disease, and cancer. Our bodies don't utilize this type of fat in any way, so most likely the body tries to incorporate it in some location where it is not vital for survival. When my first book was published, there were no laws about labeling foods for trans fat content. But now, the amount of trans fat in a food must be printed on its label. So must the amount of unsaturated fats (the "good" fats) and saturated fats (the so-called "bad" fats).

Saturated fats, which come mostly from animal products, have also been directly linked to inflammation levels and heart disease. Saturated fats, however, unlike trans fats, do have a use in the body and when eaten in moderation in a proper form can be beneficial. If you are going to eat animal products, it is much safer to consume organic, grass-fed meat that is free of added hormones and other added chemicals. According to Janet Kim in an interview with Dr. David Katz, health experts are finally realizing that not all saturated fats are created equal.[2]

Besides the quality of the saturated fat, it is also important to consider *how much* you consume. Saturated fats should only be consumed in low to moderate quantities. When using coconut oil (a saturated vegetable fat) or butter for baking, the amount you use is small when compared to how much saturated fat you get from eating a steak. One of the benefits of saturated fats is their stability when subjected to the cooking process. A monounsaturated fat like olive oil is less stable and can actually change its chemical structure when overheated, resulting in a trans fat. Don't get me wrong: I love olive oil, and it is one of the three oils I use often in my house, but I rarely heat it, and when I do I use only low to medium-low heat.

Coconut Oil: Bad or Good?

Coconut oil is largely made up of saturated fatty acids, which are still somewhat controversial because of their link to elevated levels of LDL cholesterol (the bad cholesterol), which in turn have been linked to heart disease. This is why the FDA still doesn't recommend the widespread use of coconut oil. As noted, however, not all saturated fats are necessarily bad for you, when consumed in moderation. Research shows that coconut oil has been used by Pacific Island populations for generations, at levels amounting to as much as 30–60 percent of their daily caloric intake, with no evidence of increased heart disease risk.

Coconut oil is a very special saturated fat, being one of the few dietary sources of medium-chain fatty acids. Medium-chain fatty acids help boost metabolism and help the body utilize fat for energy, often aiding in weight loss.

One important saturated fatty acid found in coconut oil is lauric acid. Lauric acid, when made into monolaurin in the body, is helpful in boosting the immune system to fight off viruses. I don't have patients consume coconut oil therapeutically during an illness; rather, I have them supplement with either lauric acid or monolaurin. Still, eating coconut oil during an infection is not a bad idea.

While there is a general lack of research on the benefits of coconut oil, lauric acid and monolaurin have been shown in the laboratory to

(cont'd.)

Coconut Oil: Bad or Good? (cont'd.)

have antifungal and antiviral properties.[3] I have used both of them for over ten years for shingles, herpes simplex outbreaks, and influenza with excellent results.

In new research involving animal studies, coconut oil has shown promising results for treating diabetes and insulin resistance.[4]

I am a purist when it comes to oils. I want to consume very pure oils in their purest state. I only use oils that are minimally processed. As stated in my first book, I don't condone the use of canola oil, mostly because it undergoes quite a bit of processing to become safe for consumption. Pure canola oil contains erucic acid, an omega-9 fatty acid that makes the oil bitter. Omega-9 fatty acids promote inflammation in the body. Canola oil is processed at high temperatures to remove the erucic acid; therefore, the processing alone causes a risk of rancidity and oxidation.

Cold-pressed oils such as cold-pressed olive oil and cold-pressed sesame oil are much better, healthier oils. If you're using cold-pressed sesame oil, add it to the food right before serving to avoid heating the oil too high. Use olive oil for light sautéing only. At moderate temperatures it does an okay job of withstanding heat. For cooking at higher temperatures or for a prolonged time, I use mostly coconut oil or, occasionally, a little organic butter. Good fats are discussed again later in the chapter.

Palm oil is still too controversial and not well enough understood for me to add it to my and my family's diet, especially because olive oil, coconut oil, and a little bit of organic butter provide all the oils we need.

Food Additives

There are several reasons why so many people experience elevated inflammation from eating certain foods. In the case of food intolerances or allergies, the body reacts to the innate nature of the food and its chemical structure. In addition, due to high-stress lifestyles, a lack of live-enzyme content in our foods, and simple aging, most people suffer from low stomach acid. Low stomach acid results in poorly digested food fermenting in the stomach, a causative factor in inflammation and illness. And finally, most processed foods now contain so many artificial additives that the additives themselves pose significant risk for increasing inflammation and provoking allergenic or intolerant-type reactions. Pesticide residues, the heavy metals found in some fish, preservatives, coloring agents, flavoring agents, man-made (trans) fats, industrial waste chemicals — all of these unnecessary additives can have an impact on health, especially when considered cumulatively. Many pose potential harm to the immune system. Most, due to their irritating nature, can stimulate inflammatory processes.[5]

Take MSG, for example. An additive that works as a flavor enhancer, it is used in many foods and has a strong reputation for provoking allergic or sensitivity responses in some people. Some food dyes are known to increase asthma attacks and to exacerbate symptoms of ADD and ADHD. Pesticide residues have been linked to childhood cancers,[6] neurological conditions,[7] and other disorders.[8]

Food Allergies and the Importance of a Healthy Digestive Tract

Some of the most problematic substances in foods are allergens, which stimulate a response from the immune system. Allergens in foods can occur naturally, or they can be the result of artificial ingredients such as those listed above. Oral tolerance develops in infants as foods are gradually introduced to the gastrointestinal tract. (See Chapter 4 for recommendations on introducing new foods to babies.) Most of the time the body makes the decision to allow foods into the digestive tract without mounting a defensive immune reaction; this is important so that a wide variety of foods can be broken down into nutrients to be used by the body for energy. If oral tolerance develops incorrectly due to environment, genetics, or improper food introduction, allergies can result.

Interestingly, food allergies are often associated with low stomach acid (hydrochloric acid). To understand why, it's important to have a basic knowledge of digestion. Digestion is dependent on a three-step process of breaking down foods. The first step, called predigestion, occurs in the mouth and esophagus. The second step takes place in the stomach and relies on stomach acid and the enzyme pepsin. The third step occurs in the small intestine, where additional digestive enzymes complete the breakdown process and nutrient absorption finally occurs.

The digestion process can be negatively affected during any of these steps. The predigestion of food in the mouth and esophagus can be compromised by the simple act of failing to chew one's food thoroughly. It can also be affected by the foods we choose. Foods that are low in enzyme content or that are highly processed can lead to insufficient predigestion, resulting in undigested food landing in the stomach. Over time, this takes a toll on how much stomach acid our bodies can produce. Aging generally reduces the amount of stomach acid we produce. This natural phenomenon, coupled with the reduction in stomach acid triggered by poorly digested food passing into the stomach, can affect the second stage of digestion. The third step of digestion can be affected by an insufficiency of pancreatic digestive enzymes, leading to compromised digestion of food particles.

Compromised digestion, no matter the cause, simply means that larger food particles and proteins are entering the bloodstream. Larger proteins in the bloodstream lead to immune response and food allergies.

Another effect of low stomach acid is fermentation of undigested food in the bowel, resulting in symptoms such as gas, bloating, and upset stomach. (This is not the same thing as consuming fermented foods.) Fermentation of undigested food provokes a response from the immune system, usually resulting in increased inflammation through rising histamine levels. As explained in Chapter 1, histamine is an important substance in regulating the immune system's response to an invasion of foreign substances. But sometimes histamine overreacts, to an exaggerated or pathological degree, resulting in an allergic response. Antihistamines reduce allergy symptoms because they counteract histamine.

Magnesium is also needed to reduce histamine levels,[9] so be sure to supplement with magnesium for any allergy issues. Tranquility, a product from Herb Fusion that contains magnesium, comes in a highly absorbable powder form that is easy to take. Magnesium is the first supplement of choice for many of my patients. (In a vicious cycle, low stomach acid can also diminish levels of beneficial intestinal bacteria, which are needed for the absorption of magnesium. Low stomach acid both heightens allergic response, caused by increased histamine levels, *and* compromises the absorption of magnesium, which keeps histamine levels under control.)

As you can see, your digestive tract plays a major role in immunity and in counteracting inflammation; therefore, improving gastrointestinal function can have a huge impact on health. In fact, autoimmune diseases, some cancers, and all diseases associated with imbalanced immune response relate in one way or another to the health of the gut. The healthier the

GI tract, the stronger the immune system's ability to distinguish "friend" from "foe." That is, a healthy GI tract helps the body's immune response get better at determining which molecules to allow in and which to allow to pass out of the system, all of which decreases unnecessary inflammation. Simply put, the gastrointestinal tract—and what we feed it, how we nurture it, and how it developed—cannot be ignored when approaching any illness holistically.[10]

How do you determine if you have any food allergies? Conventional food allergy testing consists mainly of testing for levels of the antibodies known as IgG and IgE (immunoglobulin G and E). Antibodies are proteins made by the immune system to fight antigens, such as bacteria, viruses, toxins, and allergens. When their level is elevated, it signals that the body is responding to the presence of an invasive substance. Skin scratch testing can also be done to test for food allergies, but I prefer the IgE and IgG testing. However, I warn my patients to interpret the results with caution. No one wants to find out that they can't eat twenty-odd different foods or that they have a slight reaction to them. I now often urge against food allergy testing and instead suggest that a patient try an anti-inflammation diet (AI diet) for one month and then reintroduce foods one at a time while watching for reactions. This is a much more realistic and economical way to figure out what is ailing you.

Food Intolerances or Sensitivities

Food sensitivities and food intolerances are not the same as food allergies (which involve an immune system reaction) but are still important to understand when considering a person's overall health. Many people are lactose intolerant. This means that either they lack the enzyme lactase, which is needed to break down lactose, or the functioning of their lactase is less than optimal. It is my belief that as we age, our ability to digest dairy products decreases. Most people over age twenty-five should not consume dairy in the form of milk, cream, or ice cream. They may be able to tolerate some fermented forms of dairy (e.g., yogurt) or hard cheeses that are easier to digest. Truly lactose intolerant individuals can't tolerate eating dairy in any form.

Food sensitivities can be identified by following an elimination and challenge diet, in which a person eliminates a food entirely from the diet for at least one month, and then reintroduces the food to see if they notice a specific reaction. The elimination and challenge diet, as well as food allergies and sensitivities in general, were discussed in greater depth in *The Anti-Inflammation Diet and Recipe Book*.

The Anti-Inflammation Diet: Food Choices for Reducing Inflammation

So what do I mean by an anti-inflammation diet (AI diet), and how will it benefit you? What should you eat — and avoid eating — to minimize inflammation and maximize health? That's the focus of the rest of the chapter, in which we shift our attention from defining the problem to investigating the solution.

The results of following an AI diet have been reported on by many physicians who have prescribed it to their patients and have seen significant benefit in those who've followed it. Some practitioners of conventional medicine have disputed the idea that an AI diet really can prevent illnesses, though in February 2012, at the Integrative Healthcare Symposium in New York City, a physician lecturer stood by the AI diet as the best balanced diet currently available to suggest to patients.

Studies conducted on diets that are very similar to the AI diet have shown decreased health risks. Research consistently points to the benefits of consuming vegetables and whole grains, and to the negative effects of dietary choices such as high glycemic foods and processed foods. Studies have shown that the Mediterranean diet, for example, offers cardiovascular benefits presumably due to the amount of olive oil and vegetables consumed.

Further research from the last few years supports many aspects of the AI diet:

- In one study, a healthy diet led to improvement in mental and emotional health, including decreased symptoms of anxiety and depression.[11] The researchers defined a "healthy diet" as one that included fruits and vegetables as "core food groups" (i.e., that included two or more servings of fruit per day and four or more servings of vegetables). It generally avoided processed foods such as chips, fried foods, chocolate, sweets, and ice cream.

- Elimination diets have proven to be successful in treating ADHD.[12] Using the AI diet as a starting point for an elimination diet is ideal.

✦ Eating good-quality eggs doesn't result in cardiovascular risk, as was once believed. In fact, the fat in eggs is cardio-protective, not harmful.[13]

✦ Decreasing dietary sugar has been found to reduce irritable bowel symptoms.[14]

✦ Type-2 diabetics who consumed more nuts instead of carbohydrates enjoyed improved glycemic control and serum lipid levels.[15]

✦ Two large prospective trials have associated dairy intake with acne vulgaris. In addition, other prospective trials, including randomized, controlled studies, have shown a positive association between a high-glycemic-load diet, hormonal mediators, and acne risk. Based on the findings from these multiple trials, convincing data now exist to support the role of dairy products and high-glycemic-index foods in influencing hormonal and inflammatory factors.[16]

✦ High-protein and low-glycemic diets have proven beneficial in helping maintain weight loss. The DASH diet, which has been touted for treating hypertension, has been shown to facilitate weight loss, improve HbA1c (a blood test to measure historic glucose levels), decrease blood pressure, decrease blood sugar, and improve cholesterol in type-2 diabetics.[17] The DASH diet is high in fruits and vegetables and whole grains, and low in saturated fat, total fat, cholesterol, refined grains, and sweets.

✦ Reuters Health reported on two separate studies revealing that inflammation from celiac disease was related to heart disease and asthma.[18] Celiac disease has also been shown to be more prevalent in people with psoriasis, multiple sclerosis, reproductive problems, elevated liver enzymes, and obesity. It increases a patient's risk for neurological and psychiatric disorders. Late diagnosis of celiac disease has been related to a diagnosis of cancer, presumably because of the continued ingestion of gluten when it was causing problems for the patients.

As you can see, changing your diet to exclude inflammatory foods and include health-promoting foods is an excellent way to begin improving many aspects of your health. Below is a quick summary of dietary suggestions for the AI diet.

Important: I highly recommend incorporating these changes into your diet gradually rather than all at once. That way you're more likely to stick with them. I have developed a three-month plan for introducing the AI diet into your life. You can find it in Chapter 4.

Foods to Include and Foods to Avoid on the AI Diet

The table below will help you prioritize the foods you should strictly avoid ("primary") and the foods you may be able to tolerate ("secondary"). At first, if you feel the diet will be difficult for you to follow, you may want to avoid only the primary foods. This column of the table lists the main offenders. Then, once you've become more comfortable with the AI diet, also avoid the secondary foods. Within the list of secondary foods, the main offenders are potatoes and tomatoes. For someone in ill health, I would suggest eliminating all of the foods at once. The "foods to limit" are those that may not have a direct link to inflammation but can still cause health issues or inhibit optimal body functioning. You should limit consumption of these items to special occasions.

Table 2. Foods to Include and Foods to Avoid on the AI Diet

Foods to Include	Foods to Avoid–Primary	Foods to Avoid–Secondary	Foods to Limit
Cold-water fish that are low in mercury	All fast foods	Corn	Alcohol
Dark-green, leafy veggies	All hydrogenated oils/ fats ("trans" fats)	Dried fruit**	Caffeine
Fermented beverages and foods such as kombucha, kefir, or sauerkraut	All processed foods	Irritating grains (may vary from person to person; determine any negative reactions from your personal experience)	Chocolate
Flax oil	All refined sugars	Nightshade vegetables other than to-matoes and potatoes, e.g., peppers and eggplant	Fish high in mercury, tuna

Table 2. Foods to Include and Foods to Avoid on the AI Diet (cont'd.)

Foods to Include	Foods to Avoid–Primary	Foods to Avoid–Secondary	Foods to Limit
Fresh fruits	Dairy	Peanuts	Healthy sweets
Grass-fed, hormone-free meats, eggs	Food additives and chemicals such as MSG	Soy	Tomatoes
Green tea	Foods that trigger allergies/intoler-ances***		White rice
Healthy oils such as olive oil	Gluten (contained in wheat—including kamut and spelt—barley, rye, triticale, some oats)		
Mushrooms	Juice*		
Nutritional powders, e.g., kelp powder, spirulina powder (for more examples, see list in the recipe section for Smoothies)	Meats and eggs containing added hormones		
Nuts	Potatoes		
Rainbow of vegetables each week			
Root vegetables			
Seeds, including hemp and chia seeds			
Spices such as turmeric, ginger, and cinnamon			
Vinegars such as apple cider vinegar			

* Rare use allowed for desserts only—better than sugar for a sweet treat.
** Occasional use allowed for nondiabetics, but still keep to a minimum.
*** These can be tested for in various ways, ideally through an elimination and challenge diet.

More Dietary Do's and Don'ts
for Reducing Inflammation

In addition to adopting the suggestions outlined in the table above, if you pay attention to the following simple guidelines when choosing and eating foods, you will be well on your way to incorporating the AI diet into your daily life.

Engage the Power of Visualization

First, start with visualization. See yourself eating well and enjoying the foods you eat. Visualize yourself feeling full and satisfied, with a controlled appetite and a healthy relationship to food. See your plate filled with foods that are very colorful and appetizing.

Get Rid of Processed and Unhealthy Foods

Research demonstrates that diets high in minimally processed, high-fiber, plant-based foods will markedly blunt the postmeal (postprandial) increase in glucose, triglycerides, and inflammation. Experimental and epidemiological studies indicate that eating patterns that are similar to the traditional Mediterranean and Okinawan diets reduce inflammation and cardiovascular risk and promote longevity. The AI diet should be considered for the primary and secondary prevention of coronary artery disease and type-2 diabetes.[19]

Minimally processed natural foods are low in caloric density but high in nutrient density. They include fresh, unprocessed vegetables and fruits, lean proteins, antioxidants, and healthy fats such as omega-3 fatty acids. They are low in saturated fats and trans fats, processed carbohydrates, and sugars.[20]

Follow this guideline by making fresh vegetables and fruits the centerpiece of your diet. Include whole grains (but eliminate or minimize gluten-containing grains), legumes, and nuts. Include lean protein, vinegar, fish oil, tea, and cinnamon. If you drink alcohol, consume it at only low to moderate levels. Watch your caloric intake, lose weight if necessary, and get adequate exercise (more on this suggestion in the next chapter).

Choose Carbs Carefully

Choosing the right forms of carbohydrate can be important in determining one's risk for inflammation. Excess intake of processed carbohydrates sets up a vicious cycle whereby quick spikes in blood glucose and then insulin soon after a meal trigger reactive hypoglycemia and hunger an hour or two later. On the other hand, restriction of refined carbohydrates improves post-prandial glucose levels and triglycerides and can reduce intra-abdominal fat, a response that has been especially noted in individuals with insulin resistance.[21] This is not a new concept, yet I encounter many diabetics who haven't been told by their physicians to stop consuming all high-carbohy-drate foods such as bread, white rice, juice, potatoes, alcohol, and dried fruit. "Simple carbohydrate" doesn't have to only mean "sugar." Even nondiabet-ics need to watch their carbohydrate intake. The same principles apply to everyone when considering inflammatory risk related to blood sugar levels.

Deal with Cravings

If you find yourself with cravings for high-carb, highly processed foods, care-fully increase the amount of protein and fat you are consuming. A slightly higher intake of fat will often curb any cravings for sweets you may have. But make sure it's the right kind of fat.

Eat the Right Kinds of Fats and Oils

Earlier in the chapter I introduced the topic of healthy versus unhealthy fats and oils. Good fats are an important part of the diet. The body and brain function best when they receive the proper amount of fats, especially those that are high in essential fatty acids.

EFAs are necessary fats that the human body cannot synthesize; they must be obtained through foods or supplements. EFAs are long-chain polyunsaturated fatty acids derived from linolenic, linoleic, and oleic acids. There are two families of EFAs: omega-3 and omega-6 fatty acids. (Omega-9 fatty acids are necessary but are not considered "essential" because the body can synthesize them if they are not obtained through diet.)

Omega-6 fats, found in a variety of nuts and seeds, are common in our diets. Omega-3 fats occur less commonly. In most diets nowadays omega-3 fats need to be sought out. They are in my opinion the superior type of EFA because of their direct anti-inflammatory action. Omega-6 fats feed the inflammatory pathway but play an important role in immune system bal-ance. Omega-6 fats are vital, but because they are already abundant in the diet taking more omega-6 fats may, in fact, trigger the inflammatory cascade.

EFAs are studied regularly in regard to cardiac health; a recent study demonstrated their ability to reduce the risk of stroke and heart attack.[22]

Store your cooking oils in a cool, dark place and in dark bottles if possible. Purchase organic cooking oils whenever you can because fats have a high potential to carry toxic compounds.

Table 3. Good Fats to Include in the Diet

Fat	Type of Fat	Cooking Information
Coconut oil	Saturated fat, medium-chain fatty acid	Warming and high heat are usually okay; don't allow to reach the smoking point
Cold-pressed sesame oil	High percentage monoun-saturated, low percentage saturated	Low heat is okay; don't allow to reach the smoking point
Fish oil in the form of wild, cold-water fish or fish oil supplement	Omega-3, essential fatty acid	Don't heat
Flax seed oil (nonheated)	Omega-3, essential fatty acid	Don't heat
Oils from other seeds, e.g., chia, hemp	Omega-3, essential fatty acid	Don't heat
Olive oil	Monounsaturated fat	Warming is okay; don't allow to reach the smoking point
Organic butter	Saturated fat, long-chain fatty acid	Warming and high heat are usually okay; don't allow to reach the smoking point

Consume Only Grass-Fed, Organic Meats

Make sure the animal products you consume are organic, free of added hormones (certain hormones occur naturally in animal flesh, just as they occur in your body), and grass-fed. Meats that aren't organic are more likely to contain pesticide residues, antibiotic residues, and compounds such as heterocyclic amines (HCA) and polycyclic aromatic hydrocarbons (PAH), both of which have been linked to cancer. Select animal products that have undergone the least amount of processing that is possible. Eat local products if you can. Limit your consumption of animal products overall. Even though the AI diet allows for some organic, grass-fed beef, eating it daily can increase your risk for cardiac conditions and high cholesterol (due to its saturated fat content) as well as cancer. Large studies in England and Germany from the 1990s showed that vegetarians were about 40 percent less likely to develop cancer than meat eaters. Meat also lacks the protective fiber present in vegetables.[23] Likewise, it is important to make sure the chickens you consume are free-range and free of added hormones and antibiotics. Eggs from chickens fed properly contain much more nutrient potential.

Include Plenty of Vegetables

I can't stress enough the importance of including lots of vegetables in your diet. Choose a wide variety, and aim for more veggies than you're currently getting. It's probably safe to assume that no one eats enough vegetables. We were meant to get our nutrients primarily from plants; instead, nowadays people try to get their nutrients from boxes, bags, and cans. Practice adding one new colorful vegetable to your diet each week, and keep it in the next week when you add another. Drinking green drinks and smoothies is a great, quick way to add more vegetables. Pureeing and making sauces from veggies takes a little more time, but it's another way to add some vegetable bulk to your meal.

Avoid Sugar

Please understand that your body is not meant to consume the types of sugars available to us now. I keep only natural sugars in the house, such as pure maple syrup, honey, and stevia (which is a naturally sweet leaf; I have a plant in my house off of which I pick leaves when I need it). On rare occasions I may use agave syrup or brown rice syrup. I use these less often because the verdict is still out on agave syrup, and brown rice syrup must undergo processing to get to a usable state. They're not all bad, but I prefer the sweeteners that have been around for hundreds of years. Avoid all high fructose corn syrup and other artificial sweeteners, such as aspartame, sucralose, sorbitol, Splenda, and acesulfame potassium (these will be listed on labels). Note that a lot of organic products contain cane sugar. It is a better form of sugar than many sweeteners used in packaged foods because it is less processed, but it is still sugar, so reserve it for special occasions or use it with caution.

Eat Mindfully

Practice mindfulness when eating. There is a fairly large movement toward mindfulness in our daily living practices. Mindfulness is the art of performing tasks and participating in life in a completely present way. Bring mindfulness to all your activities by really thinking about what you are doing and paying attention to how you are doing it. Mindful eating is important because it will slow you down, allowing you to enjoy your food and to become full more readily than if you are eating on the go or in front of the TV.

Sit at a table with no media distractions such as phones, computers, or TVs. Arrange the food on your plate in a visually pleasing and artful manner. Consider the plate your palette: try to include a variety of colors. When you sit down to eat, appreciate your meal; take a moment to either say a prayer or to feel thankful for the food you will eat.

Remember to continue breathing—nice and slow—throughout the meal. Take the first bite, really taste it, and enjoy it. Set your fork or spoon down between bites, and take the time to savor each morsel. Often we taste the first mouthful and shovel in the rest. This isn't good for the appetite as it fails to produce the satiety that we want from a meal. Chew each bite twenty-one to twenty-five times—more if needed. Before you swallow, make sure you have completed the digestion that is supposed to occur in the mouth. Then allow yourself another bite. Remember, the second and tenth bite should be just as slow as the first bite. When you eat this way you will notice that you get fuller quicker, and you won't find yourself standing at an open fridge after the meal looking for something sweet.

Avoid drinking while eating. If you need something to drink, enjoy a few sips of water, but drink only enough to give your mouth moisture. Don't gulp, and don't drink more than one glass of water with your meal. Water dilutes the digestive enzymes found in the mouth and the stomach, which are needed to adequately break foods down for assimilation.

Creating a mindful eating environment is not always possible with families' busy work schedules, sports schedules, and various other commitments. If you are unable to practice mindful eating at every meal, make sure to set aside time each week to do so. Soon it will become part of your normal routine. You'll find yourself practicing mindful eating even when you aren't in the "ideal" environment for it.

Enjoy Meals as a Family

Family meals are extremely important for children and teenagers. Eating together with the family has been shown to decrease behavioral problems in teens. According to the National Center on Addiction and Substance Abuse at Columbia University (CASA), children who don't regularly eat dinner with their families are almost four times more likely to consider using alcohol, tobacco, or illegal drugs.[24] Setting boundaries with your children and teaching them good habits by example is the first step in raising well-adjusted young people.

Let's face it, everyone has problems, and families struggle with time demands and commitments, but maintaining routine and rhythm whenever possible can help ensure that your children understand who they are and what type of family they come from. It is important to teach them what your family values. I commonly repeat sayings to my children such as, "As a family, we eat well." "As a family, we eat together on Wednesdays and Sundays." "As a family, we are courteous to others." "As a family, we don't eat candy." "As a family, we eat our vegetables." You get the point. Teaching children who they are is important, but we can't just say it, we have to live it if we want our children to follow our example.

Breaking the Rules: How to Cheat

Cheating is okay, sometimes. You don't want to get into the habit of cheating, but you want to allow yourself some mistakes and some occasions when you just eat for the soul. As long as you keep your cheating to a minimum, you should be able to continue the AI diet for the rest of your life. Depending on your health, cheating may or may not cause consequences.

For people who are just starting the diet I usually suggest trying to be as strict as possible at first so that you can figure out what your body can and can't handle. Here's how: Follow the AI diet exactingly for at least a month, and then begin to reintroduce some of the foods you miss the most. Reintroduce foods one at a time, and wait at least three days before you add a new food so you can understand your body's reaction, if any, to the food you've reintroduced. Pay attention to symptoms such as mood changes, sleep changes, bowel or urination changes, skin changes, headaches, or pain in the muscles or joints. Some of these may be indicators that you cannot tolerate a certain food.

Once you figure out what ails you the worst, stay away from it as much as possible, and cheat on the foods that don't bother you as much. For example, I don't tolerate wheat or dairy that well, so I avoid them most of the time. Tomatoes don't seem to bother me, so I consume them sometimes, but not daily, and usually not even weekly, other than when they are in season. On the other hand, I really don't do well with potatoes, so I avoid them almost always. I don't indulge in a French fry, I don't eat mashed potatoes at holidays, and I avoid baked potatoes. A lot of gluten-free baking mixes contain potato flour, so I don't usually buy the commercial ones; I make my own mixes instead. And I can handle a little sugar, mostly in the form of natural sugars, coconut palm sugar, or honey powder. My family consumes white sugar pretty minimally unless we are at a birthday party or at someone else's house for dinner. In my home, the only white sugar I keep around is for making kombucha (a sparkling, fermented tea). All my baking is done without the use of white flour or white sugar, and by now I've developed many easy-to-follow recipes. You have to remember that I've been experimenting with eating, baking, and cooking like this for many years.

But I love to cheat sometimes! And if I cheat, I enjoy it. I don't fret about it. I just concentrate on keeping my portions small, chewing the food well, and considering it a boost for the soul.

If you find at first that any cheating causes reactions, don't allow yourself to cheat until your health improves. If you are suffering from a serious condition like cancer, I wouldn't cheat at all, or I would keep the cheating to an *extreme* minimum.

Tips for Eating Out

When you eat out, consider ahead of time what you are willing to let yourself eat and what you want to accomplish with the meal. Most of the time, the purpose of eating out is to enjoy a party of people socially, even if it is just your family. There is no time spent preparing food or cleaning up, so use this time to enjoy the people you are with.

Here are a few pointers for eating out:

- Order salads. You can even bring your own dressing if needed. Choose salads made with rich, dark greens like spinach or mixed greens rather than iceberg lettuce.
- Order grilled meats and fish with vegetable sides. Skip the potatoes and the bread.
- Don't let them bring the fries as your side dish because you may just eat them. Order a side salad instead.
- Want a burrito or wrap but don't want the tortilla? Order the insides served like a salad.
- Ask them to leave out the bun or bread that comes with the entrée.
- Skip the "special sauces" if you can, because most likely they will contain dairy, sugar, and gluten.

‒ Many restaurants now have gluten-free options, which can be very helpful. In most places you can order a gluten-free pizza with lots of veggie toppings (skip the cheese).

‒ Eat a snack containing protein and fat thirty minutes before you go out to help you control your appetite when ordering food. Good choices include avocado, celery with nut butter, apple with nut butter, or a small handful of raw nuts.

‒ To aid digestion, supplement with one or two capsules of a digestive enzyme before going out. Taking apple cider vinegar and/or lemon juice before a meal can also help. Drinking 2 teaspoons of apple cider vinegar or 1 teaspoon of lemon juice in a little bit of water prior to a meal can stimulate digestive capability.

Adopting the AI diet will set a foundation that supports and enhances all the other steps you take to improve your health. You will feel better and look better. But it is also important to exercise and to practice simple stress-reducing techniques. Stress is a leading cause of inflammation, and techniques focused on reducing stress can benefit you immensely. The next chapter will discuss these and other lifestyle causes of inflammation and offer tools to counteract them.

CHAPTER 3

Addressing Other Inflammatory Triggers

In addition to modifying your diet, there are many other steps you can take to reduce inflammation. Following the simple suggestions outlined in this chapter can empower you to live a longer, happier, healthier life.

Exercise Regularly

A sedentary lifestyle and a lack of exercise are triggers for inflammation. As a species we were meant to move, to run, to walk long distances, to gather food with others, and to stay physically fit. Sedentary jobs have been shown to increase the risk of inflammatory diseases and insulin resistance. Adopting a consistent exercise regime can improve health outcomes and decrease risk for chronic illness.

Studies reveal that regular exercise over a period of months to years is related to lower levels of inflammatory markers and a reduced risk of cardiovascular disease and other illness.[1] Short-term changes in exercise patterns—such as the sedentary person exercising hard for one week, or the exercise buff taking a week off—don't seem to affect inflammatory markers,[2] providing further support for the conclusion that exercise needs to be a lifelong habit, not something we pick up occasionally for a few weeks or only when we feel like it. My healthiest patients are the ones who exercise consistently.

It has been suggested that I avoid placing too much emphasis on exercise because regular exercise is the lifestyle change people find hardest to embrace. But I'm confident that everyone can find some form of physical activity that works for them and that they enjoy. If you have limitations or need help determining what type of exercise plan is right for you, talk with your doctor, and consider enlisting the help of a personal trainer. Even walking outside thirty minutes a day for most days of the week can offer immense benefits. I encourage my patients to exercise outdoors any time they can because being outside exposes you to fresh air, which increases your endorphins ("feel-good" hormones), and to sunlight, which provides vitamin D. Walk at a brisk enough pace to elevate your heart rate at least a little bit. If your health or fitness level is such that thirty minutes is too much, start where you can—walking for even five to ten minutes is better than nothing. If you stick with it, you will soon see improvement in your endurance, and that will motivate you to continue. Again, if you're not used to exercising, consult with your doctor before starting any exercise program.

For healthy individuals, thirty minutes of daily exercise is ideal, and forty-five minutes is even better. If your schedule doesn't permit daily exercise, then find a way to get that forty-five minutes in at least three to four days per week.

Here is a list of exercises that can be incorporated easily into a person's daily or weekly routine:

- running, walking, jogging, hiking
- yoga, either at a class, from a video, or following a home routine if you are trained or have a yoga instructor to help you
- Pilates, either at a class, from a video, or following a home routine
- stability-ball exercises
- treadmill, elliptical machine, or other cardio equipment
- cycling, either road- or mountain-biking
- team sports such as soccer or basketball
- tennis, racquetball, and handball
- dance-based aerobics such as Zumba or Jazzercise at a class, from a video, or following a home routine
- other forms of dance, such as taking a ballroom-dance class with your partner (as long as it keeps your heart rate up)
- skiing, kayaking, other outdoor sports

Choose an activity that resonates with you so you'll stay with it. If you try something and don't like it, try something else. If no activity seems to stick, please see a doctor or hire a trainer. Get help to figure out what is going on. It may be that you are unable to tolerate activity and need to be evaluated medically.

Manage Stress

Stress and a lack of mental/emotional wellness are huge contributors to illness and inflammation. Chronic stress, cynical distrust, and depression were linked with elevated levels of inflammatory markers in a large cross-sectional study published a few years ago in the journal *Archives of Internal Medicine*.[3] Numerous other studies support the finding that negative emotions increase inflammatory markers. When we are under stress, our bodies secrete the same chemicals that trigger inflammation.

Calming the brain is important. Calming the body is important. Reducing stress is important. Almost everyone knows by now that stress can cause disease and can eventually kill, but many do nothing about it, continuing to live their day-to-day lives in turmoil. This doesn't have to be the case. There are simple solutions for stress reduction that needn't take up too much time in your busy schedule. Learning to balance your stress with lighthearted happiness is important enough to prioritize.

Here are some simple pointers for reducing stress and finding calm:

- Breathe. Concentrate on taking deep breaths into the belly. Do this throughout the day, or spend five minutes in the morning or evening sitting up straight, with good posture, breathing.
- Exercise or get outside daily.
- Obtain counseling, if needed.
- Develop a community of people you can talk to and spend time with.
- Spend one to three minutes every day thinking positive thoughts and visualizing what you want. Some spiritual traditions teach that our bodies don't distinguish between good feelings generated by our imaginations and those that come from actually experiencing something pleasant. I often suggest to my patients that they visualize themselves sitting in beautiful surroundings experiencing vibrant good health.
- Laugh out loud. Watch funny movies. Limit your TV watching to shows that make you feel good, not stressed or depressed.
- Pet your dog or cat. A companion animal's unconditional love can immediately make you feel more calm.
- Clean out the clutter from your surroundings. Make sure your bedroom is uncluttered and is simply and pleasingly decorated.

* Listen to music or sing a song. The right type of music can be very healing for some people. Listening to music that triggers memories of a very happy time in your life can often improve mood and decrease stress.

* Write in your journal. It's like venting without having to have someone around who can listen to you. Journaling forces you to process your thoughts as you are writing them down.

* Take supplements that support your adrenal glands. (Adrenal glands sit atop the kidneys and are responsible for releasing the primary stress hormones.) B vitamins and magnesium are two of the best supplements for aiding adrenal function; taking them regularly can help a person feel significantly less fatigued. (See Resources for purchasing information.)

* Have sex! I understand that sex may be the last thing from your mind, but you'll find that it helps improve feelings of well-being every time. Sex lowers blood pressure, boosts self-esteem, and increases feelings of intimacy with your partner.[4]

* Try taking alternating hot and cold showers. One of our patients shared with us a trick he learned after a few years of marriage. He takes a hot and then a cold shower right before bedtime. It revives his energy, makes his body feel tingly, and makes him want to touch his wife. He reports that this regimen has dramatically improved his sex life — as well as his marriage in general. Additionally, alternating hot and cold showers helps to increase circulation, increase lymphatic detoxification, decrease inflammation, and improve elimination through the skin. It can help to relieve sinus congestion, break up mucus in upper respiratory infections, and stimulate glandular function. You can do a similar treatment using a hot tub or sauna in place of a hot shower. Make sure to always end with a cold rinse; this will carry blood back to your vital organs and close your pores so that you don't get a chill.

Get Good Sleep

With many stimuli such as television, the internet, gaming, work, and other commitments taking the front seat to sleep these days, it is becoming clearer that sleep deprivation or lack of restful sleep may be taking an unprecedented toll on people's health. Much research has been focused on lack of sleep, revealing its connection to various illnesses such as obesity and weight gain,[5] cardiovascular disease,[6] and hypertension.[7] Sleep loss has also been directly related to inflammatory signaling,[8] which may explain its positive correlation with increased risk of cardiovascular disease.

Investigators in Finland found that inadequate sleep in children appeared to be an independent risk factor for behavioral symptoms of attention-deficit/hyperactivity disorder.[9] Short sleep duration in children is also linked to obesity and propensity for weight gain.[10] It is fairly common knowledge that in the last two decades, the incidence of obesity has increased worldwide to extreme numbers and is a major predictor of comorbidity (the presence of more than one disease condition) in later life.

It is vitally important to give our bodies time to heal, time to filter, time to detox, and time to recuperate from the day. Sleep provides that support. My guess is that many people, including children, are not getting the sleep they need for their bodies to perform all of the vital repair processes that can only occur during deep sleep.

Here are some suggestions for improving the quantity and quality of your sleep:

- Pay attention to your body and state of mind to determine how much sleep you need. Experts acknowledge that there really is no magic number of hours for adults. Most adults will know how much sleep they need and will understand when they are not getting enough. The amount of sleep you need will vary depending on things like your general state of health, whether you are recovering from illness or trauma, and how activity-filled your days are.

- Go to bed earlier. For every hour you sleep before midnight, something powerful seems to happen. For my patients who regularly don't get to sleep until after midnight, regardless of how late they sleep in the morning, healing is slower from a clinical perspective. I tell most of my adult patients that they should go to bed at 10:00 PM. For most people's schedules, that allows plenty of time to get seven or eight hours of sleep.

- Make sure your surroundings are conducive to restful sleep. If you use your cell phone as an alarm clock, make sure incoming calls and text messages are silenced, and distance the phone from your head.

- Sleep in a dark room with no nightlight to enhance sleep hormones. Keep the room cool and invest in a good mattress.

- Consider using sleep-enhancing supplements such as magnesium, GABA, L-theanine, or 5-HTP.

- Manage your stress well, include regular daily exercise, and maintain a regular routine throughout the day.

- Consider a nightly meditation or prayer to calm your nerves for a restful night.

Reduce Exposure to Environmental Toxins

Exposure to harmful chemicals can trigger inflammation. It is well known that chronic exposure to nicotine and other chemicals found in cigarettes causes significant inflammation in the lungs, eventually leading to lung cancer or chronic bronchitis in many individuals. Exposure to pesticides, aspartame (the artificial sweetener), BPA (found in some plastics), and DES (a drug prescribed for several decades in the mid-twentieth century to prevent miscarriages) has been linked to cancer. Air and traffic pollution have been linked to diabetes,[11] emphysema,[12] and rheumatoid arthritis.[13]

Many cleaning products deliver a fairly large amount of toxicity. I have seen quite a number of janitorial workers struggle with their health. Many of my fibromyalgia patients have been professional cleaners for years. I express my concern to each of them and am able to convince some of them to switch to using less-toxic products that don't risk harm. Some cleaning supplies can irritate the throat and eyes or cause headaches. Some products release dangerous fumes, including volatile organic compounds (VOCs). Others contain harmful ingredients such as ammonia and bleach. Even natural fragrances such as citrus can produce dangerous pollutants indoors. Research has connected VOCs to respiratory problems, allergic reactions, and headaches.[14] Studies have also connected the chemicals in cleaning supplies to asthma and other respiratory illnesses.[15] Don't mix cleaning products that contain bleach with ones that contain ammonia. Doing so can create harmful effects, including chronic breathing problems and even death.[16]

Products that may contain VOCs and other unhealthy chemicals are listed below:

- aerosol spray products, including health, beauty, and cleaning products
- air fresheners
- chlorine bleach

+ detergent and dishwashing liquid
+ dry-cleaning chemicals
+ furniture and floor polish
+ oven cleaners
+ rug and upholstery cleaners

To begin reducing your exposure to harmful chemicals, first consider where your exposure may be coming from. Here are some suggestions:

+ If you live in a large city with quite a bit of air pollution, you may be unable to completely avoid exposure. But perhaps you can avoid getting on your bike during rush hour, or at least change your route to choose quiet residential streets rather than heavily trafficked main thoroughfares where you'd be riding alongside lots of smog-producing cars.

+ Avoid drinking tap water at restaurants and other places. Get a filter for your tap water at home to avoid the heavy metals and harmful chemicals found in some water.

+ Reduce your exposure to fertilizers and pesticides by finding a park nearby where the maintenance crew doesn't spray. The parks with perfect green lawns most likely are heavily sprayed.

+ Avoid ordering animal products at a restaurant unless you know they're organic.

+ Avoid arsenic by not smoking.

+ Avoid other artificial chemicals by eliminating your intake of processed foods.

+ In your home, one product at a time, gradually get rid of all the bad ones. Use natural cleaners, natural shampoos and soaps, and house paint that doesn't release VOCs. Practice organic gardening and lawn-care methods.

+ Avoid using perfumes and lotions that contain artificial chemicals, as well as unnaturally scented candles, air fresheners, and plug-ins.

+ Begin the challenging process of getting rid of all of your plastic. It's okay to store food in some plastics that are BPA-free, but don't heat food in them. For water bottles, choose stainless steel or BPA-free plastic. Don't use bottled water unless you have to.

Reduce Exposure to Mercury and Other Heavy Metals

Mercury is a big subject and a controversial one. I believe it is important to speak about because even the Environmental Protection Agency (EPA) believes that overconsumption of mercury negatively affects health.

A significant source of mercury contamination for humans is related to fish consumption. Although fish are healthy to eat due to their content of essential fatty acids, some species contain dangerous amounts of mercury. Each variety needs to be considered individually.

The following comes from the EPA/FDA advisory on fish consumption for pregnant and nursing women, women who may become pregnant, and young children:

> By following the recommendations below for selecting and eating fish or shellfish, women and young children will receive the benefits of eating fish and shellfish and be confident that they have reduced their exposure to the harmful effects of mercury.
>
> + Do not eat shark, swordfish, king mackerel, or tilefish because they contain high levels of mercury.
> + Eat up to 12 ounces (two average meals) a week of a variety of fish and shellfish that are lower in mercury.
> + Five of the most commonly eaten fish that are low in mercury are shrimp, canned light tuna, salmon, pollock, and catfish.
> + Check local advisories about the safety of fish caught by family and friends in your local lakes, rivers, and coastal areas. If no advice is available, eat up to 6 ounces (one average meal) per week of fish you catch from local waters, but don't consume any other fish during that week.[17]

My recommendation regarding the consumption of tuna is to highly limit it. We generally limit our tuna consumption to eating sushi at a restaurant. If we want canned fish, we purchase salmon. Occasionally we have gotten freshly canned salmon from our patients. This is the best choice because we know how long it has been canned.

Mercury used to be prevalent as a preservative in many health and beauty products, such as contact-lens solution. In recent years, companies have reduced or eliminated their use of mercury in consumer products, mostly due to demand. Read labels, and avoid purchasing any product containing thimerosal. Thimerosal was also used as a preservative in vaccinations. It has now been removed from *most* childhood vaccinations. Make sure you educate yourself prior to vaccinating a young infant.

Other heavy metals can be found in many products, including cigarettes, canned products, water, well water, old paint, old pipes, fertilizers,[18] soil, rivers, lakes, pesticides, and more. Visit the EPA's website if you desire more information about the presence of heavy metals in your environment.

Take Care of Your Teeth and Gums

Significant research has connected periodontal disease (gingivitis, or inflammation of the gums) to various types of illness, including inflammatory heart disease, stroke, and atherosclerosis. The teeth can tell a physician so much about a person's health, because the mouth is where we consume our foods and take in other items such as cigarettes, coffee, candy, and drugs like chewing tobacco. How we take care of our teeth can directly affect our health. Many times a patient will come into our office with complaints about one side of his or her body. A look in the mouth often reveals inflamed gums, cavities, or a tooth in dire need of a root canal. If the damage is all located on, say, the left side of the mouth, there's a good chance that the patient's other symptoms are localized to the left side of the body.

It is imperative to brush teeth at least twice daily, floss daily, and visit the dentist regularly for cleanings and exams. Because of the direct connection between periodontitis, heart disease, and inflammation, it's also important to see the dentist as soon as you notice any problems with your teeth or gums. If you have a cavity, do your research about mercury versus porcelain fillings. Porcelain fillings aren't free of chemicals, but in my family, we've decided they are the better option. Minor cavities in baby teeth may not need immediate treatment if they aren't causing any problems. They should be watched and evaluated for pain or progression.

Tend to Injuries and Infections

Chronic injuries can lead to increased levels of inflammation. The injured area remains unhealed, continually stimulating the inflammatory response. Most chronic pain patients suffer from inflammation.

Chronic infections can lead to a low-grade elevation in inflammation, which can prove dangerous in later years. Low-grade infections may not seem to require immediate attention because they don't cause alarming symptoms, but over time they are a problem and can lead to undetected damage from inflammation. (Another reason why it is so important to deal with periodontal issues, which can cause low-grade, ongoing infection.)

If you have a wound or an injury that won't heal, please see a doctor to obtain appropriate medical care.

Learn About Possible Genetic Factors

Connecting inflammation to genes is a relatively new concept, but for decades we have associated many of the prime inflammation-related diseases to genetic factors such as obesity, diabetes, and heart disease. Thus, it makes sense that the susceptibility to chronic inflammation can be inherited.

Knowing your immediate family's medical history is important when you choose your self-care practices. If you're aware that several relatives had or have high cholesterol, and if there have been quite a few strokes and heart attacks in your family, then you know that your genetic risk is probably high for heart disease. In such a case, you would want to make doubly sure you're eating right to counterbalance that risk (for example, limiting consumption of red meat), getting regular cardiovascular exercise, and practicing stress-relieving strategies such as meditation.

Be Aware of Potential Fetal Exposures

A baby's environment for the nine months it is in its mother's belly will affect its immune response and its potential for developing disease and inflammation later on. Most pregnant women know the basics about what to avoid, but may not be aware of all of them. Here's a list:

- alcohol, drugs (recreational or pharmaceutical unless absolutely necessary), cigarettes
- all mercury-containing fish
- caffeine in large doses (one serving per day hasn't shown negative effects, according to recent studies)
- chemical perfumes, lotions, makeup
- cleaning supplies that are not "green"
- cleaning the cat's litter box
- emotional stress

- fast foods
- high-dose vitamin A supplements (they increase risk of birth defects)
- nail polish, unless it is considered "green" and free of formaldehyde
- pesticides, fertilizers, nonorganic foods
- processed foods, artificial chemicals, preservatives, food additives
- tap or well water (drink filtered water unless you have a well whose water has been tested for heavy metals)
- vaccinations (most vaccinations contain heavy metals and other immune-system stimulants, including human and animal tissues that may confuse the immune system)
- teeth cleaning (have your teeth cleaned as part of your pre-pregnancy preparation, or wait to visit the dentist for teeth cleanings until after pregnancy, especially if you have any amalgam [mercury-containing] fillings)
- X rays

Take Nutritional Supplements as Needed

I deem certain supplements important for prevention, despite how healthy a person is. I suggest that every patient of mine take the following (see Resources for purchasing information):

- vitamin B complex and/or adrenal support
- omega-3 fatty acid supplement, such as fish oil, cod liver oil, or flax seed oil
- a probiotic (or you can make and consume fermented foods on a daily basis)
- for patients living in northern climates, including the Pacific Northwest, where I live, vitamin D, for at least nine months of the year (can be skipped during the summer months)
- magnesium

Depending on any health problems, other supplements may be indicated.

CHAPTER 4

Focusing on Wellness: An Action Plan

Part of my responsibility as a health practitioner is looking at the big picture of my patients' lives. How can I assist them in embracing the variety of new behaviors I'm proposing? How can I help parents who want practical tips for getting their young children started on the right path toward a lifetime of healthy habits? The idea of making all those changes can seem overwhelming. In this chapter I provide strategies for putting the anti-inflammation diet and lifestyle into practice—for your children and yourself.

Promoting Wellness for Your Children

The best way to prevent chronic illness is to preserve the optimal health most of us are born with. A child's body must be supported as it develops proper responses to illnesses. It is very sensitive and will alter its functioning based on its environment, inside and out. Good diet, a supportive emotional environment within the home, healthy lifestyle modeling from parents, and wholesome daily routines are only a few aspects of an effective chronic-disease prevention program.

Environment is everything for children. They spend the first eighteen months of their lives seeking survival, security, and nurturing. The love and support a child receives during this time can set the stage for the future. What is said and done around a child molds and shapes them. We, at least partially, become our parents, in mannerisms, habits, level of self-esteem, and so much more. Confidence can be instilled or killed in a child by either parent or by another significant authority figure. Habits begin at home— around exercise, treatment of others, work ethic, drive, and positive or negative outlook. Following a healthy diet begins at home. Children observe and then copy. As much as possible, be a good example for your children and support them when needed. Let them have failure, but be there to discuss it when it happens.

Childhood environment even affects inflammation levels in later life, as shown in an article published in the *Archives of General Psychiatry*. Adults who had a history of maltreatment in childhood were more likely to experience high levels of inflammation. This confirms the fact that prolonged emotional stress can put people at risk of heart disease, which is linked to inflammation.[1]

Dietary Basics

Children may not need to consume a strict anti-inflammatory diet. We should be more concerned about what children are including in their diets rather than being hypervigilant about what they should exclude. I generally suggest keeping infants away from dairy and gluten until after they are one year old, and I advocate introducing grains later than most pediatricians suggest. In general, children's diets need to contain more vegetables, fruits, and whole foods, and fewer processed foods. Children should eat very little sugar, enjoying it only on special occasions, not for daily desserts. Children should get really good fats through foods such as cold-water fish, eggs, healthy saturated fats, flax oil, nuts, and seeds. Children need adequate amounts of iron and vitamin D. Children who live in northern latitudes should supplement with extra vitamin D, at least during the darker winter months.

Introducing Foods to Your Infant

Food introduction is extremely important. Introducing foods in the right manner can set up a better-functioning gastrointestinal tract while promoting healthy oral tolerance. Here are my suggestions for food introduction:

+ Don't introduce any foods before six months.

+ Introduce one food at a time, and wait at least three to four days before introducing a new food.

+ Watch for any changes in skin, bowel, sleep, or mood that would suggest a reaction to the food. For example, if you introduce a food for the first time and your baby begins to develop cradle cap, then stop any foods, wait three weeks, and begin the process again.

+ Start with vegetables first, for at least a couple of weeks, before introducing fruits.

+ Hold off on grains until at least age eight to nine months.

* Avoid dairy, gluten, and sugar until after one year of age.
* Always limit sugar, both in the household and in the child's diet.

Feeding the "Picky Eater"

Many children have reputations as picky eaters. First of all, refrain from calling them "picky" in front of them. Saying it will only reinforce the behavior because it gains attention. Toddlers especially are naturally picky eaters. Many parents have said to me, "When my child first started eating, she would eat anything, but as soon as she turned one, she stopped eating vegetables." Most children will grow out of this stage. Between ages one and three, children sometimes fall into the "mono stage," when they want the same food over and over. Don't fret; they won't want the same food for two years. Usually they love a food for a few months and then move on to a new love.

Children at this age don't know how to sort well, so keeping foods and snacks visually organized and uniform is extremely important. Infants grow rapidly during the first year of life and then tend to slow down a little bit as their curiosity increases and they focus on learning to walk and respond verbally. Toddlers and young children want to graze and not sit down, and that is perfectly okay. They may not be the best eaters at the family dinner table, but if you regularly put healthy, simple snacks in front of them they will eat them. Try it. Before your child is usually hungry, put out a snack of grapes, carrots, or another simple food. They may not eat it the first time, but they will get used to it.

Here are some tactics for getting a few more healthy foods into your kids:

* When offering a snack to a child under age three, put only one food on a plate at a time.
* Prepare and have snacks readily available for grazing before children ask. This minimizes drops in blood glucose, which can create moodiness in children who don't eat often enough.
* Keep foods visually simple. A toddler most likely won't understand a stir-fry because he or she can't sort it out visually.
* Stop stressing about your child's eating habits, and stop saying that he or she is picky.
* Let toddlers eat to their appetite; don't force them into eating more.

✦ Offer only nutritious foods during meal and snack times; don't have desserts readily available to your infant or toddler. In fact, don't have desserts on hand at all. Out of sight, out of mind.

✦ If you're going out for dinner, feed your infant or toddler before leaving so you don't have to stress about whether he or she eats. You'll have a much more enjoyable meal.

✦ Make porridges for your babies that have a balance between soaked grains and legumes.

✦ Purée vegetables into sauces or veggie burgers.

✦ Explain to older children that "This is the way we eat as a family" so they understand you are serious about the habits you want them to maintain. But, again, don't force them.

✦ Add vegetables to smoothies. Younger babies and some toddlers prefer to drink rather than eat. You can puree some cooked sweet potatoes with a little water, put the mixture in a bottle, cut the tip off, and serve. Babies also like the combination of mashed cooked peas, avocados, and water. Sometimes, rather than taking the time to feed them, this is a better meal on the go for a young baby. And they don't seem to mind one bit.

✦ Provide a good example by eating plenty of vegetables yourself.

✦ Get your children used to consuming the color green *very* early. My kids have consumed green beverages since they were seven or eight months old, even out of a baby bottle.

✦ Make fun names for the foods you eat, such as "Princess Noodles with King Sauce" and get your children to participate in the name-calling. "Ants on a Log" is a well-known example of this.

✦ Get children in the kitchen. They love to create with you; it makes them feel important. For older children who are beginning to learn fractions in school, get them baking and practice doubling a recipe or cutting it in half.

✦ Grow and harvest a garden, even if it is a simple container garden of herbs on your deck.

✦ For preschool- and elementary-school-age children, shapes of foods are important. Find out how they want their sandwiches cut, or use cookie cutters for foods. Create shapes together and have fun.

✦ Offer dips. Dips are very popular in my house. My children don't eat their salads the way most people do. They just want plain lettuce leaves and salad dressing in a separate bowl so they can dip each leaf and eat it. Use a variety of dips to get your children eating veggies and fruits. Serve apples with almond butter, carrot sticks with honey-mustard sauce, celery with hummus — the list goes on. Remember: For the little ones, serve only one food with one dip.

- ❧ Have toddlers and children do their own spreading. They love getting involved and love accomplishment. And if it is a nutritious spread, like hummus, and not just jam, who cares how much they put on? Let them experiment. They will find the right amount sooner or later.

- ❧ Grate zucchini and other vegetables into cookies, muffins, and sauces. It is much easier to get vegetables in than you may think. Foods that look more uniform may be more appealing. If your kids don't go for the grated vegetables, puree them instead so the mixture becomes more consistent to the eye.

- ❧ Lightly steam vegetables for little ones rather than expecting them to eat veggies raw, which can be a challenge for a toddler. My three-year-old loves what she calls "squishy carrots" and asks for them often. They are carrots that are lightly steamed so she can chew them easily.

- ❧ Add nutritious powders to their foods or drinks — for example, kelp, spirulina, nutritional yeast, probiotics, açai powder, or others.

- ❧ Have a play date with a child around the same age who is a good eater, and offer the kids a nutritional snack to share. Follow the one-food-per-plate guideline.

- ❧ Let children's feet touch the floor when they eat. Seat them at a children's table until they are able to sit at the big table without their feet dangling.

- ❧ Don't let your children get into the habit of having something sweet after a meal. This should not be a common occurrence as it can set bad habits for the future. If we have something sweet after the meal, it is special, as is obvious from my children's happy expression while they eat it. Interestingly, sometimes they don't even finish it.

- ❧ When you do consume sweets, try to make them as healthy as possible with the least amount of processing or sugars. See the sweet recipes contained in this book for ideas.

- ❧ Get input from older children on meal planning. They will be much more likely to eat a meal that they helped plan.

School Lunches

School lunches can be a challenge, both because of what is served at schools for lunch and because making lunches creates extra work on a daily basis. Neither of my kids has ever eaten the lunch provided at school. Sometimes my fourth grader asks if she can eat the school lunch, and I always say no without asking why she wants it. The other day we talked about why, and she said it was because she wanted to have chocolate milk. That's easy to solve: we can buy some chocolate hemp milk, or, better yet, make some chocolate milk of our own. Once we talked about it, she seemed to be over it. She also said that most of the food served at school looks pretty unappealing anyway.

Making lunches does create extra work for parents, and when both parents work outside the home, morning routines can get pretty busy and sometimes a little crazy. Still, I make my children's lunches because I understand the importance of nutrition and I want them to eat the foods I prepare. I feel better about their day if I know what they are consuming. And even if my daughter did sneak chocolate milk at school, as long as she eats what is in her lunch I know she is getting the nutrition she needs.

Here are some tips for packing lunches that I have found helpful. The recipe section also contains more ideas for school lunches.

- Send leftovers in a thermos the next day. I preheat the thermos first with boiling water that I pour out right before putting the food in.
- Pack soups in the winter and salads in the warmer months. Always put salad dressing on the side.
- Send veggies and dip or fruits and dip. My kids will eat lightly steamed and cooled vegetables.
- Keep frozen fruit or veggies on hand to pack in a pinch.
- Find creative ways to make sandwiches.
- Pack seaweed snacks. They are salty treats that are healthy.
- As discussed, don't pack cookies or sweets on a regular basis. Sometimes I will make a sweet bread like pumpkin or banana and send a slice of that. Don't let your children get used to having a sweet in their lunch, and don't pigeonhole yourself into saying you'll pack a sweet on a certain day of the week in case you don't have anything to send on that day. Sweets aren't a regular feature in our house, so when my kids get a treat in their lunches they are smiling from ear to

ear when I pick them up after school, and that feels great to me. And most of the time the treat I pack is pretty darn healthy anyway.

Promoting Wellness for Yourself:
A Three-Month Plan

I recommend making changes that fit your lifestyle in a time frame that works for you. Below is a three-month plan to wellness, modeled on one first presented in my book *Living with Crohn's and Colitis* and designed to help your transition be easier and more attainable. It also allows patients to really sense the amazing improvements that occur in their bodies as they eliminate the foods, one by one, that are ailing them. Most people will feel some positive changes as they progress through the plan, and some may even become symptom free.

The aim of this step-by-step process is to create a foundation for wellness and build upon it, rather than overwhelming the body by incorporating all of the changes at once. Taking new steps each week will help to keep you focused and motivated through the entire process. Just as each individual is unique, so too is her or his road to wellness. This plan is meant to be followed loosely, so feel free to adjust each step as needed for your own recovery. The introduction of new changes can be slowed down or speeded up as feels right.

Please consult your physician when beginning this program, and continue to visit your established team of specialists so that they can help you monitor your progress and make any necessary adjustments to the program.

I don't assume that the diet plan outlined in this book will work for everyone, but if a person tries at least half of the suggestions it contains, they should see improvement in their health. So what are you waiting for?

Weeks 1–2

1. Observe proper mealtime habits such as chewing your food thoroughly, not drinking while eating, and eating in a relaxed atmosphere (see Chapter 2).
2. Eliminate all dairy from your diet.
3. Include at least seven more servings of dark green, leafy vegetables per week. This only amounts to one serving per day—you can do it! If you are at a loss, just put them in a smoothie for now until you are more comfortable cooking and eating dark greens.

4. Drink filtered water, with a goal of drinking half the number of your body weight in pounds, in ounces each day (if you weigh 160 pounds, drink 80 ounces, or 10 glasses).

5. Add one supplement or herbal medicine, if you desire, such as fish oil, adrenal support, or magnesium.

6. See the change and believe in the change! Spend at least a few seconds (yes, seconds) every day visualizing optimal health. Imagine yourself happy, active, and vibrant.

Weeks 3–4

1. Continue previous points.

2. Eliminate all refined sugar from your diet, using only the natural sweeteners allowed on the anti-inflammation diet (see Table 2 on page 24). Eliminate all juice and dried fruit if you are diabetic or have heart disease.

3. Practice incorporating a rainbow of vegetables into your diet weekly.

4. Do something daily to support your stress response, such as a three-minute meditation, yoga, prayer, or a tapping routine ("tapping" involves using the fingers to rhythmically tap various acupuncture/acupressure points on the body in a certain pattern; see the Resources section at the back of the book for more information).

5. Add an additional supplement or herbal medicine, such as a high-quality probiotic.

Weeks 5–6

1. Continue previous points.

2. Eliminate all gluten from your diet.

3. Eliminate all food allergens if you know them, either by testing for them or by observing your own body's reactions.

4. Add additional good fats to the diet by consuming more cold-water fish, nuts, seeds, coconut oil, and flax oil.

5. Begin to incorporate movement/exercise. Do this at least three times per week, but daily if possible. Consult with a physician if you're completely unused to exercising. Hire a trainer if necessary.

6. Add an additional supplement or herbal medicine such as adrenal support or Strength from Herb Fusion (see Resources).

Weeks 7–8

1. Continue previous points.

2. Eliminate tomatoes, potatoes, and white rice.

3. Incorporate daily nutritional powders into your diet such as spirulina, kelp, green tea, or açai powder.

4. Add an additional supplement or herbal medicine such as magnesium, Tranquility from Herb Fusion (see Resources), or B complex.

Weeks 9–10

1. Continue previous points.

2. Eliminate all meats and animal products containing added hormones.

3. Add mushrooms, vinegars, and healthy spices (see Table 2 on page 24) to your dietary regimen.

4. Practice reading labels and eliminating all chemical food additives, especially the ones you cannot pronounce. I save this suggestion until you've been following the diet for a while because the reading of labels can seem overwhelming and you may not want to continue. By this time you are most likely feeling a little better, and you have faith in the diet and lifestyle change. Now you have to take one of the final steps by knowing everything you put in your body. Avoid packaged foods whose ingredients contain words like MSG, monosodium glutamate, sodium nitrite or nitrate, sulfur dioxide, yellow number 6 (or another color and number combination), aluminum, sodium benzoate, ethyl para-hydroxybenzoate, formic acid, butylated hydroxytoluene (BHT), aspartame, acesulfame potassium, or saccharine. The fewer processed foods you eat and the more you shop on the periphery of the grocery store, the less likely you are to see these ingredients on your food labels.

5. Begin the home elimination by getting rid of foods you haven't yet consumed that contain these chemicals. Let go of the unhealthy addictions. Again, we don't tackle this step for a few weeks because it can be hard. Maybe you need someone to come over to your house and help you. Although throwing food away can be difficult, it can also be a very enlightening move toward improved health.

Weeks 11–12

1. Continue previous points.

2. Eliminate soy, corn, and peanuts from the diet.

3. Add fermented foods to the list of foods you commonly eat. You can try to start making them, or you can buy them at first and learn how to make them later, when you are feeling more comfortable with the dietary changes.

4. Add an additional supplement if you still need more support for something specific such as arthritis or diabetes risk. See a qualified naturopathic physician if necessary.

5. Incorporate activities to enhance lymphatic flow, such as hot and cold showers or dry skin brushing. In a hot *and* cold shower, start with hot water, and then switch to cold water three times throughout the shower for at least fifteen seconds. End on cold to close your pores and shunt blood back into your vital organs. Dry skin brushing employs very short, light strokes starting at the fingertips and toes and moving toward the heart. Use a wash cloth, your hand, or a brush with soft, natural bristles. It is best done at night before going to bed to parallel your body's normal lymphatic cycle for moving waste products.

Weeks 13 and Beyond

1. Continue previous points.

2. Begin learning how to follow the anti-inflammation diet when you travel and when you eat out. Share the diet with others; begin hosting anti-inflammation potlucks to trade ideas with your friends who also want to enhance their health and live longer.

3. Find out which foods bother you the most by introducing them back into your diet. Reintroduce only one food at a time, and wait a few days to see if you have any negative reactions before reintroducing another food. If you discover that a certain food causes a reaction, aim to completely eliminate it and *only* eat it on very special occasions.

4. If there is a food on the "avoid" list, such as corn, that you are able to tolerate with no adverse effects, continue to minimize it in your diet.

5. Aim for variety. Make sure you're not eating the same foods all the time. Rotate all foods and grains regularly so you are not eating the same foods more than a few days in a row.

6. Continue with your exercise and stress-reduction programs. Keep drinking plenty of filtered water.

7. Rotate your supplements rather than taking the same ones every day. For example, use calcium for two weeks and then vitamins E and C for two weeks. Try to avoid synthetic supplements of unknown quality; these, too, have been known to contain heavy metals and artificial chemicals.

8. Now focus on eliminating harmful chemicals from your home. Replace harsh cleaning supplies with "green" ones such as Biokleen brand products. Use safe, nontoxic laundry detergent. Use natural shampoos, conditioners, and toothpaste. Get rid of aluminum-containing deodorants, even the crystal ones. Anything that says "alum" still has a form of aluminum, and I suggest getting rid of it. Use only naturally scented candles or air fresheners.

9. Get rid of all your plastic food containers, or at least commit to not heating food in them or storing anything hot in them. Purchase only BPA-free plastic containers. Stop using your microwave for heating foods, even in glass containers, because microwaving decreases foods' nutrient content.

Table 4 below summarizes this sample three-month plan to wellness in a handy chart. Remember, the plan starts with a basic foundation, and each week you build on what you already have. These changes won't feel so overwhelming if you tackle them one at a time.

Table 4. Sample Treatment Suggestions for the Three-Month Plan to Wellness

Weeks 1–2: Visualize and believe in change. Also:	
• See and believe in change • Eliminate dairy • Take 400 mg magnesium per day	• Chew food and eat in a relaxed atmosphere • Drink filtered water, half your weight in ounces per day • Include 7 more servings of dark, green leafy vegetables per week

(cont'd.)

Table 4. Sample Treatment Suggestions for the Three-Month Plan to Wellness (cont'd.)

Weeks 3–4: Continue the previous steps and add:

- Eliminate all sugar, juice, and dried fruit
- Practice incorporating a rainbow of vegetables in the diet each week
- Add a daily probiotic, at least 12 billion organisms
- Meditate 3 minutes daily for stress relief

Weeks 5–6: Continue the previous steps and add:

- Eliminate all gluten
- Add cold-water fish, nuts, seeds, coconut, and flax oil
- Begin incorporating movement/ exercise
- Eliminate foods to which you have known allergies
- Take an adrenal support

Weeks 7–8: Continue the previous steps and add:

- Eliminate tomatoes, potatoes, and white rice
- Consume nutritional powders such as spirulina, kelp, or açai on a daily basis
- Add 4000 mg fish oil per day

Weeks 9–10: Continue the previous steps and add:

- Eliminate all meats or animal products that have hormones
- Add mushroom, vinegars, and healthy spices to your foods
- Practice reading labels and eliminating food additives
- Begin home elimination and let go of unhealthy food addictions

Weeks 11–12: Continue the previous steps and add:

- Eliminate soy, corn, and peanuts
- Add fermented foods to your diet
- Take hot and cold showers daily*

* This is a hot and cold shower. Start with hot water, and then switch to cold water three times throughout the shower for at least fifteen seconds. End on cold to close your pores and shunt blood back into your vital organs.

PART II

Anti-Inflammation Recipes

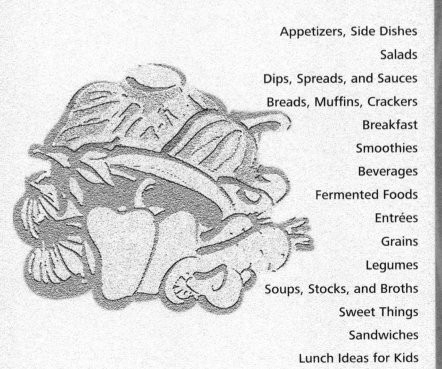

CHAPTER 5

Helpful Tips for
Anti-Inflammation Cooking

Adopting the anti-inflammation diet (AI diet) has its challenges. I know that's true from personal experience, because we as a family have followed an AI diet for quite some time now. I believe it's well worth any hassle involved. As a health-care practitioner, I find that if a patient commits to undertaking the recommended dietary changes, they see results, and often very quickly. They experience less pain, enhanced mood, and improved bowel habits. Most of the time they experience weight loss. Overall they feel much better.

Let's consider our relationship with food to be a vital part of survival. If we exist because of the nutrients we consume, our health is reflected by what we eat on a daily basis.

Be Prepared and Don't Be Afraid

Taking lunches and snacks along with you when you leave the house prevents you from getting lost in the American wasteland of fast food if you become urgently hungry. Resisting the temptations of sweets and treats at work takes willpower and backbone. Understanding creates willpower: understanding the risks involved when making poor food choices and the risk inflammation poses to your and your family's long-term health, and understanding how great it feels to enjoy vibrant health and well-being.

Know that with any change, you are bound to make mistakes! Don't be afraid to fail. Behind every success often lie a significant number of failures. Be creative. Don't think you have to follow the recipes or the lifestyle plan verbatim. Make it your own thing. Create your own meals from the ideas presented in this book, and learn to season foods in your own unique way. Experiment a lot! Your experiments may result in the occasional funny moment in your kitchen or at the dinner table with your family, but they will also force you to learn and improve your skills.

For more discussion about my and my family's experiences following an AI diet and lifestyle, please visit my blog at www.drjessicablack.com/blog.

Navigating Food Choices

Food is prepared in many ways. Sometimes the method of food preparation can interfere with the food's quality and nutrient content. Below are my suggestions for choosing foods that are as natural and nutrient dense as possible. The main goal here is to get back to our roots. That means greatly reducing or eliminating consumption of artificial additives, chemicals, preservatives, and unnatural substances, many of which have been linked to cancer and other illnesses.

* *Filter your drinking and cooking water.* Consider this a golden rule in your kitchen and for your family. Plain tap water simply contains too many chemicals that can affect your health, such as heavy metals, hormones, residues from chemicals used in treatment facilities, and farming chemicals. Furthermore, the balance of minerals in your water may be off. A filter can help remove unwanted chemicals and correct imbalances. Many different types of water filters are available; spend some time researching them before purchasing one. You can begin with a simple system, like a Brita pitcher, which utilizes a carbon filter, but for the long term, consider going with a more advanced filtration system for your entire home.

* *Organic meat is best.* Organic meat is free of toxic chemicals. If you can't always find organic meat, then look for hormone-free meat. Organic meat usually comes from animals that have been grass fed or, in the case of poultry, have been given feed free of additives such as antibiotics. Grass-fed animal proteins are better than proteins from grain-fed animals. Cattle and buffalo were meant to graze on grass, and that is what they do for most of their lives. Most commercially raised cattle will graze on grass but will be finished off in the last months of their lives with grains such as corn to increase their weight and fat content. The meat taste we have grown to love as Americans comes from this extra fat content. Grass-fed animals are leaner; they have ⅓ to ½ the fat of grain-fed animals of the same size. The meat from grass-fed animals is higher in good nutrients: Beef from a grass-fed cow has three times the vitamin E content and is higher in omega-3

fatty acids, providing a better omega-3 to omega-6 ratio, than beef from a grain-fed cow. Grass-fed beef also has a higher content of conjugated linoleic acid (CLA), a lesser-known but important group of polyunsaturated fatty acids found in beef, lamb, and dairy products. The less our farming practices adhere to an animal's natural growth and development patterns, the greater the risk of something going wrong, such as the meat being contaminated or the animal getting sick. It is also important to avoid meat from animals that have been fed antibiotics or hormones or have spent time around pesticides. Hormones fed to animals are used to increase their growth, but they are detrimental to health. Many of the common cancers, such as prostate, breast, and ovarian cancers, are often directly related to excess hormone influence.

✦ *Whenever possible, choose organic vegetables and fruits.* Produce is best purchased fresh and local. A few vegetables and fruits, such as peas and berries, may be purchased frozen for ease of use. Never buy canned vegetables and fruits, with the exception of canned tomatoes on rare occasions. If you are on a tight budget and organic produce seems out of reach cost-wise, be aware that there are a few fruits and vegetables that are more important to purchase organic because they are heavily sprayed with chemicals when grown following conventional methods. A comprehensive list of both the cleanest and the most contaminated fruits and vegetables can be found at the website of the Environmental Working Group: www.ewg.org/foodnews /summary.

✦ *Use Real Salt over other types of sea salt or table salt.* Many table salts contain added anticaking agents or dextrose, which is a potato sugar. Other types of sea salt are sometimes more processed and may not offer the variety of minerals that Real Salt does. Real Salt brand sea salt comes from Redmond, Utah, and has a distinct, rich taste. Its off-white color comes from the many trace minerals (as many as 60 different ones) that are present in the salt. Himalayan or Celtic salts are also acceptable, but I prefer using a salt local to our area rather than from other parts of the world.

✦ *Buy fresh foods over canned.* Exceptions to this guideline include coconut milk, canned wild-caught salmon, or beans (occasionally) when you are in a pinch and haven't soaked any.

- *Purchase wild-caught fish instead of farm-raised.* Wild fish contains significantly higher levels of omega-3 fatty acids, the important fats that help our bodies ward off cancer and other inflammatory illnesses. They are also extremely important in supporting brain function and helping maintain memory and cognitive ability into older age. Farmed fish such as salmon often contains dyes to make it appear rich in omega-3 fatty acids.

- *Avoid processed foods as much as possible.* Chips, boxed foods, prepared meals, cold cuts, hot dogs, frozen pizzas, frozen snacks, SpaghettiOs, and prepared macaroni and cheese are just some examples of processed foods that should be avoided.

Food Items to Keep on Hand/Shopping List

Below is a list of some helpful items to keep in your kitchen. Having these groceries on hand can minimize your trips to the store when you're planning a meal and will make it easier to throw together healthy dinners spontaneously. A meal of beans and rice is an easy staple you can prepare in a pinch, even if you haven't been able to go grocery shopping.

- sweeteners: agave syrup, raw honey, pure maple syrup, stevia, brown rice syrup, coconut palm sugar

- dried grains and legumes: brown rice, legumes/beans (e.g., black beans, white beans, kidney beans, split peas), millet, gluten-free steel-cut oats, gluten-free whole rolled oats, quinoa, wild rice

- canned goods: salmon, beans, coconut milk

- dried spices: cinnamon, ginger, basil, garlic powder, onion powder, mustard powder, cumin, turmeric, nutmeg, peppercorns or fresh-ground pepper, Real Salt

- dried goods: unsweetened coconut, dried fruits (e.g., raisins, unsulfured apricots, figs), nuts, seeds

- fresh vegetables in season, including salad greens

- fresh fruit in season

- frozen goods: homemade broths, bananas, fruits and berries for smoothies

- vinegars: apple cider vinegar, red wine vinegar, white vinegar, others as desired

* condiments: gluten-free tamari sauce, mustard, organic mayonnaise
* fresh herbs and spices: garlic, onions, ginger, parsley
* fats and oils: organic butter, coconut oil, olive oil
* milk and eggs: unsweetened almond milk, unsweetened hemp milk, organic eggs
* specifics for the recipes you want to prepare during the week

Making Healthy Eating Easier

It is important to reduce kitchen time and make your kitchen and yourself more efficient. This task is not always easy, especially with our busy lifestyles involving work, kids in sports, and other commitments. Here are a few tips for reducing kitchen time:

Food Preparation

* Pre-chop vegetables you know you will be using during the week.
* Pre-chop garlic and onions, and keep them refrigerated in airtight containers for use.
* Prepare everything for dinner when you are making lunch so that dinner is much easier to get on the table.
* Make stocks and broths ahead of time, and store them in small quantities in the freezer.
* Make large batches of soup so you have extra each time to freeze for a later date.
* Prepare extra servings when you're cooking dinner so you have leftovers for lunch the next day.
* Do not microwave food. If you microwave at all, do so sparingly because the process destroys important nutrients.

Food Equipment

* Rice cooker (gives you less to manage during the cooking of a meal)
* Small food chopper
* Coffee grinder (for grinding nuts and seeds)
* Blender or Vitamix. A Vitamix is an extremely high-powered blender that can handle a full range of tasks, from making a smoothie, to grinding nuts and seeds, to making your own flours. If you have

a Vitamix, then you generally won't need a coffee grinder or food chopper.

* Food processor. Superior to the Vitamix for grating a large quantity of an ingredient such as zucchini to make relish.

* Nonaluminum sauté pans and ovenware

Cooking Tips

* Use easy steaming procedures for simple vegetable side dishes topped with a small amount of your favorite sauce. You can use an inexpensive basket-style steamer, or just put ½ inch water in a saucepan, add your chopped vegetables, and cook over medium heat. With either method, steam until the vegetables have a bright color but are still crunchy-tender. You may need to add more water if it evaporates during steaming.

* When boiling pasta, add salt to the cooking water. This will slightly reduce the time it takes for the water to swell the noodles, helping to prevent an overcooked, mushy noodle and resulting in that perfect "al dente" texture. Pasta prepared al dente has a lower glycemic index than overcooked pasta and therefore is better for balancing blood sugar levels.

* Learn to improvise! Don't think you always need a recipe. The more you cook, the more you will learn to guess what you need, and the more you will learn about how seasonings blend together. You'll get better at substituting when you don't have the exact ingredient. Don't be afraid to experiment with new ingredients.

* Make extra servings of grain when preparing a meal, and freeze the extra in airtight containers. It is handy to be able to pull out some frozen rice and sauté it with beans for a nutritious side dish or main dish.

* Discover a few readily prepared sauces that you and your family love. Sauces make it easier to serve a very simple dinner. Here's one of our favorites: beans (sometimes soaked overnight, but sometimes from the can), rice, and steamed veggies. We make three sauces, and we each get to choose which one we want to add to our rice and beans. We call these our bento bowls. Another easy dinner idea is to roll these same ingredients into a gluten-free tortilla.

✦ Eat raw one night per week. This can be an easy meal of cut-up veggies, fruits, and dips. Often, we will throw veggies and fruit into the blender with water and have a green drink for the evening. This feels very refreshing and healthy. Make sure you are able to tolerate raw foods before incorporating "Raw Night" into your household.

Organization and Preparation

✦ Keep your pantry, refrigerator, and spice area well organized.

✦ Make lists when you run out of items that you need from the store.

✦ Plan meals before you grocery shop.

✦ Have "go to" meals that are easy and quick, but still nutritious and healthy. This helps to reduce snacking time.

✦ Have ideas for healthy snacks, and avoid buying snacks that you will feel guilty about eating.

✦ Clean the kitchen as you prepare meals. Utilize the natural gaps in time that occur when cooking to wash the dishes and utensils you have used and no longer need. That way, many of your dishes are already rinsed and placed in the dishwasher before your meal is finished.

✦ Pack your lunches, and take snacks with you everywhere you go. Don't rely on finding food while you're out. Most of the time you won't be able to find much that's healthy. Carrying snacks will also keep you and your children happier by avoiding blood sugar crashes and the resulting moodiness.

Food Attitude

✦ Have fun when you go shopping. Take the whole family so that you all participate in choosing foods. Think about foods and cooking in a new perspective. Don't fight the change; accept and appreciate it for what it will bring to you and your family.

✦ Get the children involved. Have them pick out a new vegetable at the store, and then go home and research how to cook it.

Measurement Conversion Charts

Liquid Measures
1 cup = 8 fluid ounces = 250 ml
1 tablespoon = ½ fluid ounce = 16 ml
1 teaspoon = ⅙ fluid ounce = 5⅓ ml
16 tablespoons = 1 cup
3 teaspoons = 1 tablespoon

Dry Ingredients (Approximate; Not Exact)
whole-grain flour: 1 cup = 170 grams   rolled oats: 1 cup = 90 grams
baking powder: 1 tablespoon = 15 grams   honey: 1 cup = 339 grams
baking soda: 1 tablespoon = 15 grams   raisins: 1 cup = 150 grams
vanilla: 1 tablespoon = 12 grams   sesame seeds: 1 cup = 135 grams
salt: 1 teaspoon = 7 grams   chopped nuts: 1 cup = 160 grams

Egg Sizes (Large Is the U.S. Standard for Cooking)
egg (U.S., graded size "large"): 1.5 fluid ounces = 1.75 ounces without shell =
     50 grams without shell
egg whites (U.S., graded size "large"): 1 egg white = 2 tablespoons = 32 milliliters =
     30 grams
egg yolks (U.S., graded size "large"): 1 egg yolk = 1 tablespoon = 16 milliliters =
     20 grams

Solid Fats (Butter, Cheese, Shortening, Margarine, Lard)
8 tablespoons = 4 ounces = ¼ pound = 115 grams
butter: 1 stick = 8 tablespoons = 4 ounces = ¼ pound = 115 grams

Temperatures
250°F = 120°C = very low   400°F = 200°C = hot
200°F = 150°C = low   450°F = 230°C = very hot
325°F = 165°C = moderately low   500°F = 260°C = extremely hot; most
350°F = 180°C = moderate   broilers are set at this temperature or above
375°F = 190°C = moderately hot

 Recipes with this symbol are not strictly anti-inflammatory,
therefore we suggest avoiding these recipes until you are feeling
well and are ready to introduce a little variety to see how you do.

Appetizers, Side Dishes

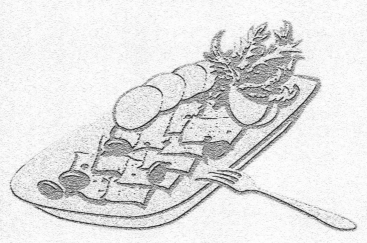

 Recipes with this symbol are not strictly anti-inflammatory, therefore we suggest avoiding these recipes until you are feeling well and are ready to introduce a little variety to see how you do.

Blanched Beans with Salt

PER SERVING: 30.9 CALORIES ~ 1.8 G PROTEIN ~ 7.0 G CARBOHYDRATE ~ 2.7 G FIBER ~
0.2 G TOTAL FAT ~ 0.1 G SATURATED FAT ~ 0.0 MG CHOLESTEROL ~ 151.0 MG SODIUM

1 pound green beans, trimmed

Salt to taste

Steam green beans in about ½ inch of water until crisp-tender, around 5 minutes. Remove from heat. Sprinkle with salt; immediately place beans in a glass container and chill in refrigerator.

Serve chilled.

Serves 4.

Substitutions

You can use this simple technique for many vegetables, such as yellow beans, asparagus, broccoli, and others. It saves time if you want to make food ahead of time for a party or potluck.

Healthy Tidbit

Green beans are high in vitamin C, which is an important antioxidant. Vitamin C is used by the body to support the immune response against infections. It speeds the healing of cuts, bruises, and injuries. It also helps to decrease blood pressure and to prevent heart disease and stroke.

Nutritional Analysis per Serving

Vitamin A	62.0 RE	Vitamin D	0.0 µg
Thiamin (B-1)	0.1 mg	Vitamin E	0.0 mg
Riboflavin (B-2)	0.1 mg	Calcium	35.2 mg
Niacin	0.6 mg	Iron	1.0 mg
Vitamin B-6	0.1 mg	Phosphorus	34.1 mg
Vitamin B-12	0.0 µg	Magnesium	23.7 mg
Folate (total)	21.4 µg	Zinc	0.2 mg
Vitamin C	9.1 mg	Potassium	189.5 mg

Roasted Vegetables

PER SERVING: 98.7 CALORIES ~ 1.6 G PROTEIN ~ 8.3 G CARBOHYDRATE ~ 2.1 G FIBER ~
7.1 G TOTAL FAT ~ 1.0 G SATURATED FAT ~ 0.0 MG CHOLESTEROL ~ 18.1 MG SODIUM

2 zucchini

2 yellow squash

1 red pepper

1 green pepper

1 purple onion

2 large carrots

¼ cup olive oil

Salt and freshly ground pepper to taste

Preheat oven to 450°F.

Cut vegetables into 1- to 2-inch pieces. Toss in large bowl with olive oil until coated. Arrange vegetables in single layer on two foil-lined sheet pans and sprinkle lightly with salt and pepper. Roast for 30–45 minutes, stirring every 10 minutes, until vegetables are crisp-tender and starting to brown.

Serves 8.

Substitutions

Many different vegetables can be used for this recipe. It is easy to roast most vegetables; even broccoli or cauliflower work.

Healthy Tidbit

Vegetables are rich in dietary fiber. Fiber can help facilitate better bowel movements by adding bulk and weight to stools. It can also help maintain balanced blood sugar levels and is therefore especially helpful for diabetics.

Nutritional Analysis per Serving

Vitamin A	334.3 RE	Vitamin D	0.0 µg
Thiamin (B-1)	0.1 mg	Vitamin E	0.0 mg
Riboflavin (B-2)	0.1 mg	Calcium	27.7 mg
Niacin	0.8 mg	Iron	0.7 mg
Vitamin B-6	0.3 mg	Phosphorus	68.3 mg
Vitamin B-12	0.0 µg	Magnesium	20.8 mg
Folate (total)	35.9 µg	Zinc	0.4 mg
Vitamin C	52.8 mg	Potassium	360.8 mg

Garlic Chard with Poached Egg

PER SERVING: 172.3 CALORIES ~ 7.0 G PROTEIN ~ 2.7 G CARBOHYDRATE ~ 0.5 G FIBER ~
15.0 G TOTAL FAT ~ 3.0 G SATURATED FAT ~ 186.0 MG CHOLESTEROL ~ 123.1 MG SODIUM

Inspired by my friend Lynn Stahr, of Portland, Oregon.

6 garlic cloves, chopped
3 tablespoons olive or coconut oil
2 bunches Swiss chard, sliced
4 cups water
1 tablespoon vinegar
4 eggs
Salt to taste (optional)

Sauté garlic in oil in large saucepan until tender, 1–2 minutes. Add chard; sauté over medium heat until chard is tender but still bright green, 3–5 minutes.

To poach eggs: Heat water and vinegar to simmering in medium saucepan or skillet. Crack eggs and gently add to water. Simmer very gently until whites are set and yolk is still somewhat soft, about 3 minutes.

Spoon chard onto four plates; top each serving with a poached egg and sprinkle with salt.

Serves 4.

Substitutions
You can prepare this recipe without the poached egg and it is still delicious. I have also served it topped with Faux Creamy Cheese Sauce (see recipe on page 111). If you can tolerate a little dairy, try shaving a few large pieces of parmesan cheese on top.

Healthy Tidbit
Chard is a lovely ingredient to keep on hand. Try it with lentils, in stir-fries, or sautéed in egg sandwiches, soups, and many other dishes. It is a great source of easily absorbable calcium and of vitamins A and C. It is also a good source of vitamin B-1 (thiamin), folic acid, zinc, dietary fiber, vitamin E (alpha tocopherol), vitamin K, vitamin B-2 (riboflavin), vitamin B-6, iron, magnesium, phosphorus, potassium, copper, and manganese. Chard is naturally high in sodium, so you need very little salt to flavor it.

Nutritional Analysis per Serving

Vitamin A	227.8 RE	Vitamin D	1.0 µg
Thiamin (B-1)	0.0 mg	Vitamin E	0.5 mg
Riboflavin (B-2)	0.2 mg	Calcium	48.5 mg
Niacin	0.2 mg	Iron	1.4 mg
Vitamin B-6	0.2 mg	Phosphorus	116.9 mg
Vitamin B-12	0.4 µg	Magnesium	26.6 mg
Folate (total)	27.0 µg	Zinc	0.8 mg
Vitamin C	8.6 mg	Potassium	178.1 mg

Baked Beans

PER SERVING: 285.8 CALORIES ~ 18.4 G PROTEIN ~ 34.9 G CARBOHYDRATE ~ 9.7 G FIBER ~
6.7 G TOTAL FAT ~ 2.2 G SATURATED FAT ~ 40.5 MG CHOLESTEROL ~ 936.2 MG SODIUM

2 cups dry Great Northern beans, washed

1 pound turkey bacon, cut into 1-inch pieces

5 cups water

1 cup minced onions

3 cloves garlic, minced

2 tablespoons molasses

2 tablespoons Dijon mustard

2 bay leaves

2 teaspoon grated fresh ginger

1 teaspoon thyme

1 teaspoon salt

1 teaspoon ground black pepper

One day ahead of time, soak the white beans according to the soaking instructions in the legume cooking section (page 221). Discard the soaking water. Cook bacon in medium skillet until partially cooked and softened; drain. Combine beans, bacon, and remaining ingredients in large slow cooker. Cook on high for 12 hours, until beans are tender and darkish red. Add additional seasonings to taste.

Serves 8.

Substitutions

Now you can enjoy baked beans with no tomato content! These are delicious, great for parties, and extremely easy to prepare. Any type of white bean will work for this recipe. Experiment with different seasonings.

Healthy Tidbit

Molasses, although it comes from the sugar cane, provides a wealth of nutrients due to its rich vitamin and iron content. One tablespoon of blackstrap molasses offers 3.5 mg of iron and 172 mg of calcium.

Nutritional Analysis per Serving

Vitamin A	0.8 RE	Vitamin D	0.0 µg
Thiamin (B-1)	0.1 mg	Vitamin E	0.0 mg
Riboflavin (B-2)	0.1 mg	Calcium	89.7 mg
Niacin	0.6 mg	Iron	2.4 mg
Vitamin B-6	0.2 mg	Phosphorus	173.6 mg
Vitamin B-12	0.0 µg	Magnesium	76.0 mg
Folate (total)	70.6 µg	Zinc	1.0 mg
Vitamin C	3.5 mg	Potassium	526.4 mg

Yum Peas

PER SERVING: 132.3 CALORIES ~ 6.8 G PROTEIN ~ 18.4 G CARBOHYDRATE ~ 5.6 G FIBER ~
3.4 G TOTAL FAT ~ 0.5 G SATURATED FAT ~ 0.0 MG CHOLESTEROL ~ 256.3 MG SODIUM

1 medium onion, chopped
2 cloves garlic, minced
1 tablespoon olive oil
16 ounces frozen green peas
Salt and freshly ground pepper to taste

Sauté onion and garlic in oil in large skillet until onions are beginning to
brown, about 5 minutes. Add peas. Cook, covered, until the peas are tender,
about 5 minutes. Season to taste with salt and pepper.
    Serves 4.

Healthy Tidbit

This makes a very quick accompaniment to many dinners. Peas are sweet, so
kids tend to like them. I use frozen peas because they are easy to obtain. When
purchasing vegetables, consider where they came from and what nutrients
they offer. Fresh vegetables are best, frozen vegetables are next best, and canned
vegetables will do in a pinch.

Nutritional Analysis per Serving

Vitamin A	51.0 RE	Vitamin D	0.0 µg
Thiamin (B-1)	0.3 mg	Vitamin E	0.0 mg
Riboflavin (B-2)	0.1 mg	Calcium	9.1 mg
Niacin	2.0 mg	Iron	1.5 mg
Vitamin B-6	0.1 mg	Phosphorus	103.3 mg
Vitamin B-12	0.0 µg	Magnesium	32.6 mg
Folate (total)	65.4 µg	Zinc	1.0 mg
Vitamin C	10.1 mg	Potassium	219.7 mg

Roasted Tempeh

PER SERVING: 267.2 CALORIES ~ 20.5 G PROTEIN ~ 28.3 G CARBOHYDRATE ~ 3.7 G FIBER ~
8.5 G TOTAL FAT ~ 0.0 G SATURATED FAT ~ 0.0 MG CHOLESTEROL ~ 2184.9 MG SODIUM

1 8-ounce package tempeh
½ cup soy sauce
¼ cup honey
¼ cup red wine vinegar
2 cloves garlic, minced
¼ teaspoon salt

Cut tempeh into 4-inch strips. Combine remaining ingredients; pour over tempeh and marinate several hours or overnight.

Preheat oven to 400°F.

Arrange tempeh on lightly greased baking sheet; bake until lightly browned, about 20 minutes, turning after 10 minutes.

Serves 2.

Substitutions

You can use this same recipe to roast extra-firm tofu. Tofu is a little harder to work with because it can break apart, so handle carefully.

Healthy Tidbit

This is delicious served over salad, quinoa, or veggies.

Soy is used heavily in the American diet. We began considering soy a "health" food by studying the low rates of cancer in Japan and relating it to their diet. But the Japanese treat soy as more of a condiment. They don't drink soy milk and they don't take soy in capsule form; they enjoy it in the form of soy sauce and tofu. Their overall consumption of soy is not excessive. I prefer the fermented forms of soy, such as tempeh, miso, and fermented soy sauce. I use and consume tofu and soy milk sparingly.

Nutritional Analysis per Serving

Vitamin A	0.0 RE	Vitamin D	0.0 µg
Thiamin (B-1)	0.1 mg	Vitamin E	0.0 mg
Riboflavin (B-2)	0.6 mg	Calcium	90.2 mg
Niacin	5.0 mg	Iron	2.9 mg
Vitamin B-6	0.1 mg	Phosphorus	256.9 mg
Vitamin B-12	0.0 µg	Magnesium	16.9 mg
Folate (total)	5.5 µg	Zinc	0.3 mg
Vitamin C	2.3 mg	Potassium	302.9 mg

Broccoli with Lemon

PER SERVING: 48.6 CALORIES ~ 2.3 G PROTEIN ~ 5.7 G CARBOHYDRATE ~ 2.1 G FIBER ~
2.5 G TOTAL FAT ~ 0.3 G SATURATED FAT ~ 0.0 MG CHOLESTEROL ~ 606.6 MG SODIUM

2 heads broccoli, separated into florets

2 teaspoons extra-virgin olive oil

2 cloves garlic, minced

1 teaspoon salt

½ teaspoon pepper

½ teaspoon lemon juice

Preheat the oven to 400°F.

In a large bowl, toss broccoli florets with olive oil, garlic, salt, and pepper. Spread the broccoli in an even layer on a foil-lined baking sheet.

Bake until florets are tender and lightly browned, about 15 minutes. Place broccoli on serving platter. Sprinkle with lemon juice.

Serves 4.

Substitutions

Also great with cauliflower, or try a combination of the two vegetables. The lemon juice adds a bright note.

Healthy Tidbit

Broccoli is my favorite vegetable. It is so versatile, can soak up sauces, and just tastes delicious any way it's prepared. Avoid overcooking broccoli. Make sure it still crunches when you eat it. Broccoli is a good source of calcium and should therefore be an important food source of calcium for people who don't consume dairy products. Getting enough calcium through food sources is important, because a few recent studies are refuting the benefits of calcium supplementation. One study revealed that calcium supplementation failed to show a decreased risk for fracture in osteoporotic women. In addition, recent studies are showing a possible risk from calcium supplementation for heart disease. Be careful with your intake of synthetic vitamins, and ask an expert if you need more advice.

Nutritional Analysis per Serving

Vitamin A	44.8 RE	Vitamin D	0.0 µg
Thiamin (B-1)	0.1 mg	Vitamin E	0.0 mg
Riboflavin (B-2)	0.1 mg	Calcium	39.8 mg
Niacin	0.5 mg	Iron	0.6 mg
Vitamin B-6	0.1 mg	Phosphorus	52.6 mg
Vitamin B-12	0.0 µg	Magnesium	16.7 mg
Folate (total)	40.6 µg	Zinc	0.3 mg
Vitamin C	58.0 mg	Potassium	248.9 mg

Carrot Rice

PER SERVING: 246.6 CALORIES ~ 4.8 G PROTEIN ~ 39.0 G CARBOHYDRATE ~ 1.9 G FIBER ~
6.2 G TOTAL FAT ~ 0.7 G SATURATED FAT ~ 0.0 MG CHOLESTEROL ~ 21.1 MG SODIUM

1 cup basmati rice, soaked (see page 218)

2 cups water

¼ cup roasted almonds

1 onion, sliced

1 tablespoon olive oil

¾ cup finely chopped carrots

1 teaspoon minced fresh gingerroot

Salt and cayenne pepper to taste

Chopped fresh cilantro

Combine rice and water in a medium saucepan. Heat to boiling over high heat. Reduce heat to low; cover and cook until tender and water is absorbed, about 20 minutes.

While rice is cooking, grind almonds in a blender or coffee grinder and set aside. Sauté onion in oil in a medium skillet until tender and golden brown, about 10 minutes. Stir in carrots and ginger. Cook, covered, 5 minutes. Stir in almonds. Stir mixture into cooked rice; season to taste with salt and cayenne pepper. Sprinkle with cilantro.

Serves 4.

Healthy Tidbit

Carrots are extremely high in antioxidants. In a ten-year study performed in the Netherlands, consumption of yellow-orange foods significantly decreased the risk of cardiovascular disease. Carrots are high in lutein, an important antioxidant for the eyes. They are very high in vitamin A, which is important in immune system functioning. Carrots are sweet and have a high glycemic index compared to some other vegetables, but when properly balanced with other veggies they can offer a significant health benefit.

Nutritional Analysis per Serving

Vitamin A	382.2 RE	Vitamin D	0.0 µg
Thiamin (B-1)	0.1 mg	Vitamin E	0.0 mg
Riboflavin (B-2)	0.1 mg	Calcium	34.2 mg
Niacin	1.3 mg	Iron	0.8 mg
Vitamin B-6	0.1 mg	Phosphorus	45.1 mg
Vitamin B-12	0.0 µg	Magnesium	22.9 mg
Folate (total)	13.7 µg	Zinc	0.3 mg
Vitamin C	4.3 mg	Potassium	273.5 mg

Mashed Cauliflower

PER SERVING: 65.2 CALORIES ~ 2.8 G PROTEIN ~ 7.1 G CARBOHYDRATE ~ 2.9 G FIBER ~
3.8 G TOTAL FAT ~ 3.0 G SATURATED FAT ~ 0.0 MG CHOLESTEROL ~ 624.5 MG SODIUM

1 head cauliflower
1 tablespoon coconut oil
1 teaspoon salt

Steam the cauliflower until nearly soft.

Transfer to a bowl; add coconut oil and salt. Mash with a fork or hand mixer to the consistency of chunky mashed potatoes.

Serves 4.

Substitutions
This recipe is also really good with a little unsweetened almond milk. Blend the mixture with a hand blender to give it more of a sauce consistency. Sauté onions and garlic in a separate pan, add the cauliflower sauce, and serve over gluten-free pasta. Very yummy.

Healthy Tidbit
Make a list, shop carefully, and try to consume all of your vegetables before you shop again. If you are not wasting food, then you are saving money. That's important when you are trying to maintain a high-quality diet. If I have some veggies left and really need to shop, I think about how I will use them first. Spend most of your time in the grocery store getting to know the produce section. Talk to someone working at the store or someone shopping who seems to know what they are doing. I almost always get questions when I am shopping in the bulk aisle because of all the different items I am purchasing. It's fun!

Nutritional Analysis per Serving

Vitamin A	0.0 RE	Vitamin D	0.0 µg
Thiamin (B-1)	0.1 mg	Vitamin E	0.0 mg
Riboflavin (B-2)	0.1 mg	Calcium	32.0 mg
Niacin	0.7 mg	Iron	0.6 mg
Vitamin B-6	0.3 mg	Phosphorus	63.3 mg
Vitamin B-12	0.0 µg	Magnesium	21.6 mg
Folate (total)	81.9 µg	Zinc	0.4 mg
Vitamin C	69.3 mg	Potassium	429.9 mg

Roasted Squash Rings

PER SERVING: 86.7 CALORIES ~ 0.4 G PROTEIN ~ 1.5 G CARBOHYDRATE ~ 0.4 G FIBER ~
9.1 G TOTAL FAT ~ 1.3 G SATURATED FAT ~ 0.0 MG CHOLESTEROL ~ 0.9 MG SODIUM

Very tasty. My kids love these.

3 delicata squash
¼ cup olive oil
Salt and freshly ground pepper to taste

Preheat oven to 400°F.

Wash squash well. Cut each squash in half, across its width. Cut off ends, and discard seeds. Cut squash into ½-inch to ¾-inch rings. Toss with olive oil. Arrange squash on foil-lined baking sheet and sprinkle lightly with salt and pepper.

Roast for 20–30 minutes until tender and lightly browned, turning halfway through cooking time.

Serves 6.

Substitutions

Other types of winter squash can be used in this recipe as long as the skins are edible, for example, acorn or butternut. You can do some research online to see which varieties of squash fit this category. If you can't cut the squash into rings, I suggest cutting them into 1–2-inch cubes, and removing seeds and pulp before roasting. Sprinkling the squash with rosemary prior to roasting adds delicious flavor.

Healthy Tidbit

Preliminary studies have shown winter squash to have anti-inflammatory benefits. Winter squash contains some fat, including the anti-inflammatory omega-3s, but is not considered a high-fat food. One cup of baked winter squash provides approximately 340 milligrams of omega-3 fats in the form of alpha-linolenic acid (ALA). Squash also fit into the yellow-orange category of plant foods that is helpful in preventing heart disease. Finally, consuming winter squash is a good way to curb your sweet tooth. They can be a delicious sweet treat.

Nutritional Analysis per Serving

Vitamin A	5.6 RE	Vitamin D	0.0 µg
Thiamin (B-1)	0.0 mg	Vitamin E	0.0 mg
Riboflavin (B-2)	0.0 mg	Calcium	7.9 mg
Niacin	0.2 mg	Iron	0.2 mg
Vitamin B-6	0.0 mg	Phosphorus	11.9 mg
Vitamin B-12	0.0 µg	Magnesium	7.5 mg
Folate (total)	7.1 µg	Zinc	0.1 mg
Vitamin C	7.2 mg	Potassium	83.0 mg

Easy Rice and Veggies

PER SERVING: 183.6 CALORIES ~ 6.2 G PROTEIN ~ 29.3 G CARBOHYDRATE ~ 7.2 G FIBER ~
6.2 G TOTAL FAT ~ 1.2 G SATURATED FAT ~ 0.0 MG CHOLESTEROL ~ 53.3 MG SODIUM

2 cups cooked short-grain brown rice (see instructions on page 218)

2 heads broccoli, cut into 1-inch pieces, steamed crisp-tender

½ head cauliflower, cut into 1-inch pieces, steamed crisp-tender

1 bunch kale, chopped small, lightly steamed

1 avocado, sliced

1 carrot, shredded

Sprouts (optional)

Place rice on a large serving platter. Arrange cooked vegetables on top of rice, and top with avocado, carrot, and sprouts (if using). Serve with your favorite sauce: teriyaki, peanut sauce, chili or spicy sauce, or gluten-free tamari.

Serves 6.

Substitutions

This is an easy "go to" meal when you want good nutrition without a lot of effort. Experiment with a variety of vegetables. If you need or want protein with it, try the Roasted Tempeh (see page 72), marinated and baked extra-firm tofu, or chicken.

Healthy Tidbit

Lightly steaming vegetables keeps them crunchy and full of enzymes and nutrients, but it demands that you chew your food thoroughly. When eating raw or near-raw foods, your digestion needs to be thorough to help you absorb as many nutrients as possible. Digestion begins in the mouth, with the saliva produced there and with the chewing process. Chewing well breaks down food and stimulates the release of gastric (stomach) juices so that by the time the food reaches the stomach, the stomach is prepared for the digestion process. Many people eat too quickly, which can result in bloating, gastric reflux or heartburn, decreased absorption of nutrients, abdominal pain, constipation, and other problems. So *slow down* when you eat. Enjoy, relax, chew, and get into the moment. Your body will thank you for it.

Nutritional Analysis per Serving

Vitamin A	696.1 RE	Vitamin D	0.0 µg
Thiamin (B-1)	0.2 mg	Vitamin E	0.0 mg
Riboflavin (B-2)	0.2 mg	Calcium	92.1 mg
Niacin	2.1 mg	Iron	1.6 mg
Vitamin B-6	0.4 mg	Phosphorus	145.1 mg
Vitamin B-12	0.0 µg	Magnesium	70.6 mg
Folate (total)	78.7 µg	Zinc	1.1 mg
Vitamin C	91.3 mg	Potassium	698.8 mg

Raw Beets

PER SERVING: 11.6 CALORIES ~ 0.4 G PROTEIN ~ 2.6 G CARBOHYDRATE ~ 0.8 G FIBER ~
0.1 G TOTAL FAT ~ 0.0 G SATURATED FAT ~ 0.0 MG CHOLESTEROL ~ 21.3 MG SODIUM

2 large red beets, raw, peeled, and thinly sliced
Juice of half lemon (optional)

Arrange the beets on a serving dish. Sprinkle with lemon juice, if desired.
Serve immediately.
Serves 6.

Substitutions
You can use golden or orange beets for this preparation, or a combination of
all three for a beautiful but simple display of color. I like to include beets in
the raw relish tray that we serve at holidays. You can also use orange or lemon
zest on top of these beets for more of a citrus kick.

Healthy Tidbit
Raw vegetables are an extremely healthy part of a good diet. Raw foods help to
keep the body alkaline. They are full of dietary fiber, which can facilitate bowel
movements and help regulate blood sugar, decreasing risk for insulin resistance. Raw veggies can easily be carried with you for lunch or while travelling.
Eating raw is not time-consuming, and it can provide significant nutritional
benefits. The cooking process results in the loss of some important nutrients
by denaturing enzymes and proteins. Make sure that your diet includes some
raw vegetables.

Nutritional Analysis per Serving

Vitamin A	0.9 RE	Vitamin D	0.0 µg
Thiamin (B-1)	0.0 mg	Vitamin E	0.0 mg
Riboflavin (B-2)	0.0 mg	Calcium	4.4 mg
Niacin	0.1 mg	Iron	0.2 mg
Vitamin B-6	0.0 mg	Phosphorus	10.9 mg
Vitamin B-12	0.0 µg	Magnesium	6.3 mg
Folate (total)	29.8 µg	Zinc	0.1 mg
Vitamin C	1.3 mg	Potassium	88.8 mg

Kiwi Cucumber Salsa

PER SERVING: 47.8 CALORIES ~ 1.1 G PROTEIN ~ 11.3 G CARBOHYDRATE ~ 1.8 G FIBER ~
0.4 G TOTAL FAT ~ 0.1 G SATURATED FAT ~ 0.0 MG CHOLESTEROL ~ 3.0 MG SODIUM

2 cups diced kiwi, peeled
1 cup diced cucumber, unpeeled
½ cup diced red bell pepper
⅓ cup chopped fresh cilantro
¼ cup diced red onion
2 tablespoons fresh lime juice
1 jalapeño, seeds removed, diced
Salt to taste

Combine all ingredients in a large glass bowl, and chill in the refrigerator. If possible, assemble at least an hour before serving to allow flavors to marry.
Serves 6.

Serving Tip
Serve with rice chips or on tacos and salads.

Healthy Tidbit
Regular eating and sleeping patterns, combined with a balanced diet, promote balanced hormone levels. Hormones control nearly all of our bodily functions, including sleep, blood sugar, blood pressure, energy, mood, and digestion.

Nutritional Analysis per Serving

Vitamin A	47.3 RE	Vitamin D	0.0 µg
Thiamin (B-1)	0.0 mg	Vitamin E	0.9 mg
Riboflavin (B-2)	0.1 mg	Calcium	18.1 mg
Niacin	0.4 mg	Iron	0.3 mg
Vitamin B-6	0.1 mg	Phosphorus	28.0 mg
Vitamin B-12	0.0 µg	Magnesium	13.7 mg
Folate (total)	30.1 µg	Zinc	0.1 mg
Vitamin C	86.3 mg	Potassium	266.3 mg

Rice Chips with Goat Cheese and Cucumber

PER SERVING: 209.3 CALORIES ~ 9.9 G PROTEIN ~ 14.3 G CARBOHYDRATE ~ 0.8 G FIBER ~
12.5 G TOTAL FAT ~ 7.8 G SATURATED FAT ~ 29.6 MG CHOLESTEROL ~ 251.7 MG SODIUM

½ cup goat cheese
16 almond rice thins crackers or other rice crackers
16 thin cucumber slices

Spread a thin layer of goat cheese on each rice cracker. Top with a cucumber slice and arrange on a serving tray.

Serves 2.

Substitutions

You can use various types of goat cheese or soft sheep cheese. You could also use Cream Cheese "Curds and Whey" (recipe on page 172). The tart flavor of the cheese when married with the fresh cucumbers makes a delicious treat. You can also serve the goat cheese on top of the cucumber slices without the crackers.

Healthy Tidbit

This recipe would make a quick, healthy treat to take to a party or potluck. You'll be surprised that among the cookies and brownies, the healthy dishes often get gobbled up first. Other ideas: a colorful tray of cut-up veggies or fruit with a fabulous dip, romaine boats filled with a topping of your choice, gluten-free cookies, gluten-free pasta salads, and so on. Labeling your contribution as "dairy-free" or "gluten-free" can be helpful and appreciated by others who are careful of what they eat.

Nutritional Analysis per Serving

Vitamin A	156.9 RE	Vitamin D	0.2 µg
Thiamin (B-1)	0.0 mg	Vitamin E	0.3 mg
Riboflavin (B-2)	0.3 mg	Calcium	220.1 mg
Niacin	0.5 mg	Iron	0.9 mg
Vitamin B-6	0.0 mg	Phosphorus	153.1 mg
Vitamin B-12	0.1 µg	Magnesium	17.6 mg
Folate (total)	4.4 µg	Zinc	0.4 mg
Vitamin C	1.5 mg	Potassium	135.7 mg

Salads

Sesame–Ginger Vinaigrette Salad

PER SERVING: 327.3 CALORIES ~ 13.4 G PROTEIN ~ 13.4 G CARBOHYDRATE ~ 3.0 G FIBER ~
25.6 G TOTAL FAT ~ 2.8 G SATURATED FAT ~ 27.0 MG CHOLESTEROL ~ 134.8 MG SODIUM

For the Salad
1 head leaf lettuce, chopped

2 tangerines, peeled and chopped

2 tablespoons slivered almonds

1 tablespoon sesame seeds

1 cup chopped cooked chicken breast

For the Dressing
5 tablespoons flax seed oil or light sesame oil

Juice of one tangerine

3 tablespoons rice vinegar

1 tablespoon toasted sesame oil

1 tablespoon toasted sesame seeds

1 garlic clove, finely minced or puréed

1 teaspoon chopped gingerroot

1 teaspoon soy sauce

1 teaspoon agave nectar

Arrange lettuce on serving platter; top with chicken, tangerines, almonds, and sesame seeds. Combine dressing ingredients in blender; purée until smooth. Pour dressing over salad, and serve immediately.

Note: You can purchase raw sesame seeds and gently toss them in a cast iron skillet over medium heat to toast. Keep the seeds moving the entire time; the toasting time should be very short. Any good-quality flax seed oil will work if you can't find light sesame oil.

Serves 4.

Substitutions
You could also use this dressing as a dipping sauce for fresh vegetables or for chicken wraps.

Healthy Tidbit
I have seen a significant amount of recurring joint pain in many of my patients, especially as they age. Arthritis, an inflammatory condition, is a

Nutritional Analysis per Serving

Vitamin A	702.6 RE	Vitamin D	0.0 µg
Thiamin (B-1)	0.2 mg	Vitamin E	0.1 mg
Riboflavin (B-2)	0.2 mg	Calcium	70.6 mg
Niacin	3.9 mg	Iron	1.6 mg
Vitamin B-6	0.3 mg	Phosphorus	143.3 mg
Vitamin B-12	0.1 µg	Magnesium	50.5 mg
Folate (total)	49.3 µg	Zinc	1.0 mg
Vitamin C	25.8 mg	Potassium	388.2 mg

common age-related problem in the United States, which is one of the reasons why it is so important to reduce inflammation in the body through diet. Many foods can trigger inflammation, and part of the anti-inflammation diet involves learning what foods cause negative reactions for you. Though citrus fruits contain a significant amount of vitamin C and other antioxidants, they can be a common trigger for many of my arthritis patients. If you are unsure about your reaction to citrus, I suggest you stop eating all citrus except small amounts of lemon and lime juice for an entire month. Then test your reaction by reintroducing citrus. Consume at least one whole orange or grapefruit. If you wake up with joint pain the next morning, you can probably be sure that citrus triggered your inflammation. In that case, simply eliminate the tangerines from this recipe, and prepare the dressing with a very small squeeze of lime or lemon juice instead.

Cucumber Salad

PER SERVING: 92.0 CALORIES ~ 1.2 G PROTEIN ~ 24.1 G CARBOHYDRATE ~ 1.0 G FIBER ~ 0.2 G TOTAL FAT ~ 0.1 G SATURATED FAT ~ 0.0 MG CHOLESTEROL ~ 4.9 MG SODIUM

2–3 small cucumbers, peeled and chopped into ½-inch pieces
½ small white onion, minced
½ cup rice vinegar
¼ cup honey
¼ cup water
1 tablespoon chopped fresh dill

Combine all ingredients in a large bowl; chill for 30 minutes or longer before serving.
    Serves 4.

Healthy Tidbit

Cucumbers are very cooling and can help to beat the summer heat. Because cucumbers are 95 percent water, they help to keep the body hydrated. They offer good nutrition with few calories.

Nutritional Analysis per Serving

Vitamin A	16.9 RE	Vitamin D	0.0 μg
Thiamin (B-1)	0.0 mg	Vitamin E	0.0 mg
Riboflavin (B-2)	0.1 mg	Calcium	29.2 mg
Niacin	0.2 mg	Iron	0.5 mg
Vitamin B-6	0.1 mg	Phosphorus	41.0 mg
Vitamin B-12	0.0 μg	Magnesium	21.6 mg
Folate (total)	13.8 μg	Zinc	0.4 mg
Vitamin C	5.5 mg	Potassium	253.4 mg

Tangy Quinoa Salad

PER SERVING: 507.3 CALORIES ~ 7.7 G PROTEIN ~ 35.1 G CARBOHYDRATE ~ 4.6 G FIBER ~
39.0 G TOTAL FAT ~ 5.3 G SATURATED FAT ~ 0.0 MG CHOLESTEROL ~ 611.1 MG SODIUM

1 cup uncooked quinoa

2 cups water

1 cup chopped broccoli florets

1 cup sliced spinach leaves

1 cup minced parsley

1 cup lemon juice

⅔ cup olive oil

3 cloves garlic, minced

3 tablespoons minced mint leaves

1 teaspoon salt

Heat water and quinoa to boiling in a medium saucepan. Reduce the heat and simmer, covered, until water is absorbed, about 15 minutes. Place broccoli in a glass bowl; spoon hot quinoa over broccoli. Cover and let sit for about 10 minutes. Broccoli will be bright green but still crunchy. Let cool to room temperature; stir in remaining ingredients. Chill.

Serves 4.

Substitutions

You can experiment with many different greens for this salad. Instead of quinoa, you could try cooked buckwheat, which imparts a very different flavor. For added color and sweet flavor, add up to ¼ cup dried goji berries.

Healthy Tidbit

Mint is one of my favorite herbs. It is extremely easy to grow and a great addition to many recipes. Mint helps ease and promote digestion and can help to relieve bloating and gas. Even the aroma of mint is known to activate the salivary glands in the mouth, as well as other glands that secrete digestive enzymes, thereby facilitating digestion. This explains its long history of use in the culinary arts.

Nutritional Analysis per Serving

Vitamin A	218.6 RE	Vitamin D	0.0 µg
Thiamin (B-1)	0.2 mg	Vitamin E	0.0 mg
Riboflavin (B-2)	0.2 mg	Calcium	74.0 mg
Niacin	1.1 mg	Iron	3.6 mg
Vitamin B-6	0.3 mg	Phosphorus	230.9 mg
Vitamin B-12	0.0 µg	Magnesium	108.4 mg
Folate (total)	143.8 µg	Zinc	1.7 mg
Vitamin C	67.3 mg	Potassium	517.6 mg

Apricot and Butternut Quinoa Salad

PER SERVING: 163.5 CALORIES ~ 3.3 G PROTEIN ~ 21.9 G CARBOHYDRATE ~ 3.7 G FIBER ~
7.8 G TOTAL FAT ~ 1.0 G SATURATED FAT ~ 0.0 MG CHOLESTEROL ~ 8.3 MG SODIUM

1 butternut squash, peeled, seeded, and cut into 1-inch cubes

1 large onion, cut into 1-inch chunks

¼ cup olive oil

Salt and pepper to taste

4 apricots, pitted, diced

3 tablespoons chopped fresh mint leaves

3 tablespoons chopped parsley

½ teaspoon ground cinnamon

½ teaspoon cumin

Grated zest of ½ lemon

2 teaspoons lemon juice

Pinch saffron

2 cups cooked quinoa, warm

Salt and pepper to taste

Preheat oven to 375°F.

Toss squash and onion with olive oil; place in roasting pan and sprinkle with salt and pepper. Roast until lightly browned and tender, about 30 minutes, stirring halfway through baking time.

Combine roasted vegetables and remaining ingredients in large serving bowl, mixing well. Season with salt and pepper. Chill and serve.

Serves 8.

Substitutions

Try different varieties of squash, and play with the other ingredients until this salad perfectly matches your tastes. It is a fun salad to serve at a potluck because it will most likely be different from other dishes. It offers a great amount of nutrition due to the squash, parsley, and quinoa. If you are unable to get fresh apricots, you can use dried. You could also try peaches. This dish is also excellent served hot.

Healthy Tidbit

Quinoa is the only grain that provides complete protein without adding a legume. Quinoa has a strong ancestral history, dating back to ancient Incan civilization. In addition to its high protein content, it is also a satisfying, low-fat source of complex carbohydrates and fiber. One cup of cooked quinoa contains 30 milligrams of calcium, qualifying it as a good source of dietary calcium. Quinoa is also a strong source of iron, which is vital in circulating oxygen to all of your bodily tissues.

Nutritional Analysis per Serving

Vitamin A	792.9 RE	Vitamin D	0.0 µg
Thiamin (B-1)	0.1 mg	Vitamin E	0.0 mg
Riboflavin (B-2)	0.1 mg	Calcium	55.2 mg
Niacin	1.2 mg	Iron	1.5 mg
Vitamin B-6	1.2 mg	Phosphorus	103.1 mg
Vitamin B-12	0.0 µg	Magnesium	58.1 mg
Folate (total)	45.8 µg	Zinc	1.0 mg
Vitamin C	22.0 mg	Potassium	409.8 mg

Romaine Boats

PER SERVING: 233.4 CALORIES ~ 8.6 G PROTEIN ~ 12.3 G CARBOHYDRATE ~ 2.2 G FIBER ~ 15.8 G TOTAL FAT ~ 4.2 G SATURATED FAT ~ 40.5 MG CHOLESTEROL ~ 586.0 MG SODIUM

For the Boats

2 8-ounce packages turkey bacon, cut into 1-inch pieces

1 tablespoon olive oil

4 cloves garlic, minced

3 green apples, peeled, cored, and diced

2 teaspoons coconut oil

½ teaspoon cinnamon

1 bunch romaine lettuce, separated into leaves

Microgreens, as garnish (see Healthy Tidbit below)

For the Dressing

¼ cup brown rice vinegar

¼ cup apple cider vinegar

¼ cup olive oil

1 tablespoon pure maple syrup

⅛ teaspoon salt

Cook bacon in olive oil in a large skillet over medium heat until crisp, about 8 minutes, stirring frequently. Add garlic during last minute of cooking time.

Sauté apples in coconut oil in medium skillet over high heat until crisp-tender, about 5 minutes; sprinkle with cinnamon. Remove from heat; spoon apples into bowl and let cool.

Whisk dressing ingredients together in a small bowl. Arrange romaine leaves on a serving plate. Fill with bacon mixture, top with apple mixture, and garnish with microgreens. Drizzle with dressing; serve immediately.

Serves 8.

Healthy Tidbit

Think of microgreens as the "adolescent" growth stage of your favorite vegetables. (Sprouts are the "baby" stage.) They are fun and easy to experiment with. You can plant your own seeds in a small amount of soil and grow your own greens. I think small-seed plants work best for microgreens because they don't get as bitter. Try alfalfa, clover, broccoli, arugula, cabbage, cress, radish, or any other tiny seeds. *The Anti-Inflammation Diet and Recipe Book* describes in detail how to grow sprouts.

Nutritional Analysis per Serving

Vitamin A	7.4 RE	Vitamin D	0.0 µg
Thiamin (B-1)	0.0 mg	Vitamin E	0.0 mg
Riboflavin (B-2)	0.1 mg	Calcium	17.3 mg
Niacin	0.1 mg	Iron	0.4 mg
Vitamin B-6	0.1 mg	Phosphorus	15.8 mg
Vitamin B-12	0.0 µg	Magnesium	7.1 mg
Folate (total)	28.5 µg	Zinc	0.1 mg
Vitamin C	8.3 mg	Potassium	132.9 mg

Growing Microgreens

I have grown seeds in the plastic containers used for salad greens. I also have larger flats that I have purchased for about a dollar each. Both work well. If you want to stay small-scale use the salad boxes, and if you want to go bigger use the larger trays. To prepare the container, simply punch five to seven drainage holes in the bottom using a sharp pair of scissors or knife. Fill the container with well-moistened, organic potting soil to within an inch or so from the top. Evenly distribute a thin layer of seeds, sprinkling them over the soil surface with about ⅛" to ¼" of space between them. Cover the seeds with a thin layer of soil, about ⅛" deep. Set the container in the sunniest window in the house; make sure you place a drip tray beneath it. (This is why salad boxes work so well. The lid can serve as the drip tray.) Water the seeds well to get them germinating, but don't overwater to the point of promoting mold growth. (I say this because I live in Oregon, which tends to be cool and gray most months of the year, and I have had mold start growing due to overwatering.) Keep the soil moist, like a wrung-out sponge—not soaking wet. To avoid overwatering, pour out any water that remains in the drip tray an hour after watering.

Grow until the greens are close to 2" tall, pluck the whole plant, sprout and all, and eat. Generally, you can't trim microgreens and regrow new plants, so I just pick them and grow more.

Microgreens can usually be grown in any season. I generally let mine grow until the moment their first set of "true leaves" begin to peek out. The first leaves you see are called "seed leaves" since they are actually a part of the seed. "True leaves" are the second set to appear and often look very different from the seed leaves. When true leaves grow the plant will start to get a little bitter, so you should harvest before this happens. Happy growing!

Coleslaw

PER SERVING: 178.9 CALORIES ~ 2.6 G PROTEIN ~ 15.0 G CARBOHYDRATE ~ 4.7 G FIBER ~
12.9 G TOTAL FAT ~ 1.9 G SATURATED FAT ~ 5.2 MG CHOLESTEROL ~ 402.8 MG SODIUM

For the Slaw
1 head cabbage, shredded or finely chopped
1 apple, peeled, cored, finely chopped
2 carrots, shredded or finely chopped
½ purple onion, thinly sliced

For the Dressing

½ cup mayonnaise

½ cup red wine vinegar

¼ cup poppy seeds

2 teaspoons honey, or stevia to taste

1 teaspoon salt

¼–½ teaspoon ground white pepper

Combine slaw ingredients in a large bowl. Whisk dressing ingredients together in a small bowl; pour over slaw, tossing until well mixed. Chill several hours or overnight.

Serves 8.

Substitutions
Sometimes, for color, I like to use half green cabbage and half red cabbage. They don't vary in flavor that much, but I love to stimulate all the senses by including a variety of colors. You can add a little purple onion to this recipe as well.

Healthy Tidbit
Poppy seeds get a bad rap due to their potential to show up as a "positive" on a drug test. The poppy seeds we buy in stores, though, come from an entirely different plant than the poppy plant that produces drugs like opium. Poppy seeds have a large variety of uses. They are good for adding flavor to baked items such as breads, rolls, cookies, and cakes. You can grind poppy seeds to include in desserts and in sauces to help thicken and color them. You can add them to cooked foods to enhance flavor and aroma. Poppy seeds contain the minerals iodine, manganese, magnesium, zinc, and copper. They are also a good source of anti-inflammatory omega-3 fatty acids. Lastly, poppy seeds aid in digestion by stimulating the secretion of many digestive enzymes. Don't be afraid to use them; they can add nutrition and flavor to your meals.

Nutritional Analysis per Serving

Vitamin A	276.1 RE	Vitamin D	0.0 µg
Thiamin (B-1)	0.1 mg	Vitamin E	0.0 mg
Riboflavin (B-2)	0.1 mg	Calcium	116.1 mg
Niacin	0.5 mg	Iron	1.1 mg
Vitamin B-6	0.3 mg	Phosphorus	80.6 mg
Vitamin B-12	0.0 µg	Magnesium	32.7 mg
Folate (total)	57.9 µg	Zinc	0.6 mg
Vitamin C	44.1 mg	Potassium	314.7 mg

Party Slaw

PER SERVING: 337.2 CALORIES ~ 8.9 G PROTEIN ~ 38.2 G CARBOHYDRATE ~ 6.5 G FIBER ~
18.7 G TOTAL FAT ~ 2.4 G SATURATED FAT ~ 0.0 MG CHOLESTEROL ~ 598.7 MG SODIUM

I had this slaw at a potluck and came up with a recipe that tasted similar. I made some changes and *voilà,* the perfect slaw to take to a potluck.

For the Slaw
1 head white cabbage, shredded or finely chopped
½ head purple cabbage, shredded or finely chopped
½ bunch kale, thinly sliced
2 carrots, shredded
1 bunch green onions, thinly sliced
½ cup minced fresh cilantro

For the Dressing
½ cup brown rice vinegar
½ cup olive oil
¼ cup sunflower seed butter
¼ cup gluten-free tamari
2 tablespoons agave syrup or honey
3 tablespoons grated fresh gingerroot
5 large cloves garlic, minced

Combine slaw ingredients in a large bowl. Whisk dressing ingredients together in a small bowl until smooth. Pour dressing over vegetables, mixing well. Chill several hours or overnight.

Serves 8.

Substitutions
This dressing is so tasty that almost any vegetable would be good with it. Try including other leafy greens, such as chard or spinach. Avoid traditional salad greens (lettuces) because they wilt too quickly, and only use spinach if the salad will be eaten the same day it is made.

Healthy Tidbit
By eating your fruits and veggies raw, you are less likely to modify them in an unhealthy way, such as overcooking or processing. However, some individuals have a difficult time digesting raw foods; they experience gas and bloating after consuming

Nutritional Analysis per Serving

Vitamin A	984.5 RE	Vitamin D	0.0 µg
Thiamin (B-1)	0.3 mg	Vitamin E	0.0 mg
Riboflavin (B-2)	0.2 mg	Calcium	218.4 mg
Niacin	1.9 mg	Iron	3.4 mg
Vitamin B-6	0.6 mg	Phosphorus	288.2 mg
Vitamin B-12	0.0 µg	Magnesium	77.8 mg
Folate (total)	141.9 µg	Zinc	1.2 mg
Vitamin C	119.5 mg	Potassium	909.9 mg

salads and other raw vegetables. Cabbage has a tendency to cause slight gas and bloating, but it should not be troublesome or severe. If you endure severe gas and bloating after eating salads, raw greens, or other raw foods, consider steaming most of your foods for a few months to see if this calms down your digestive troubles. Nearly all veggies and fruits can be steamed or baked before eating, with the exception of avocado, melons, mango, and papaya.

Fruit Salad with Jicama and Cucumber

PER SERVING: 142.7 CALORIES ~ 2.5 G PROTEIN ~ 34.9 G CARBOHYDRATE ~ 8.2 G FIBER ~
0.7 G TOTAL FAT ~ 0.2 G SATURATED FAT ~ 0.0 MG CHOLESTEROL ~ 8.5 MG SODIUM

3 medium kiwi, peeled, diced
1 small jicama, peeled, diced
1½ cups sliced or diced strawberries
1 cucumber, peeled, seeded, diced
1 mango or papaya, peeled, diced
2 cups halved grapes
1 tablespoons lime juice
1 teaspoon honey (optional)
Small pinch of cayenne pepper (optional)

Combine all ingredients in a serving bowl, mixing well. Chill.
    Serves 6.

Substitution
You can use various fruits for this salad. Consider adding pineapple or melons. For a delicious Mexican fruit salad, add a tablespoon or two of minced cilantro. I learned about putting jicama and cucumber into my salads from my good friend Rosalinda Camacho, who lives in Lafayette, Oregon.

Healthy Tidbit
Be the person who brings healthy dishes to a potluck or function. People will appreciate seeing something nutritious as an option. Kids love this salad. They may think the jicama is strange at first because it is new to them, but they usually love its crunchy flavor. Almost all kids love the cucumbers. The cayenne is a fun addition if you are serving to adults or older children who can tolerate a little spice.

Nutritional Analysis per Serving

Vitamin A	40.9 RE	Vitamin D	0.0 µg
Thiamin (B-1)	0.1 mg	Vitamin E	0.7 mg
Riboflavin (B-2)	0.1 mg	Calcium	44.8 mg
Niacin	0.9 mg	Iron	1.3 mg
Vitamin B-6	0.2 mg	Phosphorus	68.2 mg
Vitamin B-12	0.0 µg	Magnesium	37.6 mg
Folate (total)	56.1 µg	Zinc	0.4 mg
Vitamin C	105.0 mg	Potassium	586.6 mg

Radish Salad

PER SERVING: 41.0 CALORIES ~ 0.3 G PROTEIN ~ 0.7 G CARBOHYDRATE ~ 0.3 G FIBER ~
3.9 G TOTAL FAT ~ 0.3 G SATURATED FAT ~ 0.0 MG CHOLESTEROL ~ 6.4 MG SODIUM

This dish is very pleasing to the eye.

> 1 bunch radishes, thinly sliced
> 1 tablespoon pumpkinseed oil
> 1 tablespoon red wine vinegar
> 1 tablespoon sunflower seeds
> Salt to taste
> 2 tablespoons microgreens

Arrange radishes in a spiral on a serving plate. Top with sunflower seeds;
drizzle with oil and vinegar. Sprinkle with salt and top with microgreens.
   Serves 4.

Substitutions
If you are unable to find pumpkinseed oil, then use a nice truffle, walnut, or
hazelnut oil instead.

Healthy Tidbit
Radishes are a very underutilized vegetable. I love adding them to salads,
eating them raw, or drizzling them with a little dressing, as in this lovely
preparation. Radishes are extremely high in vitamin C, an antioxidant and
powerful stimulant of the immune system. As part of the cruciferous vegetable
family, along with kale, broccoli, cabbage, and brussels sprouts, radishes provide cancer-protective properties. If you have a thyroid goiter, be careful when
consuming raw cruciferous vegetables as they are goitrogenic (can promote
the formation of goiter).

Nutritional Analysis per Serving

Vitamin A	0.1 RE	Vitamin D	0.0 µg
Thiamin (B-1)	0.0 mg	Vitamin E	0.0 mg
Riboflavin (B-2)	0.0 mg	Calcium	4.2 mg
Niacin	0.1 mg	Iron	0.1 mg
Vitamin B-6	0.0 mg	Phosphorus	7.7 mg
Vitamin B-12	0.0 µg	Magnesium	3.8 mg
Folate (total)	5.0 µg	Zinc	0.1 mg
Vitamin C	2.0 mg	Potassium	37.6 mg

Lemon–Bright Chickpea Salad

PER SERVING: 144.0 CALORIES ~ 5.9 G PROTEIN ~ 19.6 G CARBOHYDRATE ~ 5.3 G FIBER ~
5.6 G TOTAL FAT ~ 0.7 G SATURATED FAT ~ 0.0 MG CHOLESTEROL ~ 588.4 MG SODIUM

From Robin Michelle Crout, a cooking instructor from Tacoma, Washington.

1 15-ounce can chickpeas, rinsed and drained
Juice of 1 lemon
1 tablespoon extra-virgin olive oil
1 medium English cucumber, diced
½ medium red onion, diced
½ teaspoon salt
Freshly ground black pepper to taste

Combine all ingredients in serving bowl. Refrigerate; serve chilled.
Serves 4.

Substitutions

Experiment with adding other vegetables, such as chopped spinach, parsley, or black olives. If you can tolerate feta cheese, it would also be an excellent addition. So would chopped sundried tomatoes, assuming you can tolerate them, for a tangy taste.

Healthy Tidbit

Chickpeas, or garbanzo beans, are legumes that are very versatile and easy to use. They are an excellent source of both soluble and insoluble fiber. Due to their high fiber content, garbanzos are a good choice for those with diabetes or insulin resistance. The protein in the garbanzos helps to decrease the undesirable spike in blood glucose that occurs after some meals. Garbanzos are also high in iron and manganese, which acts as a valuable coenzyme in a number of reactions involved in the production of energy and antioxidant defenses.

Nutritional Analysis per Serving

Vitamin A	10.2 RE	Vitamin D	0.0 µg
Thiamin (B-1)	0.1 mg	Vitamin E	0.0 mg
Riboflavin (B-2)	0.1 mg	Calcium	53.5 mg
Niacin	0.2 mg	Iron	1.6 mg
Vitamin B-6	0.6 mg	Phosphorus	108.2 mg
Vitamin B-12	0.0 µg	Magnesium	40.8 mg
Folate (total)	37.6 µg	Zinc	0.9 mg
Vitamin C	9.0 mg	Potassium	300.1 mg

Wilted Spinach Salad

PER SERVING: 480.2 CALORIES ~ 6.4 G PROTEIN ~ 34.8 G CARBOHYDRATE ~ 6.4 G FIBER ~
37.6 G TOTAL FAT ~ 4.3 G SATURATED FAT ~ 0.0 MG CHOLESTEROL ~ 298.7 MG SODIUM

For the Walnuts
1 cup walnuts
6 tablespoons water
6 tablespoons coconut palm sugar

For the Dressing
1 cup raspberries
⅓ cup olive oil
¼ cup red wine vinegar
3 tablespoons Dijon mustard
1 tablespoon lemon juice
Salt and pepper to taste

For the Salad
6 cups spinach, trimmed and washed
½ red onion, sliced thin and long
1 fresh pear, diced

To make the walnuts: Combine walnuts, water, and coconut palm sugar in a medium saucepan. Stir over medium heat until walnuts are coated and the liquid evaporates, about 5 minutes. Cool nuts on a plate.

To make the dressing: Combine dressing ingredients in a food processor or blender. Process until smooth; strain through a fine sieve to remove seeds.

To make the salad: Combine salad ingredients in a serving bowl. Heat dressing in a small saucepan until warm but not boiling. Pour dressing over salad ingredients and toss well. Sprinkle with reserved walnuts.

Serves 4.

Substitutions
Goat cheese or gorgonzola cheese can be added to this recipe if you are able to tolerate dairy. To prepare the same recipe without wilting the spinach, don't heat the salad dressing. (Conversely, you can make most salads into wilted spinach

Nutritional Analysis per Serving

Vitamin A	424.5 RE	Vitamin D	0.0 µg
Thiamin (B-1)	0.2 mg	Vitamin E	0.0 mg
Riboflavin (B-2)	0.2 mg	Calcium	93.0 mg
Niacin	1.0 mg	Iron	2.7 mg
Vitamin B-6	0.3 mg	Phosphorus	142.0 mg
Vitamin B-12	0.0 µg	Magnesium	94.9 mg
Folate (total)	128.7 µg	Zinc	0.6 mg
Vitamin C	25.3 mg	Potassium	505.9 mg

salads by using spinach in place of other greens and heating the dressing prior to pouring it over the leaves.)

The candied walnuts are also a holiday favorite. They are easy and quick to make, are healthier, and will please guests just as much as a snickerdoodle cookie. You can add cinnamon, nutmeg, ground black pepper, or other spices. If you are diabetic or avoiding sugar, use plain roasted walnuts instead of candying them.

Healthy Tidbit

Artificial sweeteners and sugar substitutes can be very appealing to people looking to cut calories or control blood sugar, but in general I advise people against using alternative sugar sources. I encourage people to break their sugar addictions and to use limited quantities of sweeteners that are naturally present, such as honey and pure maple syrup. If absolutely needed, I allow small amounts of coconut palm sugar. The verdict is still out as to the health benefits it can provide over regular white sugar.

Coconut palm sugar is being touted by some sources as a low-glycemic alternative to white sugar. I believe more research needs to be done to confirm this claim, but for now it appears to be a better alternative to cane sugar. Made from the nectar or sap of the coconut palm tree, it does have more nutrient value. Read the label when you purchase coconut palm sugar, because some "palm sugars" that are sold in Asian markets are blended with other fillers such as white sugar. Pure, certified-organic coconut palm sugar is sold in the United States under the brand name Sweet Tree and can be found at some natural-food stores. See Resources to learn where you can find this sugar. I tell my patients that if they have a recipe in which sugar is absolutely needed, then coconut palm sugar can be a viable substitute. It does have a pleasingly complex taste, and I enjoy using it sparingly.

Rainbow Salad

PER SERVING: 368.9 CALORIES ~ 2.0 G PROTEIN ~ 16.3 G CARBOHYDRATE ~ 2.8 G FIBER ~
33.8 G TOTAL FAT ~ 5.0 G SATURATED FAT ~ 13.3 MG CHOLESTEROL ~ 221.6 MG SODIUM

1½ cups chopped red and yellow bell peppers
1½ cups chopped broccoli
1 cup shredded carrots
¼ cup minced red onion

⅔ cup mayonnaise
2 tablespoons brown rice vinegar
2 tablespoons olive oil
1½ tablespoons raw honey

Combine all ingredients in a medium bowl; toss until well mixed. Refrigerate until ready to serve.

Serves 4.

Substitutions

There are myriad changes you could make to this salad. Add sprouts, jicama, parsley, cilantro, or kale; the options really are almost limitless.

Healthy Tidbit

I love the name of this salad. It makes me think of a general rule everyone should follow: aim to include a rainbow of colored vegetables and fruits in your diet each week. A helpful list follows. If you don't know what to do with some of these veggies, do an internet search for recipes using them. For example, you can make a wonderful root-vegetable soup by simmering a few of the root vegetables listed here in one of the homemade broths included in the soup section.

Red: beets, cranberries, strawberries

Orange: carrots, orange beets

Yellow: yellow squash, golden beets, wax (yellow) beans

Green: spinach, chard, kale, broccoli, salad greens, brussels sprouts, asparagus, green beans

Light green: zucchini, cucumber, cabbage, green grapes

Blue: blueberries, blue kale

Purple: purple grapes, eggplant (if you eat the skin), plums, purple cabbage, fresh figs, purple onion, blackberries

Pink: pink daikon radish, regular radishes

White: white onion, turnip, parsnip, cauliflower

Nutritional Analysis per Serving

Vitamin A	625.2 RE	Vitamin D	0.0 µg
Thiamin (B-1)	0.1 mg	Vitamin E	0.0 mg
Riboflavin (B-2)	0.1 mg	Calcium	34.0 mg
Niacin	1.1 mg	Iron	0.7 mg
Vitamin B-6	0.3 mg	Phosphorus	51.1 mg
Vitamin B-12	0.0 µg	Magnesium	19.2 mg
Folate (total)	50.7 µg	Zinc	0.4 mg
Vitamin C	132.4 mg	Potassium	352.8 mg

Shredded Chicken over Romaine

PER SERVING: 294.8 CALORIES ~ 11.5 G PROTEIN ~ 9.2 G CARBOHYDRATE ~ 4.8 G FIBER ~
24.3 G TOTAL FAT ~ 3.7 G SATURATED FAT ~ 26.2 MG CHOLESTEROL ~ 99.7 MG SODIUM

For the Salad
4 cups chopped romaine lettuce leaves
2½ cups Shredded Chicken (see recipe on page 202)
½ cup cooked black beans
1 avocado, diced

For the Dressing
½ cup olive oil
¼ cup red wine vinegar
¼ cup lemon juice
Salt to taste

Arrange lettuce on serving platter; top with chicken, black beans, and avocado.
Whisk dressing ingredients in medium bowl until blended; pour over salad.
Serve immediately.

Serves 6.

Healthy Tidbit

Reduce stress in your life by adopting these three important behaviors:

1. Change your perspective. Own your stress, but don't let it own you. Acknowledge that you may be unable to change what is happening, but you can change your reaction to it.

2. Breathe. Take time each day to remember those deep belly breaths that help to calm you down.

3. Think positively. Envision yourself feeling more calm and carefree.

Nutritional Analysis per Serving

Vitamin A	282.1 RE	Vitamin D	0.0 µg
Thiamin (B-1)	0.1 mg	Vitamin E	0.0 mg
Riboflavin (B-2)	0.1 mg	Calcium	23.8 mg
Niacin	3.9 mg	Iron	1.0 mg
Vitamin B-6	0.3 mg	Phosphorus	120.2 mg
Vitamin B-12	0.1 µg	Magnesium	36.0 mg
Folate (total)	84.7 µg	Zinc	0.7 mg
Vitamin C	14.4 mg	Potassium	443.9 mg

Refreshing Salmon Salad

PER SERVING: 338.5 CALORIES ~ 19.5 G PROTEIN ~ 7.7 G CARBOHYDRATE ~ 1.7 G FIBER ~
25.9 G TOTAL FAT ~ 4.0 G SATURATED FAT ~ 75.2 MG CHOLESTEROL ~ 604.7 MG SODIUM

2 5½-ounce cans salmon, or 10 ounces baked salmon, boneless and skinless

½ cup mayonnaise

¼ cup Zucchini Relish (see recipe on page 107)

½ cup minced carrots

½ cup frozen peas

1 tablespoon fresh minced dill

Flake salmon, removing any bones; combine salmon, mayonnaise, and
Zucchini Relish, and mix well. Stir in carrots, peas, and dill. Serve chilled.
    Serves 4.

Healthy Tidbit

I cannot stress enough the importance of eating good-quality essential fatty acids like the omega-3s found in wild salmon. Omega-3s help to reduce inflammation and decrease "bad" (LDL) cholesterol.

Nutritional Analysis per Serving

Vitamin A	337.0 RE	Vitamin D	11.4 µg
Thiamin (B-1)	0.1 mg	Vitamin E	0.0 mg
Riboflavin (B-2)	0.2 mg	Calcium	234.5 mg
Niacin	6.3 mg	Iron	1.1 mg
Vitamin B-6	0.3 mg	Phosphorus	326.2 mg
Vitamin B-12	3.9 µg	Magnesium	33.0 mg
Folate (total)	21.9 µg	Zinc	1.0 mg
Vitamin C	8.4 mg	Potassium	356.2 mg

Warm Golden Beet Salad

PER SERVING: 247.5 CALORIES ~ 7.0 G PROTEIN ~ 27.4 G CARBOHYDRATE ~ 8.6 G FIBER ~
13.9 G TOTAL FAT ~ 1.5 G SATURATED FAT ~ 0.0 MG CHOLESTEROL ~ 192.7 MG SODIUM

Dr. Matt Fisel, a naturopathic physician practicing in Guilford, Connecticut,
contributed this recipe. He also contributed a few favorites to my first cookbook, *The Anti-Inflammation Diet and Recipe Book*.

1 bunch golden beets with tops, washed

2–3 tablespoons olive oil, divided

4 cloves garlic, minced

½ cup toasted slivered almonds

Salt and freshly ground pepper to taste

Preheat oven to 425°F.
    Cut tops from beets and reserve. Place beets on a large sheet of aluminum
foil; drizzle with 2 tablespoons oil and sprinkle with salt and pepper. Wrap
beets in foil, sealing well. Bake until tender, about 1 hour. Unwrap and let cool.

When beets are cool enough to handle, remove skin by rubbing gently. Dice beets. Reserve.

Thinly slice reserved beet greens. Sauté garlic in remaining tablespoon oil in a large skillet until golden and fragrant, about 2 minutes. Stir in beet greens and sauté until tender, about 10 minutes. Stir in reserved beets and cook over medium heat until warm. Stir in almonds; season to taste with salt and pepper.

Serves 4.

Substitutions

If you are able to tolerate dairy, you can add 4 ounces of goat cheese (chèvre) or feta cheese, crumbled. If you are unable to find toasted almonds, you can buy raw slivers and toast them yourself. Spread them on a baking sheet and bake at 350°F for 5–7 minutes or until lightly browned. (Pay attention! Nuts can burn quickly.) Of course, red beets make a fine substitution if you can't find golden beets.

Healthy Tidbit

Learn from others. This recipe was given to me by a friend. Start collecting and testing as many recipes as you can, and don't hesitate to play around with them. Also play attention to entrées and salads that you taste at restaurants. I have gotten a lot of my recipe ideas from potlucks, eating out, and seeing something in a grocery store that looked appealing. If I taste something I like at a party, but don't know the people who brought it well enough to ask what is in it, I go home and try to duplicate it. The key is to do so within about a week from the time you ate it; if you wait any longer, your memory for how it tasted isn't as good. Who knows? Your new creation may turn out even better than the original dish.

Nutritional Analysis per Serving

Vitamin A	8.2 RE	Vitamin D	0.0 µg
Thiamin (B-1)	0.1 mg	Vitamin E	0.5 mg
Riboflavin (B-2)	0.2 mg	Calcium	80.5 mg
Niacin	1.3 mg	Iron	2.6 mg
Vitamin B-6	0.2 mg	Phosphorus	168.3 mg
Vitamin B-12	0.0 µg	Magnesium	93.5 mg
Folate (total)	275.0 µg	Zinc	1.3 mg
Vitamin C	13.0 mg	Potassium	906.8 mg

Mixed Green Salad

PER SERVING: 80.6 CALORIES ~ 2.9 G PROTEIN ~ 10.0 G CARBOHYDRATE ~ 3.3 G FIBER ~
4.1 G TOTAL FAT ~ 0.6 G SATURATED FAT ~ 0.0 MG CHOLESTEROL ~ 21.3 MG SODIUM

This recipe was contributed by Sara Fry, who lives in Utah.

3 cups organic mixed salad greens
¾ cup mixed sprouts (kale, kohlrabi, broccoli, pea, radish, mung bean)
1 carrot, shredded
2 plums, pitted, sliced
2 green onions, chopped
¼ cup sesame seeds

Place greens on serving platter; arrange remaining ingredients on top.
Serves 4.

Substitutions

Sara and I both enjoy this salad without dressing. Try it. You might be surprised. My friend Lynn is queen of making green salads that need no dressing; she uses a broad range of flavorful ingredients, such as celery, cucumbers, mushrooms, sunflower seeds, and garbanzo beans. If you feel you need some sort of salad dressing, try adding just a sprinkle of balsamic vinegar. If you can't find plums in season, try apples, frozen blueberries, or any other fruit.

Healthy Tidbit

Including greens in your diet *every day* is vitally important. Greens are a powerhouse of nutrition. Besides vitamins and fiber, they contain calcium, iron, and other important nutrients that support the body's metabolism and immune system. According to recent research, increasing the amount of green leafy vegetables in your diet may reduce your risk for type 2 diabetes.[2] Get creative. A good way to incorporate greens into the diet is to pack a lunch consisting of a large salad with a few other ingredients. If you make a commitment to eat a salad for lunch daily, you will find it much easier to incorporate greens into other areas of your life. Another great strategy is to make smoothies into which you toss in a handful of greens.

Nutritional Analysis per Serving

Vitamin A	312.9 RE	Vitamin D	0.0 µg
Thiamin (B-1)	0.2 mg	Vitamin E	0.3 mg
Riboflavin (B-2)	0.1 mg	Calcium	41.0 mg
Niacin	1.0 mg	Iron	1.2 mg
Vitamin B-6	0.1 mg	Phosphorus	95.8 mg
Vitamin B-12	0.0 µg	Magnesium	42.9 mg
Folate (total)	57.9 µg	Zinc	1.2 mg
Vitamin C	10.6 mg	Potassium	275.3 mg

Dips, Spreads, and Sauces

Simple Blackberry Jam

PER SERVING: 69.5 CALORIES ~ 0.5 G PROTEIN ~ 18.1 G CARBOHYDRATE ~ 1.6 G FIBER ~
1.4 G TOTAL FAT ~ 0.0 G SATURATED FAT ~ 0.0 MG CHOLESTEROL ~ 1.1 MG SODIUM

2 cups very ripe fresh (or thawed frozen) blackberries

½ cup honey

2 tablespoons cornstarch

2 teaspoons water

Process berries in a food processor, or mash in a small bowl, until smooth. Strain through a layer of cheesecloth to remove seeds; add honey.

Combine cornstarch and cold water in a medium saucepan; stir in berry mixture. Heat to boiling, stirring constantly; reduce heat and simmer until thickened, about 6 minutes, stirring frequently.

Pour into glass container and refrigerate.

Serves 10.

Substitutions
Many different berries can be used in place of the blackberries. If you are unable to tolerate cornstarch, substitute guar gum, arrowroot powder, or pectin. Please see the substitutions chart at the end of the book for appropriate proportions. To make this recipe vegan, substitute brown rice syrup for the honey, and use slightly more than ½ cup.

Healthy Tidbit
Berries are more than just tasty; they're high in antioxidants. I suggest consuming them often. Antioxidants help to ward off the oxidative damage caused by free radicals. Damage to tissues from free radicals is directly connected to cardiovascular and cancer risk; therefore, consumption of berries is truly preventive in nature. Blackberries specifically are high in vitamin C.

Nutritional Analysis per Serving

Vitamin A	6.2 RE	Vitamin D	0.0 µg
Thiamin (B-1)	0.0 mg	Vitamin E	0.0 mg
Riboflavin (B-2)	0.0 mg	Calcium	9.4 mg
Niacin	0.2 mg	Iron	0.3 mg
Vitamin B-6	0.0 mg	Phosphorus	7.2 mg
Vitamin B-12	0.0 mg	Magnesium	6.1 mg
Folate (total)	7.5 mg	Zinc	0.2 mg
Vitamin C	6.1 mg	Potassium	55.4 mg

Nutty Delicious Spread

PER SERVING: 77.9 CALORIES ~ 1.7 G PROTEIN ~ 3.2 G CARBOHYDRATE ~ 0.9 G FIBER ~
7.1 G TOTAL FAT ~ 2.1 G SATURATED FAT ~ 0.0 MG CHOLESTEROL ~ 2.2 MG SODIUM

½ cup hazelnuts

1 cup water

½ cup cashews

½ cup unsweetened shredded or ground coconut

1 teaspoon coconut oil

⅛ teaspoon stevia powder

Salt to taste

Soak the hazelnuts overnight in water; drain. Process all ingredients in a food processor or blender until smooth. Store in a glass jar in the refrigerator.

Serves 12.

Substitutions

A delicious nut butter without the peanuts! Feel free to substitute other nuts. Cashews will afford a creamier consistency, walnuts are tasty, and almonds will be a little more rough and dark if you keep the skins on.

Healthy Tidbit

Nuts offer a significant amount of nutrition. They are high in protein, high in calcium, low in carbohydrates, and contain a fair amount of essential fatty acids. Nuts have even been shown to decrease the HgA1c in diabetic patients. (HgA1c is a measure of historic blood sugar levels over a period of about three months.) Consuming nuts can also provide benefit for blood pressure, cholesterol, and triglyceride levels.

Nutritional Analysis per Serving

Vitamin A	0.1 RE	Vitamin D	0.0 µg
Thiamin (B-1)	0.0 mg	Vitamin E	0.7 mg
Riboflavin (B-2)	0.0 mg	Calcium	9.1 mg
Niacin	0.2 mg	Iron	0.7 mg
Vitamin B-6	0.0 mg	Phosphorus	45.6 mg
Vitamin B-12	0.0 µg	Magnesium	23.9 mg
Folate (total)	10.2 µg	Zinc	0.5 mg
Vitamin C	0.4 mg	Potassium	76.9 mg

Creamy White Bean Dip

PER SERVING: 82.8 CALORIES ~ 3.9 G PROTEIN ~ 10.5 G CARBOHYDRATE ~ 3.3 G FIBER ~
2.5 G TOTAL FAT ~ 0.3 G SATURATED FAT ~ 0.0 MG CHOLESTEROL ~ 164.3 MG SODIUM

1 15-ounce can cannellini beans, rinsed and drained

2 tablespoons lemon juice

1 tablespoon olive oil

2 garlic cloves, coarsely chopped

2 tablespoons chopped fresh dill weed

1 tablespoon chopped parsley

Salt to taste

Process all ingredients in a food processor or blender until smooth. Serve chilled as a dip with fresh vegetables, rice chips, or gluten-free crackers.
  Serves 6.

Substitutions

Any white bean will do for this recipe such as Great Northern or navy. You could also use garbanzo beans and it will turn out a little more yellow and not as smooth but will still taste delicious.

Healthy Tidbit

Dill weed contains many plant-derived chemical compounds that are known to have antioxidant, disease-preventing, and health-promoting properties. Dill also contains the vitamins niacin and B-6, which help to control blood cholesterol levels, as well as folic acid, vitamin B-2, vitamin A, ß-carotene, and vitamin C.

Nutritional Analysis per Serving

Vitamin A	6.8 RE	Vitamin D	0.0 µg
Thiamin (B-1)	0.0 mg	Vitamin E	0.0 mg
Riboflavin (B-2)	0.0 mg	Calcium	47.0 mg
Niacin	0.0 mg	Iron	0.9 mg
Vitamin B-6	0.0 mg	Phosphorus	2.4 mg
Vitamin B-12	0.0 µg	Magnesium	1.0 mg
Folate (total)	2.3 µg	Zinc	0.0 mg
Vitamin C	3.3 mg	Potassium	14.2 mg

Zesty Black Bean Dip

PER SERVING: 42.1 CALORIES ~ 2.9 G PROTEIN ~ 10.1 G CARBOHYDRATE ~ 3.5 G FIBER ~
0.1 G TOTAL FAT ~ 0.0 G SATURATED FAT ~ 0.0 MG CHOLESTEROL ~ 462.3 MG SODIUM

Serve with rice crackers, add to a gluten-free burrito with vegetables, add to
lettuce for a taco salad, or roll up as a lettuce wrap.

1 15-ounce can black beans, rinsed and drained, or 1½ cups cooked black beans

1 tablespoon minced onion

1 clove garlic, minced

1 teaspoon lime juice

½ teaspoon cumin

¼ teaspoon paprika

½ teaspoon salt

¼ teaspoon pepper

2 tablespoons minced cilantro

Combine all ingredients, except cilantro, in a food processor or blender
and blend until almost smooth. Spoon into a serving bowl, stir in cilantro,
and serve.

Serves 6.

Healthy Tidbit

Eating raw onion offers many health benefits. Onions have been used to fight
off infections, treat colds and flus, and balance appetite. They are also a rich
source of fructooligosaccharide (FOS), a beneficial nutrient that promotes the
growth of healthy intestinal bacteria.

Nutritional Analysis per Serving

Vitamin A	4.9 RE	Vitamin D	0.0 µg
Thiamin (B-1)	0.0 mg	Vitamin E	0.0 mg
Riboflavin (B-2)	0.0 mg	Calcium	37.3 mg
Niacin	0.0 mg	Iron	1.1 mg
Vitamin B-6	0.0 mg	Phosphorus	1.8 mg
Vitamin B-12	0.0 µg	Magnesium	0.0 mg
Folate (total)	0.5 µg	Zinc	0.0 mg
Vitamin C	1.9 mg	Potassium	213.2 mg

White Bean Hummus

PER SERVING: 58.1 CALORIES ~ 3.0 G PROTEIN ~ 7.2 G CARBOHYDRATE ~ 2.1 G FIBER ~
2.3 G TOTAL FAT ~ 0.3 G SATURATED FAT ~ 0.0 MG CHOLESTEROL ~ 98.4 MG SODIUM

Making this recipe one day ahead of time helps the flavors marry and intensify.

3 cups cooked Great Northern beans, or 2 15-ounce cans, rinsed and drained
½ cup roasted red peppers
⅓ cup tahini (sesame seed butter)
⅓ cup lemon juice
⅓ to ½ cup water
3 garlic cloves, minced
¾ teaspoon salt
Pinch cayenne pepper

Process all ingredients in a food processor until smooth.
    Serves 20.

Substitutions
Hummus is traditionally made with garbanzo beans. I love substituting any of the white beans in place of the garbanzos, because they seem to make a smoother hummus. You can omit the roasted red peppers and cayenne for a plain hummus, to which you can add various seasonings and vegetables such as roasted garlic, artichokes, spinach, or pesto. For the tahini, which is expensive, you can substitute 1 teaspoon sesame oil plus 1 teaspoon finely ground sesame seeds.

Healthy Tidbit
Consume more legumes and less animal protein. Legumes are a beneficial source of protein, and when combined with a healthy grain they supply the body with all of the amino acids needed to constitute a complete protein. Soaking legumes allows for shorter cooking time and preserves most of the nutrient value. Soaking legumes also reduces gas by removing the indigestible complex sugars (oligosaccharides) from the outer coating of the beans.

Nutritional Analysis per Serving

Vitamin A	0.3 RE	Vitamin D	0.0 µg
Thiamin (B-1)	0.1 mg	Vitamin E	0.0 mg
Riboflavin (B-2)	0.0 mg	Calcium	24.9 mg
Niacin	0.4 mg	Iron	0.8 mg
Vitamin B-6	0.0 mg	Phosphorus	76.4 mg
Vitamin B-12	0.0 µg	Magnesium	17.5 mg
Folate (total)	31.8 µg	Zinc	0.4 mg
Vitamin C	2.2 mg	Potassium	128.2 mg

Roasted Red Pepper Dip

PER SERVING: 27.8 CALORIES ~ 0.3 G PROTEIN ~ 1.7 G CARBOHYDRATE ~ 0.5 G FIBER ~
2.3 G TOTAL FAT ~ 0.3 G SATURATED FAT ~ 1.0 MG CHOLESTEROL ~ 74.8 MG SODIUM

This recipe was inspired by our friend Todd Deneffe, of Portland, Oregon.

2 red peppers, roasted (see instructions on page 234), or
1 12-ounce jar roasted red peppers, drained

2 tablespoons mayonnaise

1 clove garlic, minced

¼ teaspoon salt

¼ teaspoon ground white pepper

Combine all ingredients in blender; blend until smooth.
Serves 10.

Serving Tip

Serve with chips or veggies. This also makes an excellent sandwich spread. The consistency of the dip can vary depending on how much moisture is produced by the peppers. If your sauce is a little runny, simply place it in the refrigerator to chill and it will firm up a bit.

Healthy Tidbit

The Paleo diet recommends eating the way humans ate over the many centuries when we were hunter-gatherers. The hallmark of the Paleo diet is avoiding grain, a rule that can be challenging to follow but also rewarding. It can lead to weight loss and other health benefits. Many recipes in this book are grain free. I find it hard on my digestive system to avoid all grain entirely, so I incorporate some rice, quinoa, or gluten-free bread.

Nutritional Analysis per Serving

Vitamin A	76.1 RE	Vitamin D	0.0 µg
Thiamin (B-1)	0.0 mg	Vitamin E	0.0 mg
Riboflavin (B-2)	0.0 mg	Calcium	2.6 mg
Niacin	0.2 mg	Iron	0.1 mg
Vitamin B-6	0.1 mg	Phosphorus	7.4 mg
Vitamin B-12	0.0 µg	Magnesium	3.0 mg
Folate (total)	11.1 µg	Zinc	0.1 mg
Vitamin C	30.5 mg	Potassium	51.8 mg

Zucchini Relish

PER SERVING: 31.6 CALORIES ~ 0.3 G PROTEIN ~ 7.4 G CARBOHYDRATE ~ 0.4 G FIBER ~
0.1 G TOTAL FAT ~ 0.0 G SATURATED FAT ~ 0.0 MG CHOLESTEROL ~ 365.2 MG SODIUM

Inspired by Cindy Stuart, this recipe makes the best sweet relish. After tasting it you will find it very hard to buy commercially prepared sweet relish ever again. Plus, the recipe offers a terrific way to use up those plentiful fall zucchinis.

10 cups grated zucchini

3 cups minced onions

3 red bell peppers, finely chopped

2 yellow bell peppers, finely chopped

5 tablespoons salt

3 cups white vinegar

2 cups honey

2 tablespoons cornstarch

2 teaspoons celery seed

2 teaspoons dry mustard

2 teaspoons turmeric

1 teaspoon coarsely ground black pepper

Place vegetables and salt in a large glass bowl and refrigerate, covered, overnight.

The next morning, rinse thoroughly in a large strainer to remove most of the salt. Drain well, pressing on vegetables to remove as much water as possible. Place vegetables in a stockpot or Dutch oven; stir in remaining ingredients. Heat to boiling; reduce heat and simmer for 25 minutes.

Ladle into hot, sterilized jars. Seal according to the instructions below.

Yields 12 8-ounce jars of 8 servings per jar.

Easy Canning Instructions

1. Preparation: wash jars and rings in the dishwasher or by hand in hot soapy water. Always wash the lids in hot soapy water, not in the dishwasher.

2. Prepare the recipe that is to be canned.

3. Simmer lids in water over medium heat for

Nutritional Analysis per Serving

Vitamin A	17.7 RE	Vitamin D	0.0 µg
Thiamin (B-1)	0.1 mg	Vitamin E	0.0 mg
Riboflavin (B-2)	0.1 mg	Calcium	5.5 mg
Niacin	0.2 mg	Iron	0.2 mg
Vitamin B-6	0.1 mg	Phosphorus	9.1 mg
Vitamin B-12	0.0 µg	Magnesium	4.3 mg
Folate (total)	7.2 µg	Zinc	0.9 mg
Vitamin C	15.6 mg	Potassium	62.4 mg

5 minutes, fill the clean jars with your recipe, and secure the lids onto the jars with the rings, using a pot holder.

4. Submerge sealed jars in boiling water. This can be done with a canner or can be done in 9×13-inch baking pans filled to the brim with water and brought to a boil in the oven. Soup pots can also work as long as you can submerge the jars in boiling water. The boiling time may vary per recipe.

Substitutions

Instead of the cornstarch, you may be able to use arrowroot powder or pectin. I haven't yet tried either of those ingredients in this recipe because organic cornstarch has worked fine for me. Note that there is very little cornstarch in each bite.

Healthy Tidbit

When you are under stress, do something you love. I happen to love being in my kitchen, so spending half the day making zucchini relish and canning helps me get out of my head and forget my stress for a few hours. Another way I like to deal with stress is to get outside and do some exercise. An outing for walking, hiking, skiing, running, or biking seems to help immensely. Other techniques for reducing stress include baking (something healthy, of course), journaling, reading, and enjoying the company of friends and loved ones. For my patients who are not well enough to exercise outside, I have them move a rocking chair or another comfortable chair onto their porch and sit in it for at least an hour. In the winter, I just tell them to bundle up. Being outside, no matter the season, offers our bodies a stimulation they can't get inside. And if it is sunny, being outdoors gives us that much needed vitamin D!

Vegetarian Chickpea Filling

PER SERVING: 77.5 CALORIES ~ 5.0 G PROTEIN ~ 14.5 G CARBOHYDRATE ~ 3.8 G FIBER ~
2.6 G TOTAL FAT ~ 0.3 G SATURATED FAT ~ 0.9 MG CHOLESTEROL ~ 336.8 MG SODIUM

This recipe is yummy for a dip with crackers or in sandwiches.

1 19-ounce can garbanzo beans,
rinsed and drained

1 stalk celery, chopped

½ small onion, chopped

1 tablespoon mayonnaise

1 tablespoon lemon juice

1 teaspoon dried dill weed

Salt and freshly ground pepper to taste

Coarsely mash the chickpeas with a fork in a medium mixing bowl. Mix in remaining ingredients, seasoning with salt and pepper.

Serves 6.

Substitutions

This recipe is kind of like chunky hummus. It's fun to use in lettuce wraps, in sandwiches, or on crackers, and offers an excellent amount of protein in each bite.

Healthy Tidbit

How do you determine how much of a bad thing is too much? This is an important question to consider when we are bombarded daily with toxic chemicals in our air, our food, and our water supply. It is safe to say that we all should be able to tolerate some chemical exposure; otherwise we would struggle to survive in modern society. My family's general rule of thumb is that we keep our home as free of chemicals as possible and make some exceptions when we are out. For example, we don't use plastic, we don't use the microwave, we use all-natural cleaning supplies, we don't use perfumes or other synthetically made personal-care products, we use natural soap, shampoo, and toothpaste, and we mostly eat an anti-inflammation diet. When we are out, we try not to stress if someone wants our children to use hand sanitizer or if we are served warm food in plastic. The amount of stress you have also affects your overall well-being, so you have to choose your battles and be willing to let some go. After all, we can't live in a bubble. A healthy person is able to withstand some toxicity but should limit overall exposure as part of a preventive lifestyle.

Nutritional Analysis per Serving

Vitamin A	5.3 RE	Vitamin D	0.0 µg
Thiamin (B-1)	0.0 mg	Vitamin E	0.0 mg
Riboflavin (B-2)	0.0 mg	Calcium	21.9 mg
Niacin	0.0 mg	Iron	0.9 mg
Vitamin B-6	0.0 mg	Phosphorus	5.9 mg
Vitamin B-12	0.0 µg	Magnesium	2.6 mg
Folate (total)	5.0 µg	Zinc	0.0 mg
Vitamin C	2.8 mg	Potassium	39.1 mg

Teriyaki Sauce

PER SERVING: 24.9 CALORIES ~ 0.4 G PROTEIN ~ 3.1 G CARBOHYDRATE ~ 0.3 G FIBER ~
1.4 G TOTAL FAT ~ 0.1 G SATURATED FAT ~ 0.0 MG CHOLESTEROL ~ 11.3 MG SODIUM

1 cup plus ¼ cup water

¼ cup gluten-free tamari

3 tablespoons honey

1 tablespoon sesame oil

1 tablespoon chopped gingerroot

1 garlic clove, chopped

2 tablespoons arrowroot powder

¼ cup cold water

¼ cup sesame seeds

Combine 1 cup water, tamari, honey, sesame oil, gingerroot, and garlic in a
blender; blend until smooth. Whisk arrowroot into ¼ cup cold water in a
medium saucepan until smooth; pour in tamari mixture. Whisk over medium-
low heat until slightly thickened, about 3 minutes. Stir in sesame seeds; cool.
Transfer to a glass container with an airtight lid; store in refrigerator.

Yields about 2 cups (32 1-tablespoon servings).

Substitutions

Try using a little pineapple juice instead of some of the water. Add a little dried
mustard powder. Add cayenne to provide some spice. Using more or less ginger
or garlic will change the taste significantly. For a lower glycemic index, you can
replace the honey with xylitol.

Healthy Tidbit

Thickeners are helpful in sauces and spreads. Cornstarch is most commonly
used, but in most cases we can substitute arrowroot powder or guar gum
instead. The benefit of arrowroot powder is that is doesn't need to be heated
as much as corn starch to activate its thickening properties; guar gum doesn't
need to be heated at all. Using alternative thickeners such as these helps you
prepare less-rich versions of
many of the food items that
normally call for butter and
flour.

Nutritional Analysis per Serving

Vitamin A	1.3 RE	Vitamin D	0.0 µg
Thiamin (B-1)	0.0 mg	Vitamin E	0.0 mg
Riboflavin (B-2)	0.0 mg	Calcium	12.9 mg
Niacin	0.1 mg	Iron	0.2 mg
Vitamin B-6	0.0 mg	Phosphorus	7.8 mg
Vitamin B-12	0.0 µg	Magnesium	4.3 mg
Folate (total)	2.7 µg	Zinc	0.1 mg
Vitamin C	0.1 mg	Potassium	9.7 mg

Faux Creamy Cheese Sauce

PER SERVING: 45.2 CALORIES ~ 1.5 G PROTEIN ~ 2.8 G CARBOHYDRATE ~ 0.4 G FIBER ~
3.5 G TOTAL FAT ~ 0.6 G SATURATED FAT ~ 0.0 MG CHOLESTEROL ~ 66.5 MG SODIUM

There are many versions of this recipe. I have found this one to work the best. I
love how creamy and cheeselike the sauce becomes. It's a great treat for vegans!

1 cup raw cashews

1 cup water

1 2-ounce jar pimentos, drained

1 teaspoon garlic powder

½ teaspoon onion powder

½ teaspoon salt

¼ teaspoon turmeric

¼ teaspoon cayenne pepper (optional)

2 teaspoons lemon juice

Combine all ingredients except lemon juice in a blender or food processor;
blend until smooth. Pour into a small saucepan; stir constantly over medium
heat until thickened. Stir in lemon juice. Cool; store in a glass jar in the refrigerator.

Yields 2¼ cups (18 2-tablespoon servings).

Substitutions

I have prepared this sauce without the lemon juice, and it turned out fine.
The original version I encountered contained thyme, but I prefer it without. I
include the turmeric for color and added health benefit, but the sauce doesn't
strictly need it. If you want less spice you can substitute a little ground white
pepper for the cayenne. I pour this sauce over sautéed greens such as spinach
or chard, but you can also use it as a dip.

Healthy Tidbit

Turmeric is a powerful anti-inflammatory spice. Consuming turmeric daily
could yield significant benefit for inflammatory conditions. In addition,
turmeric can be taken in tincture and dried herb form. Curcumin, the active
anti-inflammatory constituent
of turmeric, has been studied
extensively for its use in treating arthritis, cancer, and other
inflammatory conditions. It has
a long history of safe medicinal
use for many ailments. Turmeric
is one of my favorite spices.

Nutritional Analysis per Serving

Vitamin A	8.4 RE	Vitamin D	0.0 µg
Thiamin (B-1)	0.0 mg	Vitamin E	0.0 mg
Riboflavin (B-2)	0.0 mg	Calcium	4.0 mg
Niacin	0.1 mg	Iron	0.6 mg
Vitamin B-6	0.0 mg	Phosphorus	48.2 mg
Vitamin B-12	0.0 µg	Magnesium	23.6 mg
Folate (total)	2.4 µg	Zinc	0.5 mg
Vitamin C	3.0 mg	Potassium	60.9 mg

Muhammara

PER SERVING: 69.6 CALORIES ~ 0.5 G PROTEIN ~ 2.6 G CARBOHYDRATE ~ 0.5 G FIBER ~
6.5 G TOTAL FAT ~ 0.8 G SATURATED FAT ~ 0.0 MG CHOLESTEROL ~ 8.2 MG SODIUM

2 red bell peppers, roasted, peeled (see instructions on page 234)

½ cup extra virgin olive oil

Seeds from ¼ pomegranate

¼ cup walnuts

1 slice gluten-free bread, toasted crisp and crumbled

3 cloves garlic

1 tablespoon lemon juice

2 teaspoons blackstrap molasses

1½ teaspoon ground cumin

Process all ingredients in a blender or food processor until almost smooth.
Serves 20.

Substitutions

Serve with rice crackers or veggies.

This recipe is typically made with sun-dried tomatoes, but it works wonderfully with the roasted red peppers. I also think it would work really well with Mediterranean olives, which would make it into a kind of olive tapenade.

Healthy Tidbit

Cumin, one of my favorite spices because of its piquant flavor, contains a high concentration of antioxidants. The primary job of antioxidants is to protect cells against the oxidative stress triggered by free radicals, considered to be the leading cause of the aging process and cancer. Cumin also aids digestion, prevents digestive disorders, enhances immunity, and stimulates metabolism. It is perfect for Middle Eastern and Mexican dishes, and delicious added to eggs.

Nutritional Analysis per Serving

Vitamin A	37.5 RE	Vitamin D	0.0 µg
Thiamin (B-1)	0.0 mg	Vitamin E	0.0 mg
Riboflavin (B-2)	0.0 mg	Calcium	10.3 mg
Niacin	0.1 mg	Iron	0.3 mg
Vitamin B-6	0.1 mg	Phosphorus	9.2 mg
Vitamin B-12	0.0 µg	Magnesium	5.3 mg
Folate (total)	7.1 µg	Zinc	0.1 mg
Vitamin C	15.7 mg	Potassium	53.9 mg

Mushroom Gravy

PER SERVING: 104.7 CALORIES ~ 3.0 G PROTEIN ~ 6.8 G CARBOHYDRATE ~ 1.5 G FIBER ~
8.0 G TOTAL FAT ~ 4.5 G SATURATED FAT ~ 19.3 MG CHOLESTEROL ~ 477.3 MG SODIUM

Wonderful as a Thanksgiving gravy served over rice or vegetables.

6 tablespoons butter, divided
4 tablespoons oat flour or other gluten-free flour
1 medium yellow onion, finely chopped
½ medium green bell pepper, finely chopped
1 rib celery, finely chopped
2 cloves garlic, minced
½ bunch green onions, sliced, green tops reserved
2 cups chicken broth
½ cup unsweetened almond milk
1 pound button or crimini mushrooms
2 tablespoons Teriyaki Sauce (see recipe on page 110)
1 teaspoon salt
Freshly ground pepper to taste

Melt 4 tablespoons butter in a medium saucepan. Whisk in flour; cook over medium heat, whisking constantly until golden brown, about 15 minutes. Add onion, bell peppers, celery, garlic, and white part of the green onions, and cook until vegetables are softened but not browned, about 5 minutes. Whisk in broth and almond milk, and simmer until thickened, about 10 minutes, stirring occasionally.

While sauce is simmering, melt remaining 2 tablespoons butter in a medium skillet over medium-high heat. Add mushrooms and sauté until tender and lightly browned, about 5 minutes. Add mushrooms, Teriyaki Sauce, and salt to vegetable mixture and simmer 5 minutes. Season to taste with pepper; stir in green onion tops.

Serves 10.

Substitutions

Substitute any broth, such as vegetable broth or beef broth, and any type of mushroom or a combination of types. My favorite is chanterelles, when they're in season. Here in the Northwest we can forage

Nutritional Analysis per Serving

Vitamin A	77.1 RE	Vitamin D	0.2 µg
Thiamin (B-1)	0.1 mg	Vitamin E	0.2 mg
Riboflavin (B-2)	0.2 mg	Calcium	22.1 mg
Niacin	1.8 mg	Iron	0.7 mg
Vitamin B-6	0.1 mg	Phosphorus	65.8 mg
Vitamin B-12	0.0 µg	Magnesium	13.5 mg
Folate (total)	19.4 µg	Zinc	0.4 mg
Vitamin C	8.6 mg	Potassium	238.5 mg

for chanterelles in the fall to prepare our Thanksgiving gravy. If you want a smooth gravy, purée before serving.

Healthy Tidbit

Mushrooms contain almost 90 percent water, and at 100 calories per ounce are very low in calories. They contain very little sodium and fat, and 8–10 percent of their dry weight is fiber. Mushrooms are an ideal food for weight management, diabetes, and hypertension. They are high in potassium, riboflavin, niacin, and selenium. They have shown promise in supporting the immune system and have also been studied for their inhibitory effects on the enzyme aromatase, which may prove promising in the prevention of certain kinds of breast and prostate cancer.

Honey Mustard

PER SERVING: 51.3 CALORIES ~ 0.1 G PROTEIN ~ 13.9 G CARBOHYDRATE ~ 0.1 G FIBER ~ 0.0G TOTAL FAT ~ 0.0 G SATURATED FAT ~ 0.0 MG CHOLESTEROL ~ 138.7 MG SODIUM

Serve with fresh vegetables or salads.

½ cup honey
¼ cup Dijon-style mustard
¼ teaspoon guar gum

Whisk all ingredients in a small bowl.
Serves 10.

Substitutions

You can easily turn this dip into a delicious salad dressing by adding a little olive oil, vinegar, and salt.

Healthy Tidbit

According to Chinese medicine, mustard is warming to the system and can promote circulation, improving many health complaints. Because of these properties it makes a great metabolism booster for people hoping to lose weight. Mustard seeds are a very good source of omega-3 fatty acids as well as calcium, dietary fiber, iron, manganese, magnesium, niacin, phosphorus, protein, selenium, and zinc.

Nutritional Analysis per Serving

Vitamin A	0.0 RE	Vitamin D	0.0 µg
Thiamin (B-1)	0.0 mg	Vitamin E	0.0 mg
Riboflavin (B-2)	0.0 mg	Calcium	1.0 mg
Niacin	0.0 mg	Iron	0.1 mg
Vitamin B-6	0.0 mg	Phosphorus	0.7 mg
Vitamin B-12	0.0 µg	Magnesium	0.3 mg
Folate (total)	0.3 µg	Zinc	0.0 mg
Vitamin C	0.1 mg	Potassium	8.7 mg

Vegetable Gravy

PER SERVING: 64.1 CALORIES ~ 1.4 G PROTEIN ~ 7.3 G CARBOHYDRATE ~ 1.7 G FIBER ~
3.7 G TOTAL FAT ~ 0.5 G SATURATED FAT ~ 0.0 MG CHOLESTEROL ~ 452.8 MG SODIUM

This dish is tasty served over brown rice or quinoa.

2 large leeks, white parts chopped	2 teaspoons garlic powder
½ red onion, chopped	1 teaspoon onion powder
2 tablespoons olive oil	½ teaspoon dried paprika
½ head of cauliflower, chopped	½ teaspoon dried mustard powder
1 red bell pepper, chopped	1½ teaspoons salt
1½ cups water	

Sauté leeks and onion in olive oil in a stockpot or Dutch oven until tender, about 5 minutes. Stir in remaining ingredients. Heat to boiling; reduce heat and simmer for 15–20 minutes.

Serves 8.

Substitutions

Serve the gravy over rice, pasta, or meat. You can experiment with substituting various vegetables. You can make the sauce thinner by adding chicken or vegetable broth, or you can make it thicker by adding arrowroot powder or organic corn starch. To add the arrowroot or corn starch: dissolve it in 1 tablespoon cold water prior to adding it to the gravy. Whisk into the gravy while it's simmering.

Healthy Tidbit

Getting vegetables into your children can sometimes be a struggle. Making gravies and sauces can be a great way of doing so. It is easy to make a gravy like this one that can be served over meat or rice. Remember, children learn by example. If they are in that "mono food stage," when they want only one food all the time, continue to eat an array of vegetables and make those same veggies available for their consumption. As they get older, they will make healthy decisions on their own as long as they consistently see you making healthy decisions.

Nutritional Analysis per Serving

Vitamin A	90.6 RE	Vitamin D	0.0 µg
Thiamin (B-1)	0.1 mg	Vitamin E	0.0 mg
Riboflavin (B-2)	0.1 mg	Calcium	26.1 mg
Niacin	0.5 mg	Iron	0.8 mg
Vitamin B-6	0.2 mg	Phosphorus	34.5 mg
Vitamin B-12	0.0 µg	Magnesium	15.6 mg
Folate (total)	43.6 µg	Zinc	0.2 mg
Vitamin C	39.5 mg	Potassium	203.8 mg

Sun Sauce

PER SERVING: 40.4 CALORIES ~ 1.3 G PROTEIN ~ 5.6 G CARBOHYDRATE ~ 0.8 G FIBER ~
1.9 G TOTAL FAT ~ 0.3 G SATURATED FAT ~ 0.0 MG CHOLESTEROL ~ 588.2 MG SODIUM

Serve over veggies, meat, fish, or brown rice.

1 yellow bell pepper, chopped
½ large carrot, chopped
1 cup water
2 tablespoons raw cashews
1½ tablespoons lemon juice
1 teaspoon salt
½ teaspoon turmeric

Simmer the bell pepper and carrot in water in a small saucepan until very tender, about 15 minutes. In a food processor or blender, combine the vegetable mixture with the remaining ingredients; process until smooth.

Serves 4.

Substitutions

To achieve the beautiful yellow color that gives this sauce its name, make no substitutions. For a different appearance, try other vegetables. To keep your sauce from turning a less-appetizing brown, follow the rules of combining color as you would with paint. For example, using red pepper, green pepper, and eggplant may create a sauce that's unappealing to the eye.

Healthy Tidbit

Make up fun names for your foods and vitamins. My kids have always loved to name things. When my first daughter was very young, we gave her fish oil and acidophilus every morning, and we termed them "princess oil and sugar." She took them right down. Having fun in the kitchen is important even if you don't have children. Think about your energy level when you are preparing a meal. The mood you are in will help determine how well the meal is executed and how it will taste. A rushed meal prepared by a stressed cook will be no fun for anyone. Enjoy yourself and the food you prepare. Happier moods are better for your health anyway!

Nutritional Analysis per Serving

Vitamin A	136.7 RE	Vitamin D	0.0 µg
Thiamin (B-1)	0.0 mg	Vitamin E	0.0 mg
Riboflavin (B-2)	0.0 mg	Calcium	10.3 mg
Niacin	0.6 mg	Iron	0.6 mg
Vitamin B-6	0.1 mg	Phosphorus	39.1 mg
Vitamin B-12	0.0 µg	Magnesium	19.3 mg
Folate (total)	15.8 µg	Zinc	0.2 mg
Vitamin C	88.1 mg	Potassium	162.8 mg

Vegan Cashew Sauce

PER SERVING: 195.5 CALORIES ~ 7.3 G PROTEIN ~ 13.9 G CARBOHYDRATE ~ 4.1 G FIBER ~
13.5 G TOTAL FAT ~ 2.1 G SATURATED FAT ~ 0.0 MG CHOLESTEROL ~ 301.3 MG SODIUM

Use in place of an alfredo sauce for noodles, or serve over a bento bowl of freshly steamed veggies and quinoa.

½ yellow onion, minced

2 cloves garlic, minced

3 tablespoons olive oil

2 cups unsweetened almond milk

1 cup raw cashews

1 cup cooked or canned navy beans (rinse and drain if using canned)

2 tablespoons arrowroot powder

1 teaspoon salt

⅛ teaspoon nutmeg

Sauté onion and garlic in oil in a medium saucepan until tender; do not brown. Stir in almond milk and heat to simmering. Combine almond milk mixture and remaining ingredients in a food processor or blender, and process until smooth. Return mixture to saucepan and simmer until thickened, about 10 minutes.

Serves 8.

Substitutions

If you want a cream sauce and cannot tolerate dairy, try this versatile sauce instead. Any type of white bean will work. You can use it as a gravy by thinning it out a little bit and serving it over meat or a whole grain. You could try other nuts, but cashews seem to be the best as an alternative to dairy because when they are blended they become so smooth.

Healthy Tidbit

Don't heat olive oil to the smoking point. As a monounsaturated fatty acid olive oil is relatively stable for low to medium heating, but it cannot handle high heat for long. Watch carefully and turn down the heat before you see smoke. Overheating can denature the molecules, causing them to break down and convert into unhealthy fats. Olive oil offers significant health benefits and can be used safely with and without heating, so don't let this consideration prevent you from using it. Just exercise caution when heating it.

Nutritional Analysis per Serving

Vitamin A	0.1 RE	Vitamin D	0.0 µg
Thiamin (B-1)	0.1 mg	Vitamin E	0.0 mg
Riboflavin (B-2)	0.3 mg	Calcium	35.9 mg
Niacin	0.4 mg	Iron	2.2 mg
Vitamin B-6	0.1 mg	Phosphorus	135.1 mg
Vitamin B-12	0.1 µg	Magnesium	61.2 mg
Folate (total)	44.2 µg	Zinc	1.2 mg
Vitamin C	1.3 mg	Potassium	297.1 mg

Delicious Whole Cranberry Sauce

PER SERVING: 62.1 CALORIES ~ 0.2 G PROTEIN ~ 16.7 G CARBOHYDRATE ~ 2.0 G FIBER ~
0.1 G TOTAL FAT ~ 0.0 G SATURATED FAT ~ 0.0 MG CHOLESTEROL ~ 2.7 MG SODIUM

1 12-ounce package fresh cranberries

1½ cups water

⅓ cup honey

Wash and pick over the cranberries, discarding stems and soft berries. Combine cranberries, water, and honey in large saucepan; heat to boiling. Reduce heat and simmer until berries have burst and sauce is slightly thickened, about 5 minutes. Cool; refrigerate. Sauce will thicken as it cools.

Serves 8.

Substitutions

You can choose different sweeteners for this recipe, but I find that honey is amazingly sweet, even with the very tart cranberries. Generally, you should need less honey than other sweeteners.

Healthy Tidbit

Cranberries are a wonderful source of antioxidants. Antioxidants are responsible for warding off oxidative damage and helping promote a graceful aging process. In fact, research reveals that an antioxidant-rich diet leads to a decreased risk of dementia, type 2 diabetes, and stroke. Unsweetened cranberry juice, extract, or capsules can also help in preventing urinary-tract infections, especially in children. Make sure you include berries, and especially cranberries, in your monthly diet. Who says you should only eat cranberries at the holidays?

Nutritional Analysis per Serving

Vitamin A	2.1 RE	Vitamin D	0.0 µg
Thiamin (B-1)	0.0 mg	Vitamin E	0.0 mg
Riboflavin (B-2)	0.0 mg	Calcium	5.6 mg
Niacin	0.1 mg	Iron	0.2 mg
Vitamin B-6	0.0 mg	Phosphorus	6.1 mg
Vitamin B-12	0.0 µg	Magnesium	3.3 mg
Folate (total)	0.7 µg	Zinc	0.1 mg
Vitamin C	5.7 mg	Potassium	43.9 mg

Raw Holiday Relish

PER SERVING: 103.6 CALORIES ~ 0.5 G PROTEIN ~ 27.7 G CARBOHYDRATE ~ 3.1 G FIBER ~
0.2 G TOTAL FAT ~ 0.0 G SATURATED FAT ~ 0.0 MG CHOLESTEROL ~ 2.3 MG SODIUM

I had never experimented with making a raw fruit relish until a patient recommended this recipe. Thank you to all of my patients who have taught me so much over the years!

1 12-ounce package cranberries

1 orange, half the peel removed, cut into chunks

2 green apples, peeled and cored and cut into chunks

½ small pineapple, peeled, cored, cut into chunks

½ cup water

½ cup honey

Combine fruit in a large bowl. Process in batches in the food processor until coarsely chopped. Transfer to a serving bowl; stir in water and honey. Refrigerate; served chilled.

Serves 10.

Substitutions

Because this relish contains raw cranberries, it may be hard for some people to digest. I usually make sure that all of the cranberries are processed before adding the other ingredients; that way, you preserve the desirable chunkiness while eliminating any whole cranberries. Besides experimenting with different fruits, try adding ground cloves and toasted nuts, another terrific suggestion from a patient.

Healthy Tidbit

Pineapples are high in a nutrient called bromelain, a proteolytic enzyme. "Proteolytic" means "breaks down protein," which is why pineapple is considered a digestive aid. Bromelain in supplement form is extremely beneficial in reducing inflammation. It has been studied extensively for aiding in relief from arthritis and other inflammatory complaints. Regular ingestion of at least ½ cup of fresh pineapple daily is purported to provide mild relief from the joint pain of osteoarthritis. Pineapple is also high in manganese, a mineral that is critical to development of strong bones and connective tissue.

Nutritional Analysis per Serving

Vitamin A	10.0 RE	Vitamin D	0.0 µg
Thiamin (B-1)	0.0 mg	Vitamin E	0.1 mg
Riboflavin (B-2)	0.0 mg	Calcium	14.6 mg
Niacin	0.2 mg	Iron	0.3 mg
Vitamin B-6	0.1 mg	Phosphorus	12.8 mg
Vitamin B-12	0.0 µg	Magnesium	8.5 mg
Folate (total)	10.0 µg	Zinc	0.1 mg
Vitamin C	24.5 mg	Potassium	126.2 mg

Spiced Veggie Almond Spread

PER SERVING: 70.5 CALORIES ~ 1.7 G PROTEIN ~ 2.3 G CARBOHYDRATE ~ 1.0 G FIBER ~
6.5 G TOTAL FAT ~ 0.7 G SATURATED FAT ~ 0.0 MG CHOLESTEROL ~ 8.9 MG SODIUM

This recipe was given to me by one of our wonderful patients, Andrea Wyckoff, of Willamina, Oregon.

½ cup blanched almonds
1 rib celery, chopped
1 jalapeño pepper, chopped
1 carrot, chopped
Fresh herbs such as chives, thyme, mint, or cilantro
2 tablespoons olive oil
1 tablespoon lemon juice
Pinch of salt

Process almonds in a food processor or blender until finely chopped. Add remaining ingredients and process until finely chopped.

Spread on bread, rice cakes, or crackers. It also tastes wonderful on top of a bed of fresh greens with an avocado. It has a pleasing crunchy consistency yet still spreads well.

Serves 10.

Note: If you remove the seeds from the jalapeno, the flavor is milder than if you leave the seeds in. With the seeds, this dish may be too spicy for children or for people who don't like or can't tolerate spice.

Substitutions

Try adding some red onion and/or pickles. For a slightly heartier option, use Vegenaise or mayonnaise instead of the olive oil and lemon juice. It will remind you of a tuna salad without the tuna.

Healthy Tidbit

Friendship promotes inspiration and sharing. It is a gift to have like-minded friends and associates who can help you create and experiment in the kitchen. My patients have taught me a significant amount over the years. They are always introducing me to new recipes, new ways to ferment foods, and new ideas for saving time in the kitchen. I am very thankful to have them in my life. I also appreciate all of my friends who have shared many dinners and new ideas with me.

Nutritional Analysis per Serving

Vitamin A	104.9 RE	Vitamin D	0.0 µg
Thiamin (B-1)	0.0 mg	Vitamin E	0.0 mg
Riboflavin (B-2)	0.1 mg	Calcium	21.0 mg
Niacin	0.4 mg	Iron	0.3 mg
Vitamin B-6	0.0 mg	Phosphorus	38.5 mg
Vitamin B-12	0.0 µg	Magnesium	20.9 mg
Folate (total)	6.8 µg	Zinc	0.2 mg
Vitamin C	2.7 mg	Potassium	82.8 mg

Sun Butter

PER SERVING: 25.4 CALORIES ~ 0.8 G PROTEIN ~ 1.0 G CARBOHYDRATE ~ 0.2 G FIBER ~
1.9 G TOTAL FAT ~ 0.5 G SATURATED FAT ~ 0.0 MG CHOLESTEROL ~ 66.2 MG SODIUM

3 cups raw sunflower seeds

1 teaspoon agave syrup

1 teaspoon raw honey

¾ teaspoon salt

1 tablespoon olive oil

Place seeds in a large skillet; cook over medium heat, stirring constantly, until lightly toasted, about 5 minutes. Process seeds and agave syrup in a food processor or blender until mixture appears smooth and oily, about 10 minutes. Add honey and salt, and process until mixture is the consistency of smooth peanut butter, about 5 minutes. With food processor running, slowly drizzle in olive oil, processing until very smooth. Spoon into jar.

Warning: the long processing time can leave the mixture hot enough to burn the skin. Use caution when handling.

Serves 30.

Nutritional Analysis per Serving

Vitamin A	0.0 RE	Vitamin D	0.0 µg
Thiamin (B-1)	0.0 mg	Vitamin E	0.0 mg
Riboflavin (B-2)	0.0 mg	Calcium	0.1 mg
Niacin	0.0 mg	Iron	0.0 mg
Vitamin B-6	0.0 mg	Phosphorus	0.0 mg
Vitamin B-12	0.0 µg	Magnesium	0.0 mg
Folate (total)	0.0 µg	Zinc	0.0 mg
Vitamin C	0.1 mg	Potassium	0.1 mg

Breads, Muffins, Crackers

Organic 5-Grain Cereal Mix

PER SERVING: 168.6 CALORIES ~ 5.5 G PROTEIN ~ 32.3 G CARBOHYDRATE ~ 3.3 G FIBER ~
2.2 G TOTAL FAT ~ 0.4 G SATURATED FAT ~ 0.0 MG CHOLESTEROL ~ 2.1 MG SODIUM

½ cup organic quinoa

½ cup organic millet

½ cup organic buckwheat

½ cup organic long grain or basmati brown rice

½ cup organic amaranth

Process each grain separately in a food processor, blender, or coffee grinder until coarsely ground, but not as smooth as flour. Combine all grains in a glass jar or storage container.

To make cereal, combine ½ cup grain mixture and 1½–2½ cups water in small saucepan. (For thicker cereal use less water; for thinner cereal use more.) Heat to boiling; reduce heat and simmer, stirring occasionally, until thickened, about 10 minutes.

Yields 2½ cups (10 ¼-cup servings).

Note: You can save cooking time and improve digestive ability by putting all of these ingredients together at least an hour ahead of time and allowing them to soak prior to cooking.

Substitutions

Any grains are useful for this recipe. This blend does well as a cereal mix but not as a gluten-free bread or baking mix on its own. It can, however, be added to baked goods. For muffins, add ½–1 cup to your regular muffin recipe and increase your liquid by just a little bit. Also add to pancakes, soups, and breads.

Healthy Tidbit

Many of my patients were suffering terribly prior to eliminating gluten from their diets. I strongly urge you to consider going strictly gluten-free, at least for a trial period of thirty days, especially if you are of European descent. The main problems that I see associated with gluten are autism and ADD; arthritis, especially rheumatoid arthritis; Hashimoto's thyroiditis and other autoimmune conditions; stunted growth in children; and many other nervous-system–related conditions. Many conditions that affect the nervous system respond very well to a gluten-free diet. It gets easier to be gluten free the longer you do it. You even figure out how to eat out, so don't get discouraged if it is hard at first.

Nutritional Analysis per Serving

Vitamin A	0.1 RE	Vitamin D	0.0 µg
Thiamin (B-1)	0.1 mg	Vitamin E	0.0 mg
Riboflavin (B-2)	0.1 mg	Calcium	24.0 mg
Niacin	1.8 mg	Iron	1.8 mg
Vitamin B-6	0.2 mg	Phosphorus	182.0 mg
Vitamin B-12	0.0 µg	Magnesium	85.2 mg
Folate (total)	36.5 µg	Zinc	1.1 mg
Vitamin C	0.4 mg	Potassium	176.6 mg

Gluten-Free Pancake and Baking Mix

PER SERVING: 158.5 CALORIES ~ 2.9 G PROTEIN ~ 33.5 G CARBOHYDRATE ~ 3.0 G FIBER ~
1.5 G TOTAL FAT ~ 0.3 G SATURATED FAT ~ 0.0 MG CHOLESTEROL ~ 239.1 MG SODIUM

2 cups brown rice flour

1 cup gluten-free oat flour

1 cup tapioca flour

2 teaspoons baking powder (aluminum free)

1 tablespoon plus 1 teaspoon guar gum,
xanthan gum, or arrowroot powder

1 teaspoon salt

Combine all ingredients; store in glass jar or storage container.

Yields 4 cups (12 ⅓-cup servings).

For pancakes: in a mixing bowl, mix together 1 cup of mixture with 1 large egg and ¾–1 cup rice milk, almond milk, or water. Prepare mixture into 4-inch pancakes.

Kitchen Tip

It's a good idea to familiarize yourself with the basics of making a gluten-free mix. You can use various grains besides the ones listed here. I select 4–5 types of grains, and I grind most of them myself. Three of the flours can be any normal gluten-free flour, such as teff, buckwheat, brown rice, millet, or quinoa, but 1–2 of the flours should have some binding power. I use tapioca, arrowroot powder, and guar or xanthan gum. I don't use potato flour. Most of these mixes do very well in muffins, cookies, and sweet breads. A satisfactory gluten-free loaf of bread is a bit harder to accomplish.

Nutritional Analysis per Serving of Mix

Vitamin A	0.0 RE	Vitamin D	0.0 µg
Thiamin (B-1)	0.2 mg	Vitamin E	0.0 mg
Riboflavin (B-2)	0.0 mg	Calcium	27.2 mg
Niacin	1.7 mg	Iron	0.9 mg
Vitamin B-6	0.2 mg	Phosphorus	96.9 mg
Vitamin B-12	0.0 µg	Magnesium	29.7 mg
Folate (total)	4.2 µg	Zinc	0.6 mg
Vitamin C	0.0 mg	Potassium	104.9 mg

Rice Crackers

PER SERVING: 52.0 CALORIES ~ 0.8 G PROTEIN ~ 7.4 G CARBOHYDRATE ~ 0.6 G FIBER ~
2.2 G TOTAL FAT ~ 1.6 G SATURATED FAT ~ 0.0 MG CHOLESTEROL ~ 40.0 MG SODIUM

⅔ cup cooked brown rice

1½ cups brown rice flour

1 tablespoon chia, sesame, or flax seeds

¼ cup coconut oil

1 clove garlic, minced

1 teaspoon minced fresh rosemary

1 teaspoon honey

½ teaspoon sea salt

¼–½ cup water

Preheat oven to 300°F.

Combine all ingredients except water in a medium bowl. Stir in water gradually, adding just enough to form a dough. Turn onto floured surface, and knead several times until dough is smooth. Press or roll dough onto a greased baking sheet, spreading to an even thickness. Score with a sharp knife into 1½-inch squares. Bake for 25–30 minutes, or until bottoms are golden brown. Cool before removing from pan.

Yields 30 crackers.

Substitutions

You can use other grains, add cooked quinoa or buckwheat, or try other types of flours for these crackers. The trick is to get them thin enough.

Healthy Tidbit

It's common knowledge that avoiding fried foods is an important aspect of a healthy diet. But that doesn't just mean French fries and chicken fingers. Take a look at your consumption of chips. Most chips — including tortilla chips, potato chips, taro chips, and even many "gluten-free" items — are fried. Even when a food company uses a healthier oil, if the oil is heated too high during the frying process it has the potential to turn into a "trans fat" or to create other byprod-ucts that can be harmful to health. In our house we have a one-time-per-month fried-food rule. On a special occasion, if we are out with another family, my kids are able to order a fried

Nutritional Analysis per Cracker

Vitamin A	0.1 RE	Vitamin D	0.0 µg
Thiamin (B-1)	0.0 mg	Vitamin E	0.0 mg
Riboflavin (B-2)	0.0 mg	Calcium	4.2 mg
Niacin	0.6 mg	Iron	0.2 mg
Vitamin B-6	0.1 mg	Phosphorus	33.8 mg
Vitamin B-12	0.0 µg	Magnesium	12.1 mg
Folate (total)	1.7 µg	Zinc	0.2 mg
Vitamin C	0.0 mg	Potassium	27.0 mg

treat. This guideline works well for our family. I want my girls to enjoy some foods that are usually off limits so that when they are not in my presence they don't find themselves gorging on all of the foods they never get.

Sun Butter Bread

PER SERVING: 116.6 CALORIES ~ 3.0 G PROTEIN ~ 10.5 G CARBOHYDRATE ~ 0.3 G FIBER ~ 7.2 G TOTAL FAT ~ 4.2 G SATURATED FAT ~ 62.0 MG CHOLESTEROL ~ 196.4 MG SODIUM

1 cup Sun Butter (see recipe on page 121)
½ cup honey
¼ cup coconut oil
¾ teaspoon baking soda
½ teaspoon cinnamon
¼ teaspoon nutmeg
¼ teaspoon salt
5 eggs

Preheat oven to 275°F.

Combine all ingredients, except eggs, in a food processor or blender; blend well. Add eggs and blend until smooth.

Pour mixture into a parchment-lined or heavily greased loaf pan. Bake for 1½ hours or until a fork inserted in bread comes out clean. Remove from the oven; allow to cool before removing from pan.

Serves 15.

Kitchen Tip

This recipe provides a terrific "bread" option for people avoiding grain. It yields a dense loaf, similar in consistency to pumpkin bread. People are amazed to learn that you can make a bread with no flour or grain of any sort. The secret is the eggs.

Substitutions

You can try almond butter or other nut butters for this recipe. One of my patients converted the bread into hamburger buns by omitting most of the honey, cinnamon, and nutmeg and using a little less coconut oil. She just formed the dough into buns and baked them. I have also experimented successfully

Nutritional Analysis per Serving

Vitamin A	27.0 RE	Vitamin D	0.3 µg
Thiamin (B-1)	0.0 mg	Vitamin E	0.2 mg
Riboflavin (B-2)	0.1 mg	Calcium	10.9 mg
Niacin	0.0 mg	Iron	0.4 mg
Vitamin B-6	0.0 mg	Phosphorus	33.6 mg
Vitamin B-12	0.2 µg	Magnesium	2.4 mg
Folate (total)	8.1 µg	Zinc	0.2 mg
Vitamin C	0.2 mg	Potassium	29.4 mg

with toasting and grinding hazelnuts and walnuts, and using the ground nut meal in place of the Sun Butter. Try the same technique with other nuts and seeds.

Healthy Tidbit

Peanuts can cause significant problems in some people and is one of the most common food allergens. The peanut is a legume (rather than a true nut) that is notorious as a host for aflatoxins, a toxic substance that grows mainly on grains and legumes. Chronic ingestion of aflatoxins can affect the liver and cause immune deficiency. Eating sunflower butter and other nut butters is a good way to increase your consumption of protein and healthy fats while avoiding the potentially troublesome peanut.

Kale Chips

PER SERVING: 63.3 CALORIES ~ 2.2 G PROTEIN ~ 6.7 G CARBOHYDRATE ~ 1.3 G FIBER ~ 3.8 G TOTAL FAT ~ 0.5 G SATURATED FAT ~ 0.0 MG CHOLESTEROL ~ 222.7 MG SODIUM

1 bunch kale

1½ tablespoons olive oil

½ teaspoon salt

Preheat oven to 350°F.

Remove thick stems from kale, and cut leaves into 2-inch pieces. Wash and dry kale completely with a salad spinner. Toss kale with olive oil in a large bowl until well coated. Arrange on a greased baking sheet; sprinkle with salt. Bake at 350°F until the edges are just browned and the kale is crisp, about 10–15 minutes. Do not overcook.

Serves 6.

Substitutions

You can try this recipe with other hearty greens, such as chard.

Kitchen Tip

If you don't have a salad spinner, don't fret. Turn a clean pillowcase inside out, put the kale into the bottom of the pillowcase, go outside, and spin it around your head. This will remove a lot of the moisture from the kale without a salad spinner.

Nutritional Analysis per Serving

Vitamin A	1030.2 RE	Vitamin D	0.0 µg
Thiamin (B-1)	0.1 mg	Vitamin E	0.0 mg
Riboflavin (B-2)	0.1 mg	Calcium	90.6 mg
Niacin	0.7 mg	Iron	1.2 mg
Vitamin B-6	0.2 mg	Phosphorus	37.5 mg
Vitamin B-12	0.0 µg	Magnesium	22.8 mg
Folate (total)	19.4 µg	Zinc	0.3 mg
Vitamin C	80.4 mg	Potassium	299.6 mg

Gingerbread Bars

PER BAR: 114.3 CALORIES ~ 1.9 G PROTEIN ~ 17.5 G CARBOHYDRATE ~ 1.2 G FIBER ~
4.3 G TOTAL FAT ~ 0.6 G SATURATED FAT ~ 23.3 MG CHOLESTEROL ~ 118.5 MG SODIUM

½ cup unsweetened, organic applesauce

¼ cup grapeseed oil

¼ cup organic pure maple syrup

2 large eggs

½ cup warm water

½ cup unsulfured blackstrap molasses

¾ cup teff flour

⅓ cup brown rice flour

¼ cup arrowroot starch

1½ teaspoons ground (dried) ginger

1 teaspoon baking soda

1 teaspoon baking powder

1 teaspoon cinnamon

¾ teaspoon guar gum

¼ teaspoon ground cloves

¼ teaspoon ground nutmeg

Preheat oven to 350°F.

Prepare an 8×8-inch square baking pan by lining with parchment paper.

Combine applesauce, oil, and agave nectar in a large bowl, and mix with an electric mixer for about 2 minutes; add the eggs and mix for 3–4 more minutes until mixture becomes airy.

Process brown rice flour in a clean coffee grinder or blender for 3 minutes to create a superfine flour. In a separate bowl, combine all dry ingredients.

Mix molasses with warm water and add to liquid ingredients; mix well. Add dry ingredients to wet and mix well. Pour into the prepared baking pan. Bake for 30–35 minutes, or until fork inserted in center comes out clean.

Makes 16 bars.

Healthy Tidbit

Cinnamon is considered the antidiabetic spice. Numerous studies have shown cinnamon to have a positive effect on helping to reduce glucose and improve insulin levels.[3] I recently prescribed cinnamon and chromium supplements to a diabetic patient, and we saw a significant reduction in her bodily swelling. Studies show that doses of cinnamon as large as 3–6 grams may be needed to achieve benefits related to blood sugar. Cinnamon should not take the place of your current diabetic medication and should be used under the direction of a physician, especially if your hope is to reduce pharmaceutical medications.

Nutritional Analysis per Bar

Vitamin A	10.5 RE	Vitamin D	0.1 µg
Thiamin (B-1)	0.0 mg	Vitamin E	0.0 mg
Riboflavin (B-2)	0.1 mg	Calcium	126.7 mg
Niacin	0.4 mg	Iron	2.5 mg
Vitamin B-6	0.1 mg	Phosphorus	58.7 mg
Vitamin B-12	0.1 µg	Magnesium	28.1 mg
Folate (total)	10.2 µg	Zinc	0.4 mg
Vitamin C	0.1 mg	Potassium	291.8 mg

Pumpkin Bread

PER MUFFIN: 140.8 CALORIES ~ 2.5 G PROTEIN ~ 21.7 G CARBOHYDRATE ~ 1.8 G FIBER ~
5.3 G TOTAL FAT ~ 2.8 G SATURATED FAT ~ 41.2 MG CHOLESTEROL ~ 234.2 MG SODIUM

1¾ cup baked or steamed pumpkin (or 1 15-ounce can pumpkin)

4 eggs

½ cup plus 2 tablespoons honey

½ cup butter or coconut oil, melted

3 cups Gluten-Free Pancake and Baking Mix (see recipe on page 124)

2 teaspoons ground cinnamon

1 teaspoon ground nutmeg

1 teaspoon ground allspice

½ teaspoon ground cardamom

1 teaspoon salt

1 teaspoon guar gum (optional)

Preheat oven to 375°F.

Whisk together pumpkin, eggs, honey, and butter in medium bowl until smooth. In a separate bowl, combine dry ingredients. Stir into liquid ingredient mixture until well mixed. Pour batter into a greased loaf pan. Bake for 15 minutes; reduce heat to 350°F and bake for 30–35 minutes, until toothpick inserted in bread comes out dry.

This batter can be baked in muffin pans. Bake muffins at 350°F for 10–15 minutes.

Makes 24 muffins.

Substitutions

You can try this recipe with cooked mashed yams or sweet potatoes in place of the pumpkin. Any gluten-free mix can be used.

Healthy Tidbit

Pumpkin is an excellent addition to the diet that should be considered even when it is not holiday season. We make pumpkin curries in the fall and pumpkin bread from September well into January. Freshly steamed pumpkin offers nutrients such as vitamin A and fiber and is very low in fat, making it a healthful food to consume regularly. You can eat pumpkin all year long, but I suggest using fresh pumpkin when it is in season because the taste of the bread is so much better than with canned pumpkin.

Nutritional Analysis per Muffin

Vitamin A	327.1 RE	Vitamin D	0.2 µg
Thiamin (B-1)	0.1 mg	Vitamin E	0.2 mg
Riboflavin (B-2)	0.1 mg	Calcium	24.0 mg
Niacin	0.7 mg	Iron	0.8 mg
Vitamin B-6	0.1 mg	Phosphorus	61.1 mg
Vitamin B-12	0.1 µg	Magnesium	17.0 mg
Folate (total)	8.1 µg	Zinc	0.4 mg
Vitamin C	0.8 mg	Potassium	95.8 mg

Basic Gluten-Free Bread

PER SERVING: 212.2 CALORIES ~ 5.0 G PROTEIN ~ 33.3 G CARBOHYDRATE ~ 3.2 G FIBER ~
6.8 G TOTAL FAT ~ 4.4 G SATURATED FAT ~ 46.5 MG CHOLESTEROL ~ 218.1 MG SODIUM

3 eggs, lightly beaten
¾ cup water
¾ cup almond milk
¼ cup coconut oil
¼ cup honey
2 teaspoons apple cider vinegar
1 cup teff flour
1 cup tapioca flour

1 cup brown rice flour
⅓ cup arrowroot powder
2 tablespoons Organic 5-Grain Cereal Mix (see recipe on page 123)
1 tablespoon plus 1 teaspoon guar gum
1 teaspoon salt
1 package active dry yeast

Put ingredients into a bread machine as directed by the manufacturer, adding liquid ingredients first and followed by dry ingredients, except yeast. Make a shallow well in the center of the dry ingredients, and pour yeast into the well. Set bread machine for a sweet bread with a light crust.

Serves 12.

To make bread by hand: Preheat oven to 350°F. Combine dry ingredients, except yeast, in a large bowl. Mix yeast with ¼ cup warm water and let stand several minutes. Combine the remaining ingredients and the yeast mixture into the flour mixture, and beat until smooth. Spoon dough into 2 greased loaf pans. Bake for 30–40 minutes, or until internal temperature of bread reaches 205–210°F. Remove bread from oven; cool on wire racks.

Substitutions

If you don't get a satisfactory loaf using the bread maker, check your machine's settings and try again. You may want to decrease or increase the amount of water. A common problem with baking gluten-free breads is that they can tend to sink in the middle. Another common problem is that they don't get cooked all the way through, leaving the inside gummy. If you can't get this recipe to work in the bread maker, try it without. See if dividing the recipe into 2 loaf pans makes it less gummy.

Healthy Tidbit

A lot of prepared mixes for gluten-free foods or gluten-free breads contain potato flour or potato starch. Because potatoes can increase inflammation, I avoid mixes that include it. Just because a label says

Nutritional Analysis per Serving

Vitamin A	20.3 RE	Vitamin D	0.3 µg
Thiamin (B-1)	0.1 mg	Vitamin E	0.1 mg
Riboflavin (B-2)	0.1 mg	Calcium	30.1 mg
Niacin	1.2 mg	Iron	1.6 mg
Vitamin B-6	0.1 mg	Phosphorus	84.0 mg
Vitamin B-12	0.1 µg	Magnesium	21.3 mg
Folate (total)	34.5 µg	Zinc	0.6 mg
Vitamin C	0.1 mg	Potassium	107.4 mg

"gluten-free," doesn't necessarily mean it's healthy. Make sure you continue to check ingredients and read labels. Sometimes, gluten-free items are high in sugars, natural or otherwise, contain potato, or have very little true nutrient value. For example, who needs gluten-free donuts?

Toasted Squash Seeds or Pumpkin Seeds

PER SERVING: 209.8 CALORIES ~ 8.9 G PROTEIN ~ 5.2 G CARBOHYDRATE ~ 0.7 G FIBER ~ 21.2 G TOTAL FAT ~ 3.3 G SATURATED FAT ~ 0.0 MG CHOLESTEROL ~ 6.8 MG SODIUM

1 cup cleaned seeds from winter squash or pumpkin (see note on cleaning, below)

2 teaspoons olive oil

1 teaspoon garlic granules

1 teaspoon onion powder

Salt to taste

Preheat oven to 375°F.

To clean the seeds, separate them from the stringy membrane of the cut squash. Rinse in a colander until they are free of any membrane. This may take several rinses. Dry with paper towels.

Arrange the seeds and any remaining fibers on a baking sheet. Bake until they are well dried, about 20 minutes. Remove from oven; seeds should easily separate from any remaining fibers. Discard fibers and reserve seeds. Wipe any remaining fibers off the baking sheet.

Reduce oven to 250°F.

Toss seeds with oil, granulated garlic, and onion powder in a medium bowl; arrange on the baking sheet and sprinkle lightly with salt. Bake, stirring every 15 minutes, for about 1 hour, or until light brown.

Note: Roasting and drying times may vary by a few minutes.

Serves 4.

Substitutions

Some other ideas for seasonings are Cajun seasoning, soy sauce, Worcestershire sauce, or garlic salt. You can also add brewer's yeast or nutritional yeast before serving. If you do this, you could omit the salt as the yeast has its own sodium flavor. Paprika adds color and a distinct earthy flavor to these seeds.

Nutritional Analysis per Serving

Vitamin A	3.6 RE	Vitamin D	0.0 µg
Thiamin (B-1)	0.1 mg	Vitamin E	0.3 mg
Riboflavin (B-2)	0.1 mg	Calcium	18.9 mg
Niacin	0.7 mg	Iron	3.4 mg
Vitamin B-6	0.1 mg	Phosphorus	350.2 mg
Vitamin B-12	0.0 µg	Magnesium	185.4 mg
Folate (total)	20.4 µg	Zinc	2.6 mg
Vitamin C	1.0 mg	Potassium	286.2 mg

Storing
Store baked squash seeds or pumpkin seeds in an airtight container. Substitute them in your diet for your usual nut or seed topping.

Healthy Tidbit
Toasting seeds is a great way to avoid wasting those crunchy and healthful nuggets from your squashes and pumpkins. Toasted seeds are yummy and nutritious throughout the winter squash season, not only at Halloween.

Crêpe Flour Blend

PER SERVING: 344.7 CALORIES ~ 9.0 G PROTEIN ~ 73.2 G CARBOHYDRATE ~ 8.0 G FIBER ~
3.1 G TOTAL FAT ~ 0.3 G SATURATED FAT ~ 0.0 MG CHOLESTEROL ~ 6.9 MG SODIUM

2 cups tapioca flour

1 cup oat flour

1½ cups buckwheat flour

1 cup teff flour

¾ cup arrowroot powder

Combine all ingredients; store in airtight container until use.

Yields 6¼ cups flour (6¼ 1-cup servings).

Substitutions
For a gluten-free mix, purchase gluten-free oats and process them to a fine powder before use. You can use a combination of various grains to make flour for this recipe, such as brown rice flour, millet, or quinoa flour. Use at least 3 different flours; the more varieties you include, the more you will round out the flours' characteristics.

Healthy Tidbit
Buckwheat's name is misleading because there's no wheat in buckwheat. It is a gluten-free grain. Try it as a cereal or as a grain for a delightful taste. Buckwheat is very underutilized when you consider its health benefits. It contains linoleic acid, making it a good source of essential fatty acids. It is also high in vitamins (B-1, B-2, B-3, B-5, folic acid, and E), essential amino acids, and the minerals chromium, copper, manganese, and magnesium. Buckwheat has shown anti-tumor activities, boosts metabolism, and is liver protective.

Nutritional Analysis per Serving

Vitamin A	0.3 RE	Vitamin D	0.0 µg
Thiamin (B-1)	0.1 mg	Vitamin E	0.0 mg
Riboflavin (B-2)	0.0 mg	Calcium	52.2 mg
Niacin	0.2 mg	Iron	3.6 mg
Vitamin B-6	0.0 mg	Phosphorus	14.1 mg
Vitamin B-12	0.0 µg	Magnesium	3.6 mg
Folate (total)	48.7 µg	Zinc	0.1 mg
Vitamin C	0.3 mg	Potassium	119.5 mg

Breakfast

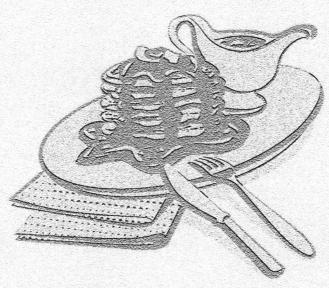

 Recipes with this symbol are not strictly anti-inflammatory, therefore we suggest avoiding these recipes until you are feeling well and are ready to introduce a little variety to see how you do.

Cashew Oat Waffles

PER SERVING: 411.6 CALORIES ~ 16.7 G PROTEIN ~ 65.2 G CARBOHYDRATE ~ 9.3 G FIBER ~
13.4 G TOTAL FAT ~ 2.7 G SATURATED FAT ~ 46.5 MG CHOLESTEROL ~ 191.6 MG SODIUM

½ cup raw cashews

2 cups water

4 whole dates

2 cups gluten-free oats

1 egg

1 teaspoon vanilla

½ teaspoon cinnamon

¼ teaspoon baking powder

¼ teaspoon salt

Preheat waffle iron. Process the cashews in a blender with 1 cup water. Add the dates and process until smooth. Add remaining ingredients and the additional 1 cup water, and process until smooth. Pour enough batter into the waffle iron to fill to edges. Cook until waffles are browned and no longer moist inside, about 12 minutes.

This waffle batter will not flow as easily as you are used to, and the batter can thicken if left to sit. Add more water if necessary. Sometimes these waffles remain a little moist in the middle; cooking them longer can help improve that.

Serves 4.

Substitutions

You could use other nuts instead of cashews, but if they have skins you will need to blanch them first and pinch off the skins. If you are diabetic, you should omit the dates. Experiment with other whole grains such as quinoa, buckwheat groats, or amaranth. Process them into flour and use about 1½ cups of the flour mixture you create. (There's no need to process rolled oats into a flour before using them in this recipe. They will easily blend when added to the blender with other ingredients. The other grains suggested here are still in their whole form; that's why they need to be ground into flour before use in this recipe.)

Healthy Tidbit

Eat breakfast *every* day. Eating breakfast regularly has

Nutritional Analysis per Serving

Vitamin A	80.4 RE	Vitamin D	0.3 µg
Thiamin (B-1)	0.1 mg	Vitamin E	0.1 mg
Riboflavin (B-2)	0.1 mg	Calcium	83.6 mg
Niacin	0.3 mg	Iron	5.0 mg
Vitamin B-6	0.1 mg	Phosphorus	154.3 mg
Vitamin B-12	0.1 µg	Magnesium	53.6 mg
Folate (total)	11.3 µg	Zinc	1.1 mg
Vitamin C	0.1 mg	Potassium	175.1 mg

been associated with weight loss, improved glucose levels, and increased metabolism. Not all breakfasts are created equal, however. A shocking new study shows that some breakfast cereals offer more sugar than three chocolate chip cookies. As many as eighty-four common breakfast cereals were evaluated, and some were found to contain more sugar than a Hostess Twinkie![4] Breakfast is not dessert. It sets the stage for the rest of the day. Starting the day with a sugary cereal will leave you with very little energy by the afternoon, more cravings, and a sluggish metabolism. Making a habit of eating a sugary breakfast can nudge you on your way toward diabetes and weight gain.

Crêpes

PER SERVING: 112.9 CALORIES ~ 3.7 G PROTEIN ~ 18.8 G CARBOHYDRATE ~ 2.3 G FIBER ~ 3.2 G TOTAL FAT ~ 1.2 G SATURATED FAT ~ 58.9 MG CHOLESTEROL ~ 150.2 MG SODIUM

1⅓ cup Crêpe Flour Blend (see recipe on page 132)

½ teaspoon salt

3 large eggs

1½ cups water

1 tablespoon butter

4 peaches, peeled, sliced

1 tablespoon cinnamon

2 tablespoons pure maple syrup

Combine Crêpe Flour Blend and salt in a medium bowl. Whisk together eggs and water; whisk into flour mixture. Pour batter through a fine strainer to remove lumps. Refrigerate at least 30 minutes; batter will appear thin at first but will thicken after standing.

Preheat oven to 350°F.

Combine peaches, cinnamon, and syrup in a baking dish. Bake until peaches are tender, about 20 minutes. Keep warm.

Add enough butter to coat the bottom of an 8- or 10-inch nonstick skillet or well-seasoned cast-iron skillet; heat over medium heat. When pan is hot, add about ¼ cup crêpe batter, or just enough to coat the pan in a thin layer. Immediately rotate pan so batter forms an even, thin layer. Cook until browned on bottom, about 1 minute; turn and brown

Nutritional Analysis per Serving

Vitamin A	54.7 RE	Vitamin D	0.3 µg
Thiamin (B-1)	0.0 mg	Vitamin E	0.2 mg
Riboflavin (B-2)	0.1 mg	Calcium	31.4 mg
Niacin	0.5 mg	Iron	1.0 mg
Vitamin B-6	0.0 mg	Phosphorus	44.4 mg
Vitamin B-12	0.1 µg	Magnesium	9.3 mg
Folate (total)	16.0 µg	Zinc	0.4 mg
Vitamin C	4.0 mg	Potassium	162.7 mg

on the other side, about 1 minute. Quickly remove crêpe from pan and place on a platter or baking sheet. Repeat with remaining batter, using additional butter as needed to prevent crêpes from sticking.

Fill crêpes with warm peach mixture.

Makes 10 crêpes (10 servings).

Kitchen Tip

Making crêpes is easy once you have the technique down. Here are some troubleshooting points. I use a well-seasoned cast iron skillet. I start with a little butter in the pan; most of the time I add another small amount halfway through the cooking process. If you put the batter in the pan and it doesn't fill the pan but the crêpe is properly thin, add more batter. If you put the batter in and it doesn't fill the pan but the crêpe is thick and clumpy, then your pan may be too hot to allow the batter to spread evenly. If as you rotate the pan, the crêpe batter flows, but holes develop, the pan is still too hot to allow the batter to spread. For the perfect crêpe, you want to pour the batter into the middle of the pan and then rotate the pan to create a thin, even layer of batter. Flipping the crêpe should be easy. You can either flip it with a spatula or carefully use your fingers to grab an edge of the crêpe.

Substitutions

For cool crêpes, make the peach filling in advance and chill in the refrigerator until serving.

You can fill crêpes with nearly anything you want. Below is a list of possibilities. You could add cinnamon and a little vanilla extract to the batter. I am sure the cinnamon would complement even a savory crêpe well.

Crêpe Fillings

- blueberries with lactose-free yogurt or coconut yogurt
- strawberries
- kiwi
- bananas and sun butter topped with honey
- jelly or jam
- smoked salmon and capers
- sautéed onions, green peppers, black beans, and avocado (for a Mexican crêpe)
- chicken sausage or pork sausage with sliced apple
- honey with lemon juice
- sautéed onions and mushrooms, with or without bacon
- Homemade Chocolate Spread (see recipe on page 258) with cherries
- diced chicken and avocado with teriyaki sauce

Sweet Potato Pancakes

PER SERVING: 267.7 CALORIES ~ 13.6 G PROTEIN ~ 15.3 G CARBOHYDRATE ~ 2.6 G FIBER ~
16.4 G TOTAL FAT ~ 9.0 G SATURATED FAT ~ 372.0 MG CHOLESTEROL ~ 178.9 MG SODIUM

1 cup cooked mashed sweet potato

4 eggs

1 teaspoon cinnamon

1 teaspoon vanilla

1 tablespoon coconut oil, melted

Process all ingredients in a blender or food processor until smooth.

Heat pancake griddle or large skillet over medium heat. Spoon sweet potato mixture onto hot nonstick griddle, using about ¼ cup batter for each pancake. Cook until browned on bottom, about 2 minutes; turn and cook until brown, about 2 minutes.

Yields 4 pancakes (2 servings).

Kitchen Tip

If you add oil to a pancake batter and cook the pancakes on a nonstick skillet, you shouldn't need to use much, if any, oil on the surface of the skillet.

Substitutions

You can also make these pancakes with mashed winter squash, peas, or carrots. They require no syrup and make a nice alternative to sweets or grain in the morning. I often pack them as snacks because they travel well.

Healthy Tidbit

Watching television has proven to lead to sedentary habits, which may put people at risk for various diseases, including colon cancer. But does watching specific types of TV shows cause more harm than just a reduction in activity? A recent study looked at the effect of watching *SpongeBob SquarePants* and similar cartoons on young children's behaviors. After only a few minutes of the fast-paced cartoon, the four-year-old children were observed to perform significantly worse on executive function tasks compared to children who were not exposed to the fast-paced cartoon. The authors of this study noted that not all television programs for children were evaluated. They state that this particular cartoon is currently the most watched television program among two- to eleven-year-olds. They write, "Perhaps Big Bird, Bert and Ernie, and Oscar the Grouch are more benign than SpongeBob, but that will require definitive testing."[5]

Nutritional Analysis per Serving

Vitamin A	1105.8 RE	Vitamin D	2.0 µg
Thiamin (B-1)	0.1 mg	Vitamin E	1.1 mg
Riboflavin (B-2)	0.5 mg	Calcium	87.7 mg
Niacin	0.5 mg	Iron	2.3 mg
Vitamin B-6	0.3 mg	Phosphorus	230.1 mg
Vitamin B-12	0.9 µg	Magnesium	29.6 mg
Folate (total)	54.4 µg	Zinc	1.5 mg
Vitamin C	1.6 mg	Potassium	370.2 mg

Savory Egg Crêpes

PER SERVING: 322.5 CALORIES ~ 40.8 G PROTEIN ~ 4.0 G CARBOHYDRATE ~ 0.8 G FIBER ~
15.8 G TOTAL FAT ~ 6.4 G SATURATED FAT ~ 465.0 MG CHOLESTEROL ~ 527.1 MG SODIUM

This is the perfect alternative to a flour crêpe. It turns out much like an omelet, but is fun because you get to roll the filling up in the egg patty.

½ small onion, minced	1 teaspoon thyme
3 cloves garlic, minced	½ teaspoon salt
2 teaspoons coconut oil	1 teaspoon ground pepper
1 pound ground buffalo	10 eggs, lightly beaten
1½ cups chopped spinach	Chopped cilantro, as garnish
1 bunch cilantro, chopped	

Sauté onion and garlic in coconut oil in a large skillet until softened, about 3 minutes; add buffalo. Cook over medium heat until lightly browned, about 8 minutes, crumbling meat with fork. Stir in spinach, cilantro, and thyme, and cook mixture until spinach wilts, about 2 minutes. Season to taste with extra salt and pepper if desired.

Heat a small, lightly greased nonstick skillet over medium heat until hot; spoon in about ¼ cup eggs. Cook until browned on bottom and set, about 2 minutes; turn and brown on other side. Repeat with remaining eggs.

Spoon meat mixture onto egg "crêpes," and arrange on serving plates. Sprinkle with cilantro.

Serves 4.

Substitutions

Most vegetable combinations will work well in this recipe. You can easily make a vegetarian version if desired. Serve with a hot sauce or any favorite sauce.

Healthy Tidbit

I love cilantro for its significant cleansing properties. Cilantro can aid in detoxification from mercury, cadmium, lead, and aluminum in both bones and the central nervous system. Consuming a lot of cilantro or taking it in tincture or tea form can help mobilize these toxins. Be careful not to overdo the cilantro if you are high in heavy metals because mobilizing heavy metals without giving them a way out can be a

Nutritional Analysis per Serving			
Vitamin A	309.5 RE	Vitamin D	2.5 µg
Thiamin (B-1)	0.2 mg	Vitamin E	1.3 mg
Riboflavin (B-2)	1.0 mg	Calcium	100.9 mg
Niacin	8.1 mg	Iron	6.0 mg
Vitamin B-6	1.2 mg	Phosphorus	488.8 mg
Vitamin B-12	2.4 µg	Magnesium	52.4 mg
Folate (total)	84.3 µg	Zinc	5.2 mg
Vitamin C	5.1 mg	Potassium	676.8 mg

problem. This retoxification can be avoided by using an intestinal absorbing nutrient such as chlorella. Chlorella has been used extensively in the heavy metal detoxification process. Be aware that eating small amounts of cilantro will not cause you problems. Significant heavy metal mobilization would only occur from consuming high levels of cilantro in concentrated forms such as juices, teas, or tinctures.

Warm Brown Rice Cereal

PER SERVING: 150.4 CALORIES ~ 2.7 G PROTEIN ~ 33.3 G CARBOHYDRATE ~ 3.2 G FIBER ~
1.2 G TOTAL FAT ~ 0.3 G SATURATED FAT ~ 0.0 MG CHOLESTEROL ~ 8.9 MG SODIUM

1 cup brown rice

5 cups water

1 tablespoon cinnamon

1 teaspoon nutmeg

2 apples, peeled, chopped

Combine all ingredients in a slow cooker. Cook on low for at least 8 hours, or overnight.

Serves 6.

Substitutions
You can try this with other gluten-free cereal blends or other grains.

Healthy Tidbit
Brown rice figures heavily in the macrobiotic diet, which emphasizes eating without changing the structure of foods to the point where you cannot recognize them. Focusing on grains, vegetables, and minimal animal proteins, the macrobiotic diet avoids the use of any processed foods. The macrobiotic diet strongly urges against overeating and encourages chewing foods well before swallowing. It generally fits with the anti-inflammation diet, though for some people it contains too much grain for good digestion. Any diet that focuses on whole foods and the elimination of processed foods will benefit most people rather quickly.

Nutritional Analysis per Serving

Vitamin A	6.9 RE	Vitamin D	0.0 µg
Thiamin (B-1)	0.1 mg	Vitamin E	0.0 mg
Riboflavin (B-2)	0.1 mg	Calcium	28.9 mg
Niacin	1.7 mg	Iron	0.6 mg
Vitamin B-6	0.2 mg	Phosphorus	110.9 mg
Vitamin B-12	0.0 µg	Magnesium	50.5 mg
Folate (total)	8.3 µg	Zinc	0.7 mg
Vitamin C	2.9 mg	Potassium	141.9 mg

Gluten-Free French Toast

PER SERVING: 331.3 CALORIES ~ 8.6 G PROTEIN ~ 41.3 G CARBOHYDRATE ~ 3.5 G FIBER ~
14.3 G TOTAL FAT ~ 7.6 G SATURATED FAT ~ 139.5 MG CHOLESTEROL ~ 477.1 MG SODIUM

3 eggs	1 teaspoon cinnamon
½ cup almond milk	¼ teaspoon salt
½ cup coconut milk	8 slices gluten-free bread
1 tablespoon raw honey, warm	

Preheat oven to 350°F.

Whisk all ingredients, except bread, in a medium bowl until well blended. Pour the mixture into a flat pan or pie pan.

Dip bread into egg mixture and allow to soak for 15–30 seconds on each side; cook bread in a lightly greased large skillet until golden brown, about 4 minutes on each side. Remove from skillet and place on a baking sheet in the oven for at least 5 minutes, or until serving. Repeat with remaining bread. Serve with topping of your choice.

Serves 4.

Substitutions

You can try various gluten-free breads, and you can add to or change the spice content. Sometimes you want cinnamon and sometimes you don't. Using nutmeg and allspice will add a pumpkin pie note.

Healthy Tidbit

Remember the bad rap that eggs used to get due to their relatively high levels of cholesterol? Turns out that fear was based on poor information, and that eggs are not as bad for the heart as was once believed. A new study shows that eggs are lower in cholesterol and higher in vitamin D than originally thought. Eggs are also high in choline, a nutrient important in adrenal function, memory, muscle control, and stimulation of the parasympathetic nervous system, which acts to calm everyday stress.

Studies also reveal that consuming eggs as part of a weight-loss diet improved weight loss by more than 65 percent compared to consuming the same number of calories in the form of carbohydrates. Protein can be an important part of regulating weight loss.

Nutritional Analysis per Serving

Vitamin A	60.9 RE	Vitamin D	0.8 µg
Thiamin (B-1)	0.0 mg	Vitamin E	0.4 mg
Riboflavin (B-2)	0.2 mg	Calcium	37.0 mg
Niacin	0.3 mg	Iron	2.9 mg
Vitamin B-6	0.1 mg	Phosphorus	104.8 mg
Vitamin B-12	0.3 µg	Magnesium	16.1 mg
Folate (total)	22.6 µg	Zinc	0.7 mg
Vitamin C	0.9 mg	Potassium	173.4 mg

Gluten-Free Eggless French Toast

PER SERVING: 229.6 CALORIES ~ 3.0 G PROTEIN ~ 41.9 G CARBOHYDRATE ~ 3.0 G FIBER ~
4.1 G TOTAL FAT ~ 0.2 G SATURATED FAT ~ 0.8 MG CHOLESTEROL ~ 272.5 MG SODIUM

5 pitted dates	½ cup apple cider
1 tablespoon raw cashews	1 tablespoon gluten-free flour mix
1 tablespoon raw sunflower seeds	1 teaspoon cinnamon
1 tablespoon raw pumpkin seeds	12 slices of gluten-free bread
1 cup water, divided	

Preheat oven to 350°F.

Blend dates, cashews, and seeds with ½ cup water in blender until chopped; add remaining ½ cup water and blend until smooth. Add remaining ingredients, except bread, and blend until smooth.

Pour mixture into flat pan or pie pan.

Dip bread into liquid mixture and allow to soak for 15–30 seconds on each side; cook bread in lightly greased large skillet until golden brown, about 4 minutes on each side. Remove from skillet and place on baking sheet in oven for at least 5 minutes, or until serving. Repeat with remaining bread.

Serves 6.

Substitutions

This recipe allows people who must avoid eggs to enjoy a version of French toast. Try adding a banana to the mixture for a different flavor profile.

Healthy Tidbit

Calories do not have to be your enemy! Don't fall into the trap of counting calories. If you are overweight and interested in weight loss and you want to watch your calories, then doing so for a period of time is perfectly fine. But on a day-to-day basis, if you are eating the right kinds of foods, eliminating most of the bad foods, controlling your serving sizes, and being careful to stop eating when you're satisfied (that is, before you're stuffed), you should not have to count calories to maintain a consistent weight. Eating should not be about numbers; it should be about nutrition and providing your body with what it needs for survival. We often eat to please our emotions without thinking about what our body needs. When you learn to tune into that part, there will be no need to count calories.

Nutritional Analysis per Serving

Vitamin A	0.4 RE	Vitamin D	0.0 µg
Thiamin (B-1)	0.0 mg	Vitamin E	0.3 mg
Riboflavin (B-2)	0.0 mg	Calcium	11.9 mg
Niacin	0.2 mg	Iron	1.8 mg
Vitamin B-6	0.0 mg	Phosphorus	16.8 mg
Vitamin B-12	0.0 µg	Magnesium	12.3 mg
Folate (total)	4.5 µg	Zinc	0.2 mg
Vitamin C	0.2 mg	Potassium	94.6 mg

Banana Split Breakfast

PER SERVING: 303.2 CALORIES ~ 13.7 G PROTEIN ~ 42.4 G CARBOHYDRATE ~ 11.2 G FIBER ~
10.5 G TOTAL FAT ~ 1.2 G SATURATED FAT ~ 2.5 MG CHOLESTEROL ~ 105.2 MG SODIUM

1 banana

⅓ cup blueberries

⅓ cup cut peeled kiwi

⅓ cup sliced strawberries

1 cup Almost Lactose-Free Yogurt (see recipe on page 171) or coconut yogurt

⅓ cup flax seeds, ground in coffee grinder

Optional toppings: brown rice syrup, agave syrup, or cocoa syrup

Cut banana in half lengthwise and place in an oval dish. Layer remaining fruit over banana; top with yogurt, and sprinkle with flax seeds.

Add optional toppings if desired.

Serves 2.

Substitutions

This is an attractive treat that is fun to serve to guests. You can use a variety of fruits, granolas, or yogurts. It also works will as a dessert after dinner, especially for those who are wanting to watch their figure or maintain an anti-inflammation diet.

Healthy Tidbit

Kiwis are a powerhouse of nutrition. Like citrus, they are high in vitamin C and carotenes, and they contain as much potassium as a banana. Enjoy a kiwi fruit before or after exercise to balance your electrolytes.

Nutritional Analysis per Serving

Vitamin A	10.1 RE	Vitamin D	0.0 µg
Thiamin (B-1)	0.1 mg	Vitamin E	0.5 mg
Riboflavin (B-2)	0.4 mg	Calcium	329.2 mg
Niacin	0.8 mg	Iron	1.5 mg
Vitamin B-6	0.3 mg	Phosphorus	222.9 mg
Vitamin B-12	0.8 µg	Magnesium	48.1 mg
Folate (total)	44.2 µg	Zinc	1.4 mg
Vitamin C	55.3 mg	Potassium	676.7 mg

Sweet Millet Biscuits and Sausage Gravy

PER SERVING: 696.0 CALORIES ~ 21.0 G PROTEIN ~ 109.0 G CARBOHYDRATE ~ 4.8 G FIBER ~
20.8 G TOTAL FAT ~ 7.7 G SATURATED FAT ~ 112.9 MG CHOLESTEROL ~ 950.2 MG SODIUM

For the Biscuits

½ cup almond milk

½ cup honey

1 egg

3 tablespoons butter or coconut oil, melted

2 cups Gluten-Free Pancake and Baking Mix (see recipe on page 124) or gluten-free flour blend

1 teaspoon baking powder

½ teaspoon baking soda

½ teaspoon guar gum

½ teaspoon salt

1 cup uncooked millet

For the Gravy

1 pound chicken or turkey breakfast sausage

¼ cup gluten-free flour or ground gluten-free oats

1 cup almond milk

1 cup hemp milk

Salt and freshly ground pepper to taste

To make the biscuits: Preheat oven to 350°F.

Whisk together almond milk, honey, egg, and butter in a medium bowl until smooth. In another medium bowl, combine remaining ingredients, except millet, mixing well. Add almond milk mixture to dry ingredients, stirring until smooth; stir in millet.

Spoon biscuits onto two greased baking pans, allowing about 2 table-spoons of dough per biscuit, or spoon into greased muffin tins. Bake for 18–20 minutes, or until a toothpick inserted in the center of a biscuit comes out clean.

To make the sausage gravy: Cook sausage in a large skillet over medium heat, crumbling it with a fork, until browned, about 10 minutes. Sprinkle with flour; add milks over medium heat ¼ cup at a time, allowing sauce to thicken after each addition. Simmer until thick, about 5 minutes; season to taste with salt and pepper. Serve over biscuits.

Serves 6.

Kitchen Tip

These biscuits turn out a little soft; if you want them firmer, reduce or eliminate the almond milk. If you desire less sweetness, you can reduce the honey by half.

Nutritional Analysis per Serving

Vitamin A	83.4 RE	Vitamin D	0.6 µg
Thiamin (B-1)	0.1 mg	Vitamin E	0.5 mg
Riboflavin (B-2)	0.2 mg	Calcium	132.7 mg
Niacin	1.6 mg	Iron	2.9 mg
Vitamin B-6	0.2 mg	Phosphorus	229.9 mg
Vitamin B-12	0.3 µg	Magnesium	46.6 mg
Folate (total)	34.4 µg	Zinc	0.8 mg
Vitamin C	0.1 mg	Potassium	213.0 mg

Healthy Tidbit

Adding millet to baked goods results in a candylike crunch that is delicious in muffins and cookies of all sorts. Millet is high in iron and is a non-animal source of amino acids.

Quick Avocado Breakfast

PER SERVING: 371.5 CALORIES ~ 6.9 G PROTEIN ~ 25.9 G CARBOHYDRATE ~ 17.1 G FIBER ~ 30.7 G TOTAL FAT ~ 6.0 G SATURATED FAT ~ 0.0 MG CHOLESTEROL ~ 6.4 MG SODIUM

1 ripe avocado, halved, seeded, and sliced

Juice of ½ lemon

Salt to taste

Sprinkle avocado with lemon juice and salt.

Serves 1.

Substitutions

This makes a satisfying, quick breakfast, especially if you're pressed for time and are tempted to skip breakfast. Sometimes I use a little gluten-free tamari instead of salt. My kids love avocados and will eat them in most any fashion, even plain.

Healthy Tidbit

Avocados are the perfect fatty fruit. They are easy to prepare and can be used in savory or sweet dishes. Avocados provide nearly 20 essential nutrients, including fiber, potassium, vitamin E, B vitamins, and folic acid. They also help the body absorb more fat-soluble nutrients, such as alpha- and beta-carotene and lutein, from foods that are eaten with the fruit. Avocados are low in saturated fat and high in monounsaturated fat, the good kind of fat that helps to lower cholesterol. Don't be scared of the fat content in avocados. Enjoy more of them with your meals.

Nutritional Analysis per Serving

Vitamin A	42.7 RE	Vitamin D	0.0 µg
Thiamin (B-1)	0.1 mg	Vitamin E	0.0 mg
Riboflavin (B-2)	0.2 mg	Calcium	32.2 mg
Niacin	2.1 mg	Iron	0.5 mg
Vitamin B-6	0.3 mg	Phosphorus	124.0 mg
Vitamin B-12	0.0 µg	Magnesium	74.8 mg
Folate (total)	112.5 µg	Zinc	1.2 mg
Vitamin C	64.7 mg	Potassium	1098.5 mg

Sunflower Butter Pancakes

PER SERVING: 177.3 CALORIES ~ 8.5 G PROTEIN ~ 16.4 G CARBOHYDRATE ~ 1.7 G FIBER ~
9.4 G TOTAL FAT ~ 2.6 G SATURATED FAT ~ 186.0 MG CHOLESTEROL ~ 71.9 MG SODIUM

The texture of these isn't like what you are used to in a pancake, but the flavor is delicious and they don't contain any grain.

1 banana

2 eggs

1 tablespoon sunflower butter

¼ teaspoon coconut oil, melted

¼ teaspoon nutmeg

¼ teaspoon cinnamon

Blend all ingredients in a blender until smooth. Pour about ¼ cup batter onto a lightly greased nonstick griddle or skillet. Cook over medium heat until browned on bottom and bubbly, about 2 minutes; turn and brown on other side. Repeat with remaining batter.

Serves 2.

Substitutions

You can use any kind of nut butter for this recipe. Remember that you can process nuts in a food processor to make your own nut butter.

Healthy Tidbit

This recipe satisfies GAPS diet requirements. The GAPS (Gut and Psychology Syndrome) diet is helpful for people who struggle with skin conditions or severe gastrointestinal disorders. GAPS concentrates on fruits, vegetables, and healthy fats and deemphasizes grains. Many people may benefit from going completely grain-free for a while and then working some whole grains back into the diet once better health is established. Many of my eczema patients are asked to start on GAPS, and they do significantly better rather quickly if they stick to it. The diet is strict at first, but with support, patients can usually begin reintroducing foods without reactions.

Nutritional Analysis per Serving

Vitamin A	84.9 RE	Vitamin D	1.0 µg
Thiamin (B-1)	0.1 mg	Vitamin E	0.5 mg
Riboflavin (B-2)	0.3 mg	Calcium	44.1 mg
Niacin	0.9 mg	Iron	1.4 mg
Vitamin B-6	0.4 mg	Phosphorus	171.6 mg
Vitamin B-12	0.4 µg	Magnesium	52.1 mg
Folate (total)	54.5 µg	Zinc	1.2 mg
Vitamin C	5.4 mg	Potassium	288.2 mg

Fried Egg with Sautéed Zucchini

PER SERVING: 445.3 CALORIES ~ 15.9 G PROTEIN ~ 23.8 G CARBOHYDRATE ~ 3.0 G FIBER ~
31.9 G TOTAL FAT ~ 6.1 G SATURATED FAT ~ 372.0 MG CHOLESTEROL ~ 293.1 MG SODIUM

2 small zucchinis, chopped

3 tablespoons olive oil, divided

Salt and freshly ground pepper to taste

4 eggs

2 slices of gluten-free toast

Sauté zucchini in 1 tablespoon oil in a large skillet until lightly browned, about 5 minutes. Season with salt and pepper. While zucchini is cooking, heat remaining 2 tablespoons oil in another large nonstick skillet over medium heat until hot. Carefully crack 4 eggs into skillet and cook until whites are set, about 2 minutes. Turn eggs and cook for another minute on the other side until whites are cooked but yolks remain runny.

Spoon zucchini onto two serving plates, top each serving with 2 eggs; sprinkle with salt and pepper to taste. Serve with toast.

Serves 2.

Substitutions

You could sauté many vegetables and top them with a fried egg. It is a great way to get vegetables first thing in the morning. Experiment with spinach, chard, yellow squash, or others. I prefer using only one vegetable to complement the egg. A whole stir-fry would overpower the simplicity of the egg and toast.

Healthy Tidbit

As much as possible, don't drink while you eat. Drinking large amounts of liquids while eating can dilute your digestive juices, making it harder for you to digest your meal. If you sometimes feel nauseous or have no appetite in the morning, and especially if eggs make you nauseated, this may indicate that you are low in stomach acid (hydrochloric acid, or HCL). Taking a digestive enzyme that includes HCL prior to meals will help you digest proteins better. You can easily find one in a health-food store. If you take any form of HCL and it gives you heartburn, discontinue use.

Nutritional Analysis per Serving

Vitamin A	201.2 RE	Vitamin D	1.1 µg
Thiamin (B-1)	0.1 mg	Vitamin E	1.1 mg
Riboflavin (B-2)	0.6 mg	Calcium	87.6 mg
Niacin	1.0 mg	Iron	3.3 mg
Vitamin B-6	0.5 mg	Phosphorus	272.5 mg
Vitamin B-12	0.9 µg	Magnesium	47.3 mg
Folate (total)	94.0 µg	Zinc	1.9 mg
Vitamin C	35.1 mg	Potassium	649.8 mg

Simple Buckwheat (Kasha) Breakfast

PER SERVING: 319.4 CALORIES ~ 10.2 G PROTEIN ~ 67.2 G CARBOHYDRATE ~ 8.7 G FIBER ~
3.5 G TOTAL FAT ~ 1.1 G SATURATED FAT ~ 2.5 MG CHOLESTEROL ~ 26.8 MG SODIUM

2 cups water

1 cup buckwheat groats

1 tablespoon apple cider vinegar or whey

2 tablespoons almond milk

2 teaspoons agave syrup

½ teaspoon butter

½ teaspoon cinnamon (optional)

Dash of salt

Combine, water, groats, and vinegar in a medium saucepan and let stand, covered, overnight. The next morning, remove any grains that have floated to the top. Heat to boiling; reduce heat and simmer, covered, until the groats have absorbed all water, about 10 minutes. Remove from heat; stir in remaining ingredients.

Serves 2.

Substitutions

You can use buckwheat in various dishes for a unique flavor. You can add it to salads, burritos, and soups, but first try it as a cereal so you understand the complexity of flavor it offers. Our family likes to just cook it and snack on it plain.

Healthy Tidbit

Sweeteners other than sugar can offer satisfaction to your taste buds without wreaking havoc on your insulin response. Agave syrup or nectar is a good alternative sweetener. Make sure you get it from a reliable source. You can order organic agave nectar by the gallon from Amazon.com. Agave nectar, with a glycemic index of 30, falls in the category of low glycemic foods. It can be a suitable option for diabetics. By contrast, pure maple syrup has a glycemic index of 54, making it still a better choice than cane sugar, which has a glycemic index of 100.

Nutritional Analysis per Serving

Vitamin A	8.9 RE	Vitamin D	0.0 µg
Thiamin (B-1)	0.2 mg	Vitamin E	0.0 mg
Riboflavin (B-2)	0.2 mg	Calcium	24.4 mg
Niacin	4.2 mg	Iron	2.2 mg
Vitamin B-6	0.3 mg	Phosphorus	262.4 mg
Vitamin B-12	0.0 µg	Magnesium	184.0 mg
Folate (total)	34.5 µg	Zinc	2.0 mg
Vitamin C	2.8 mg	Potassium	289.2 mg

Smoothies

Smoothies are surprisingly easy to prepare. You can usually default to making a smoothie when you or your children are hungry. I almost always have some frozen fruits and some greens on hand that I can throw in the blender. Add water and a little lemon and honey and *voilà*, you have a smoothie. What an excellent way to get your children to eat raw greens!

 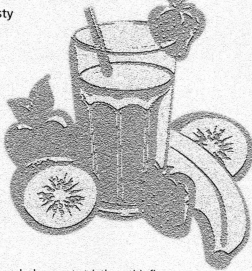
 Recipes with this symbol are not strictly anti-inflammatory, therefore we suggest avoiding these recipes until you are feeling well and are ready to introduce a little variety to see how you do.

Yummy Smoothie with Spinach

PER SERVING: 168.8 CALORIES ~ 4.2 G PROTEIN ~ 35.5 G CARBOHYDRATE ~ 5.0 G FIBER ~
2.6 G TOTAL FAT ~ 1.4 G SATURATED FAT ~ 8.0 MG CHOLESTEROL ~ 51.4 MG SODIUM

You may want to serve this smoothie in fun dishes with spoons or in decorative cups with straws to increase children's enjoyment. It makes a great nutritious snack for grown-ups too.

2 frozen bananas, cut into chunks *

1 cup spinach leaves **

½ cup frozen blueberries ***

½ cup plain whole milk yogurt, kefir,
dairy-free coconut yogurt, or almond milk

Water or almond milk, as needed

Blend all ingredients in a blender until smooth, adding water if needed.
    Serves 2.

Kitchen Tips
If the smoothie is too runny, add more banana or frozen berries. If you are having trouble getting it to blend, add more liquid.

    * It is simple to store bananas in the freezer, making them easy to use for smoothies. First, peel the banana and cut it into quarters. (Cutting them allows for easier blending once they're frozen.) Store in a zipper-lock freezer bag.

    ** I buy already-washed, prepackaged organic baby spinach.

    *** Organic frozen berries are cheaper than fresh ones, and they make the smoothie cold without having to use ice.

Nutritional Analysis per Serving

Vitamin A	212.2 RE	Vitamin D	0.1 µg
Thiamin (B-1)	0.1 mg	Vitamin E	0.4 mg
Riboflavin (B-2)	0.2 mg	Calcium	109.8 mg
Niacin	1.0 mg	Iron	1.3 mg
Vitamin B-6	0.5 mg	Phosphorus	88.4 mg
Vitamin B-12	0.2 mg	Magnesium	61.2 mg
Folate (total)	83.9 mg	Zinc	0.6 mg
Vitamin C	19.5 mg	Potassium	538.3 mg

Chia Green Smoothie

PER SERVING: 199.1 CALORIES ~ 2.8 G PROTEIN ~ 45.2 G CARBOHYDRATE ~ 7.2 G FIBER ~
2.7 G TOTAL FAT ~ 0.3 G SATURATED FAT ~ 0.0 MG CHOLESTEROL ~ 16.1 MG SODIUM

½ cup chopped collard greens, or 1 large
collard green leaf, chopped

1 cup chopped green-leaf lettuce

1 apple, chopped

1 kiwi, cubed

½ cup frozen strawberries

2 tablespoons chia seeds

2 tablespoons honey

1 teaspoon green tea powder

1¼ cup water

Blend all ingredients in a
blender until smooth.
    Serves 2.

Nutritional Analysis per Serving

Vitamin A	245.2 RE	Vitamin D	0.0 µg
Thiamin (B-1)	0.1 mg	Vitamin E	0.8 mg
Riboflavin (B-2)	0.1 mg	Calcium	92.6 mg
Niacin	1.2 mg	Iron	1.6 mg
Vitamin B-6	0.2 mg	Phosphorus	98.5 mg
Vitamin B-12	0.0 µg	Magnesium	45.6 mg
Folate (total)	62.6 µg	Zinc	0.6 mg
Vitamin C	74.3 mg	Potassium	414.3 mg

Chia Raspberry Smoothie

PER SERVING: 147.8 CALORIES ~ 3.6 G PROTEIN ~ 23.3 G CARBOHYDRATE ~ 10.3 G FIBER ~
4.8 G TOTAL FAT ~ 0.5 G SATURATED FAT ~ 0.0 MG CHOLESTEROL ~ 30.3 MG SODIUM

2 cups frozen raspberries

1½ cups water

¼ cup plus 1 tablespoon chia seeds

1 teaspoon kelp powder

Blend all ingredients in a blender until smooth.
    Serves 2.

Substitutions:

This smoothie is very seedy. If
you would like to reduce the
seed texture, use a different
fruit in place of the raspberries
and keep the chia seeds in for
health. In a pinch, you could try
small amounts of nori instead
of the kelp powder. Nori is the
seaweed sheets used to make
sushi rolls. They will still provide some iodine.

Nutritional Analysis per Serving

Vitamin A	10.6 RE	Vitamin D	0.0 µg
Thiamin (B-1)	0.1 mg	Vitamin E	0.0 mg
Riboflavin (B-2)	0.0 mg	Calcium	138.1 mg
Niacin	1.4 mg	Iron	2.4 mg
Vitamin B-6	0.1 mg	Phosphorus	133.3 mg
Vitamin B-12	0.0 µg	Magnesium	59.2 mg
Folate (total)	7.6 µg	Zinc	0.7 mg
Vitamin C	15.2 mg	Potassium	148.2 mg

Tangy Green Smoothie

PER SERVING: 73.5 CALORIES ~ 1.9 G PROTEIN ~ 15.4 G CARBOHYDRATE ~ 1.4 G FIBER ~
1.2 G TOTAL FAT ~ 0.6 G SATURATED FAT ~ 3.2 MG CHOLESTEROL ~ 26.8 MG SODIUM

2 cups water

1 frozen banana, cut into chunks

1 cup frozen green grapes

½ cup Almost Lactose-Free Yogurt
(see recipe on page 171),
coconut yogurt, or kefir

1½ cups fresh spinach leaves

Blend all ingredients in a blender until smooth.

Serves 4.

Nutritional Analysis per Serving

Vitamin A	119.2 RE	Vitamin D	0.3 µg
Thiamin (B-1)	0.1 mg	Vitamin E	0.0 mg
Riboflavin (B-2)	0.1 mg	Calcium	54.9 mg
Niacin	0.4 mg	Iron	0.5 mg
Vitamin B-6	0.2 mg	Phosphorus	45.9 mg
Vitamin B-12	0.1 µg	Magnesium	23.9 mg
Folate (total)	30.1 µg	Zinc	0.3 mg
Vitamin C	7.0 mg	Potassium	283.4 mg

Strawberry Banana Romaine Smoothie

PER SERVING: 75.8 CALORIES ~ 1.2 G PROTEIN ~ 19.3 G CARBOHYDRATE ~ 2.9 G FIBER ~
0.3 G TOTAL FAT ~ 0.1 G SATURATED FAT ~ 0.0 MG CHOLESTEROL ~ 7.1 MG SODIUM

2 cups sliced romaine lettuce

1 cup frozen strawberries

2 frozen bananas, cut into chunks

2 cups water

Blend all ingredients in a blender until smooth.

Serves 4.

Nutritional Analysis per Serving

Vitamin A	210.7 RE	Vitamin D	0.0 µg
Thiamin (B-1)	0.1 mg	Vitamin E	0.2 mg
Riboflavin (B-2)	0.1 mg	Calcium	23.1 mg
Niacin	0.7 mg	Iron	0.8 mg
Vitamin B-6	0.3 mg	Phosphorus	27.2 mg
Vitamin B-12	0.0 µg	Magnesium	26.5 mg
Folate (total)	53.2 µg	Zinc	0.2 mg
Vitamin C	28.2 mg	Potassium	352.2 mg

Pear Kale Mint Smoothie

PER SERVING: 230.5 CALORIES ~ 3.7 G PROTEIN ~ 59.0 G CARBOHYDRATE ~ 12.1 G FIBER ~
0.9 G TOTAL FAT ~ 0.1 G SATURATED FAT ~ 0.0 MG CHOLESTEROL ~ 41.2 MG SODIUM

4 ripe pears, cored and quartered   ½ cup fresh mint leaves

2 cups sliced kale   2 cups water

Blend all ingredients in a blender until smooth.
Serves 2.

Nutritional Analysis per Serving

Vitamin A	1065.0 RE	Vitamin D	0.0 µg
Thiamin (B-1)	0.1 mg	Vitamin E	0.0 mg
Riboflavin (B-2)	0.2 mg	Calcium	143.0 mg
Niacin	1.3 mg	Iron	2.0 mg
Vitamin B-6	0.3 mg	Phosphorus	78.7 mg
Vitamin B-12	0.0 µg	Magnesium	53.5 mg
Folate (total)	50.0 µg	Zinc	0.7 mg
Vitamin C	96.4 mg	Potassium	733.3 mg

Pear Avocado Smoothie

PER SERVING: 226.4 CALORIES ~ 3.0 G PROTEIN ~ 35.8 G CARBOHYDRATE ~ 9.5 G FIBER ~
10.4 G TOTAL FAT ~ 2.0 G SATURATED FAT ~ 0.0 MG CHOLESTEROL ~ 7.7 MG SODIUM

2 large frozen pears, cored,
cut into chunks   2 teaspoons honey

¾ cup frozen green grapes   1 teaspoon lemon juice

1 small avocado, peeled and pitted   1½ cups water

Blend all ingredients in a blender until smooth.
Serves 3.

Nutritional Analysis per Serving

Vitamin A	19.2 RE	Vitamin D	0.0 µg
Thiamin (B-1)	0.1 mg	Vitamin E	0.0 mg
Riboflavin (B-2)	0.1 mg	Calcium	27.8 mg
Niacin	0.9 mg	Iron	0.5 mg
Vitamin B-6	0.1 mg	Phosphorus	60.6 mg
Vitamin B-12	0.0 µg	Magnesium	36.1 mg
Folate (total)	44.4 µg	Zinc	0.5 mg
Vitamin C	24.2 mg	Potassium	564.8 mg

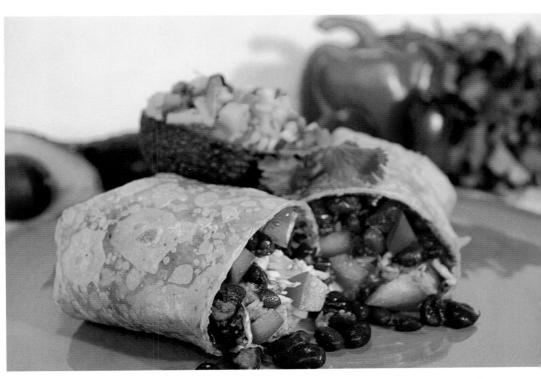

Crunchy Burritos (p. 191) with Kiwi Cucumber Salsa (p. 79)

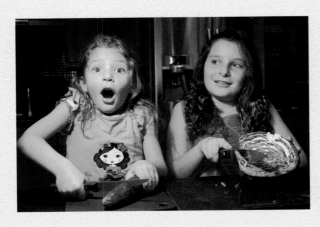

Once upon a time a mother fed her children only healthy food.

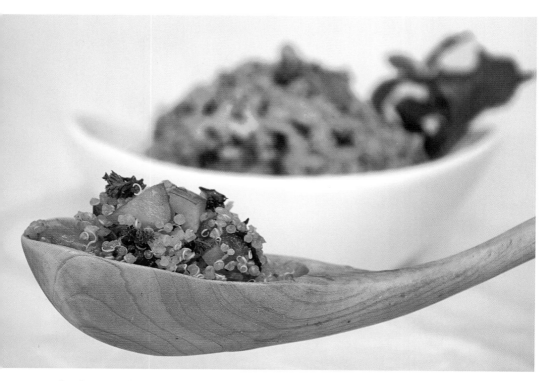

Apricot and Butternut Quinoa Salad (p. 85)

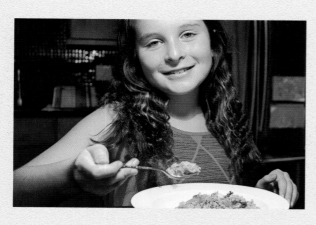

Each day, she tried out new recipes for her family's enjoyment.

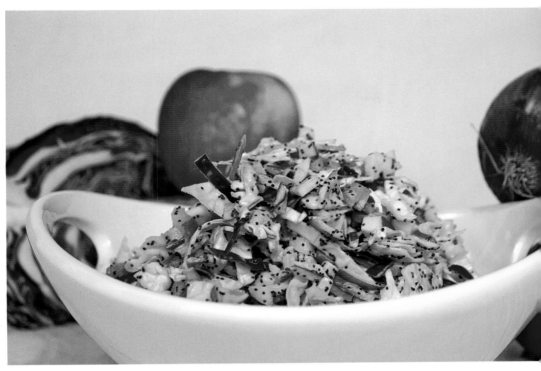

Coleslaw (p. 88)

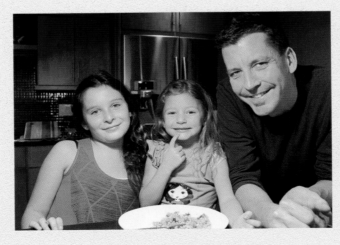

The healthy food brought her family inner and outward peace and beauty.

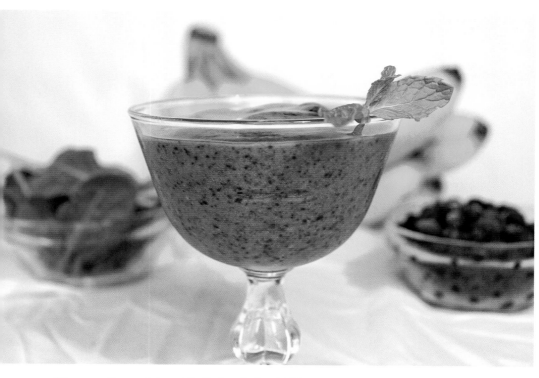

Yummy Smoothie with Spinach (p. 149)

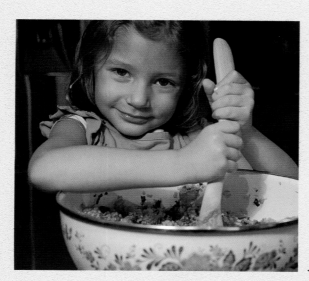

Not all of the recipes turned out exactly right the first time!

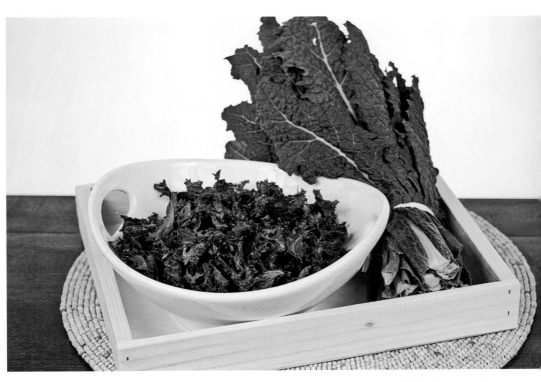

Kale Chips (p. 127)

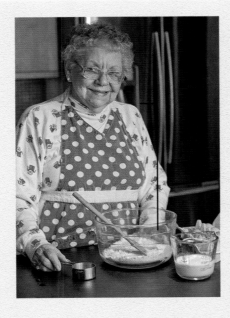

Even Great-Grandma Ruth joined the fun and changed her diet.

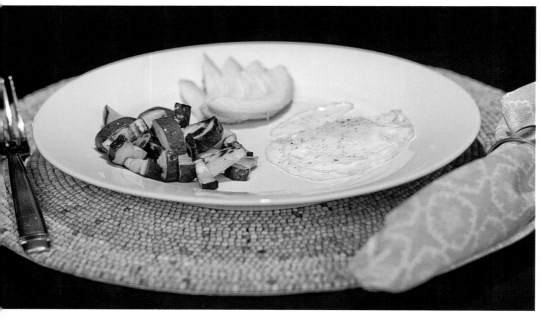

Fried Egg with Sautéed Zucchini (p. 146) with a side of avocado

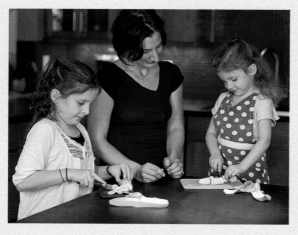

Now everyone in the family knows what foods to eat and what to avoid (although they might not always follow the rules).

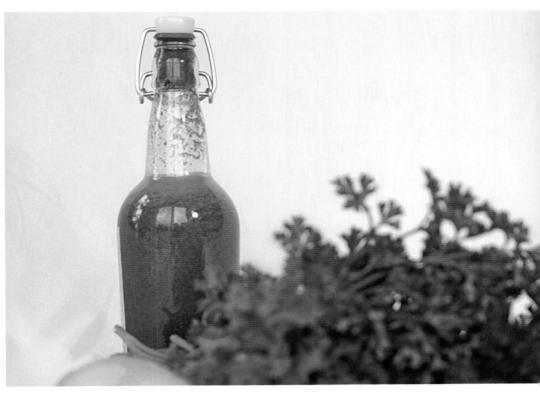

Green "Lemonade" (p. 158)

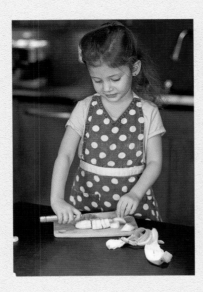

Zienna, the little one, loves to bake and has experimented with ingredients since she was two.

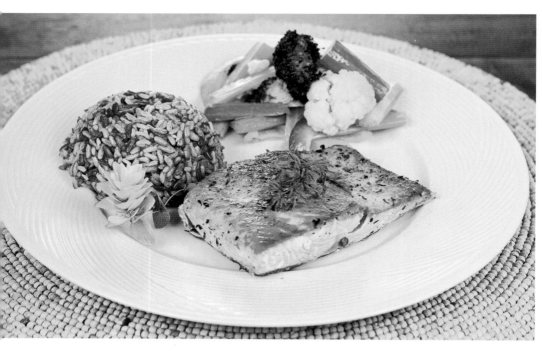

Easy Teriyaki Salmon (p. 200) with Roasted Vegetables (p. 68)

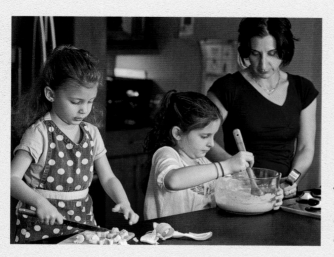

[P.S. Both girls will make wonderful roommates, house guests, wives, and mothers because of their exquisite cooking.]

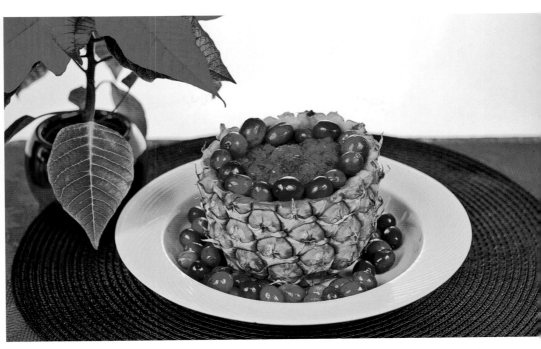

Raw Holiday Relish (p. 119)

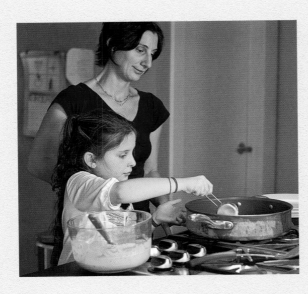

Sadie, the older one, loves mixing flavors, often generating "never-before-tasted" creations in the kitchen.

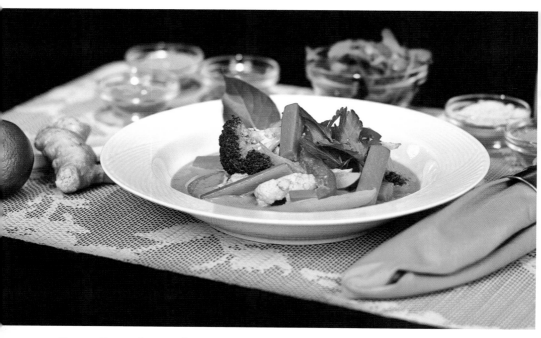

Green Curry (p. 204)

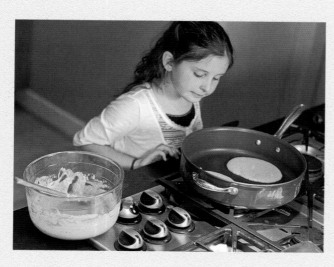

One day the mother shared her recipes in **The Anti-Inflammation Diet and Recipe Book**—*and people loved them!*

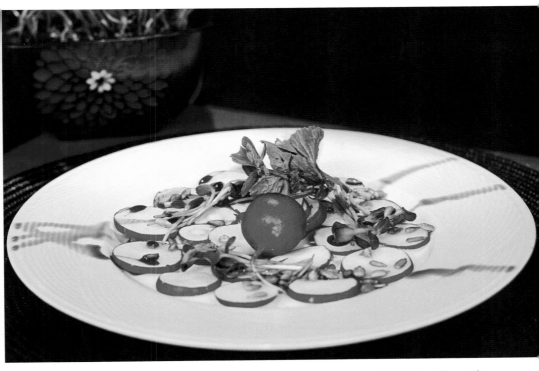

Radish Salad (p. 91)

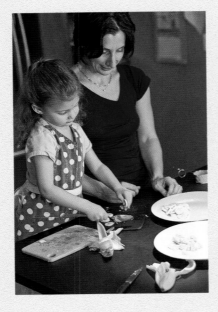

Now she continues to create new recipes for her family, patients, and many, many readers.

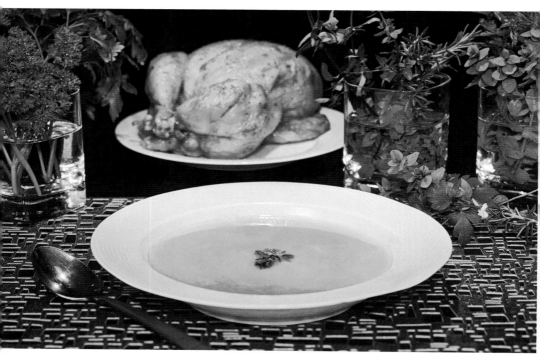

Chicken Broth (p. 225) with Spiced Chicken (p. 209)

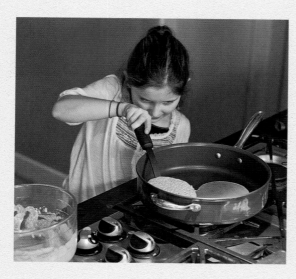

Who doesn't love the pure enjoyment you get from every bite of a delicious and healthy meal?

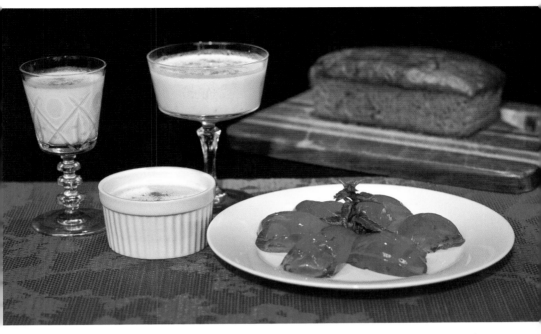

Tapioca Pudding (p. 238) with Fruit Juice Jell-O (p. 250)

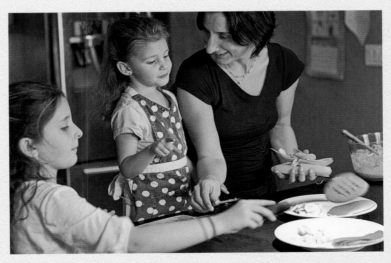

Most important, though, the mother taught her family the importance of sitting and eating meals together.

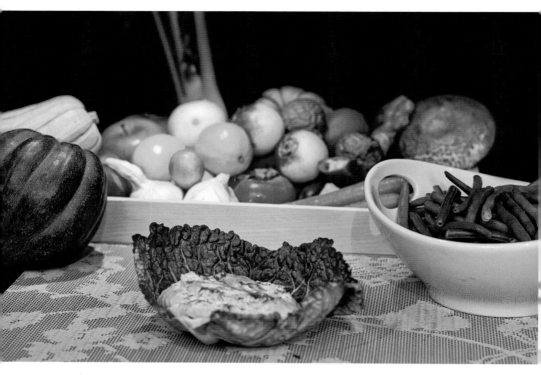

White Bean Hummus (p. 105) and Blanched Beans with Salt (p. 67)

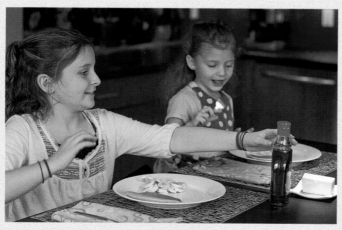

This allows conversation to flow easily in the household and healthy food habits to get established.

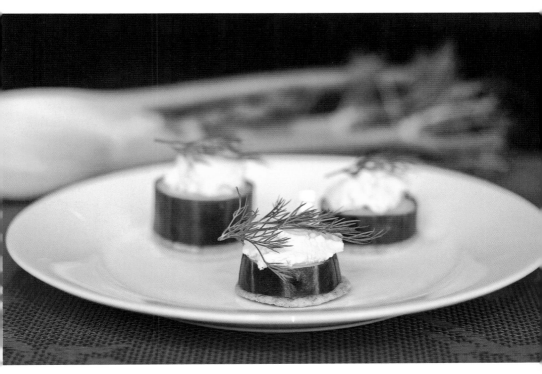

Rice Chips with Goat Cheese and Cucumber (p. 80)

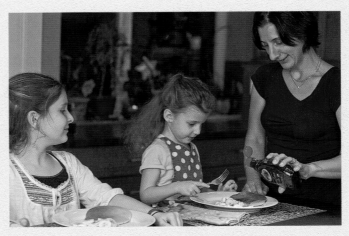

Sadie's life advice is: "Choose chocolate over vanilla" and "Never stop stirring (in life)."

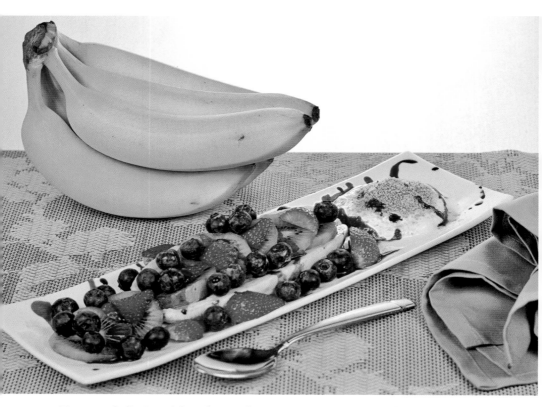

Banana Split Breakfast (p. 142) with Chocolate Syrup (p. 257)

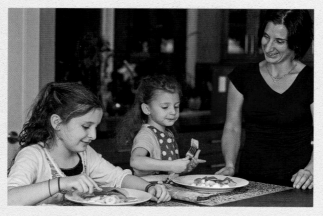

Zienna's life advice is: "Squishy carrots make everything better" and "Eat when you are hungry."

Gingerbread Smoothie

PER SERVING: 140.4 CALORIES ~ 6.3 G PROTEIN ~ 25.1 G CARBOHYDRATE ~ 5.4 G FIBER ~
2.6 G TOTAL FAT ~ 0.4 G SATURATED FAT ~ 0.0 MG CHOLESTEROL ~ 26.8 MG SODIUM

½ 15-ounce can pumpkin

1 cup unsweetened almond milk

1½ tablespoons pure maple syrup

1 teaspoon molasses

½ teaspoon cinnamon

¼ teaspoon ground ginger

6 ice cubes

Blend all ingredients in a
blender until smooth.
Serves 2.

Nutritional Analysis per Serving

Vitamin A	1654.7 RE	Vitamin D	0.0 µg
Thiamin (B-1)	0.0 mg	Vitamin E	0.0 mg
Riboflavin (B-2)	0.3 mg	Calcium	75.9 mg
Niacin	0.5 mg	Iron	2.6 mg
Vitamin B-6	0.1 mg	Phosphorus	39.2 mg
Vitamin B-12	0.0 µg	Magnesium	36.4 mg
Folate (total)	12.9 µg	Zinc	0.4 mg
Vitamin C	4.5 mg	Potassium	454.6 mg

Cool Wheatgrass Pineapple Smoothie

PER SERVING: 154.1 CALORIES ~ 1.9 G PROTEIN ~ 40.2 G CARBOHYDRATE ~ 1.8 G FIBER ~
0.3 G TOTAL FAT ~ 0.0 G SATURATED FAT ~ 0.0 MG CHOLESTEROL ~ 9.2 MG SODIUM

1 cup frozen pineapple chunks

½ cup fresh orange juice

½ cup water

½ cup fresh lime juice

¼ cup wheatgrass juice

¼ cup packed fresh mint leaves

2 tablespoons honey

Blend all ingredients in a blender until smooth.
Serves 2.

Kitchen Tip

You can usually find wheatgrass juice at a local health-food store or juice bar. If you can't find it, you can usually find wheatgrass growing in containers at a health-food store. You can either juice it yourself or simply add ¼ cup lightly packed wheatgrass to the blender.

Nutritional Analysis per Serving

Vitamin A	45.7 RE	Vitamin D	0.0 µg
Thiamin (B-1)	0.2 mg	Vitamin E	2.9 mg
Riboflavin (B-2)	0.1 mg	Calcium	43.2 mg
Niacin	0.8 mg	Iron	0.8 mg
Vitamin B-6	0.7 mg	Phosphorus	49.9 mg
Vitamin B-12	0.0 µg	Magnesium	31.4 mg
Folate (total)	51.0 µg	Zinc	0.4 mg
Vitamin C	88.7 mg	Potassium	351.9 mg

Banana Carob Frosty

PER SERVING: 295.3 CALORIES ~ 6.9 G PROTEIN ~ 53.2 G CARBOHYDRATE ~ 7.3 G FIBER ~
8.7 G TOTAL FAT ~ 6.0 G SATURATED FAT ~ 0.0 MG CHOLESTEROL ~ 9.6 MG SODIUM

3 frozen bananas, cut into chunks
½–1 cup almond milk
¼ cup unsweetened carob chips
1 teaspoon carob powder
Stevia, or other sweetener, to taste

Blend bananas, almond milk, carob chips, and carob powder in a blender until almost smooth; do not overblend. Use only enough almond milk as needed to blend. Add stevia.

Serves 2.

This smoothie is meant to be very thick, almost like a shake. Be careful not to oversweeten with stevia.

Other Smoothie Ideas

- Kale*, spinach, blueberries
- Kale, spinach, watermelon
- Kale, spinach, kiwi, grapes, orange juice
- Kale, strawberries, blackberries or raspberries, pineapple
- Kale, peach, yogurt
- Basil, lime, cucumber
- Mint, lime, cucumber
- Ginger, lemon, spinach, green grapes

* Baby kale can now be found in easy-to-use prewashed bags or plastic containers.

Nutritional Analysis per Serving

Vitamin A	13.4 RE	Vitamin D	0.0 µg
Thiamin (B-1)	0.1 mg	Vitamin E	0.3 mg
Riboflavin (B-2)	0.3 mg	Calcium	120.5 mg
Niacin	1.5 mg	Iron	1.0 mg
Vitamin B-6	0.7 mg	Phosphorus	50.6 mg
Vitamin B-12	0.3 µg	Magnesium	57.9 mg
Folate (total)	35.7 µg	Zinc	0.4 mg
Vitamin C	15.4 mg	Potassium	908.8 mg

Smoothie Additives Other than Fruits and Veggies and Their Benefits

Additive	Benefit
Açai powder or smoothie packet	Antioxidant
Acidophilus	Source of probiotics
Berries	Source of antioxidants
Brewer's yeast	B vitamins, beneficial yeast
Chia seeds	EFAs, hydrating, fiber
Chlorella powder	Blood cleansing, heavy metal detoxification, source of many EFAs
Coconut butter or flaked coconut	Good source of fat, good source of protein
Coconut milk	Healthy fat source, helpful for weight maintenance
Coconut oil	Lauric acid, good source of fats
Coconut water	Hydrating, electrolytes
Flax oil	EFAs, regulation of hormones
Flax seeds	Fiber, EFAs, regulation of hormones
Fresh nettles	Support for the kidney and adrenal glands, antistress and antiallergy
Fresh organic raw eggs, washed well	Better than protein powders, good source of protein, healthy fats
Ginger	Warming, cleansing, immune stimulating
Kefir or kombucha	Source of probiotics
Kelp powder	Supports thyroid, natural source of iron
Lucuma powder, sweetener	Antioxidants, carotene, niacin
Milk thistle seeds, ground	Liver support and detoxification
Matcha green tea powder	Antioxidant, stimulates brain function
Maqui powder	Antioxidants, fiber, vitamin C
Mesquite powder, sweetener	Fiber, lysine, zinc, protein, potassium, iron, calcium, and helps balance blood sugar levels
Nut butters	Good source of protein and fat
Nutritional yeast	B vitamins, beneficial yeast
Protein powders	Good way to increase protein consumption

(cont'd.)

Smoothie Additives Other than Fruits and Veggies and Their Benefits (cont'd.)

Additive	Benefit
Raw honey	Good sweetener, antimicrobial, helpful with seasonal allergies
Salba seeds	Fiber, EFAs, powerhouse of nutrition
Spirulina powder	Blood cleansing, heavy metal detoxification, increases energy, source of complete protein (contains all essential amino acids), source of many EFAs
Sunflower, pumpkin, sesame seeds	Good source of protein and healthy fats

Beverages

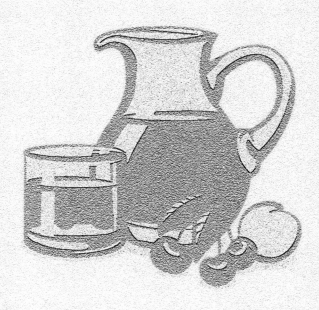

Green "Lemonade"

PER SERVING: 23.0 CALORIES ~ 0.3 G PROTEIN ~ 5.7 G CARBOHYDRATE ~ 0.4 G FIBER ~
0.1 G TOTAL FAT ~ 0.0 G SATURATED FAT ~ 0.0 MG CHOLESTEROL ~ 12.4 MG SODIUM

2–3 cups water

1 bunch parsley

2 teaspoons molasses

2 teaspoons fresh lemon juice

1 teaspoon pure maple syrup

Blend all ingredients together in blender until smooth.

Serves 3.

Note: Some separation does occur and foam will form at the top. Make sure to shake well before serving. This drink will keep for up to 3 days in the refrigerator.

Substitutions

You can use various greens for this drink. I have used a combination of fresh parsley, cilantro, basil, mint, kale, spinach, and others. My favorite is still the parsley. You can omit the sweeteners or use stevia if you don't consume sugars. If you reduce the level of sweetness, you could also reduce the lemon juice. The molasses is included due to its iron content.

Healthy Tidbit

Parsley, my favorite herb, is so underused. How often do you ignore the sprig of parsley on your plate at a restaurant? What a shame to leave this important source of nutrients uneaten. Parsley is an excellent source of vitamin A, B vitamins, vitamin K, and calcium, and it contains more vitamin C than many fruits. Besides containing a wealth of nutrients, parsley aids digestion and cleanses the blood by supporting kidney function.

Nutritional Analysis per Serving

Vitamin A	85.4 RE	Vitamin D	0.0 µg
Thiamin (B-1)	0.0 mg	Vitamin E	0.0 mg
Riboflavin (B-2)	0.0 mg	Calcium	30.3 mg
Niacin	0.2 mg	Iron	0.8 mg
Vitamin B-6	0.0 mg	Phosphorus	7.6 mg
Vitamin B-12	0.0 µg	Magnesium	18.1 mg
Folate (total)	16.1 µg	Zinc	0.2 mg
Vitamin C	14.8 mg	Potassium	130.9 mg

Hydration Drink

PER SERVING: 9.1 CALORIES ~ 0.0 G PROTEIN ~ 2.4 G CARBOHYDRATE ~ 0.0 G FIBER ~
0.0 G TOTAL FAT ~ 0.0 G SATURATED FAT ~ 0.0 MG CHOLESTEROL ~ 903.5 MG SODIUM

This is a helpful blend for children during fevers or diarrhea. Also helpful for adults if they are trying to hydrate or kick a cold or cough.

2 cups water

1 teaspoon pure maple syrup

1 teaspoon fresh lemon juice or lemon juice concentrate

½ teaspoon baking soda

½ teaspoon salt

Combine all ingredients in pitcher; serve at room temperature or chilled. Serves 2.

Substitutions

You can add minced garlic to this drink for added immune support. You can add a little cayenne pepper for sore throats and for increasing warmth on a cold day. This drink can be consumed at room temperature for fevers, warm for chills, and cold for sore throats.

Healthy Tidbit

Food dyes are not good for you, and most commercial hydration drinks, such as Pedialyte and Gatorade, contain them. I prefer this drink to any hydration drink, and it offers the same amount of balancing electrolytes without the added dyes. I always keep these ingredients in my kitchen so I can whip up this remedy whenever it's needed.

Nutritional Analysis per Serving

Vitamin A	0.0 RE	Vitamin D	0.0 µg
Thiamin (B-1)	0.0 mg	Vitamin E	0.0 mg
Riboflavin (B-2)	0.0 mg	Calcium	11.0 mg
Niacin	0.0 mg	Iron	0.0 mg
Vitamin B-6	0.0 mg	Phosphorus	0.3 mg
Vitamin B-12	0.0 µg	Magnesium	3.2 mg
Folate (total)	0.5 µg	Zinc	0.1 mg
Vitamin C	1.0 mg	Potassium	12.1 mg

Runner's Blend (Chia Fresca)

PER SERVING: 69.9 CALORIES ~ 1.7 G PROTEIN ~ 10.0 G CARBOHYDRATE ~ 3.5 G FIBER ~
3.1 G TOTAL FAT ~ 0.3 G SATURATED FAT ~ 0.0 MG CHOLESTEROL ~ 12.4 MG SODIUM

1½ cups water
1 tablespoon chia seeds
1 teaspoon lime juice
1 teaspoon agave syrup

Combine all ingredients in a pitcher or water bottle.

Serves 1.

Drink after running. When running long distances, you may want to prepare this ahead of time and take it with you to drink halfway through your run. If necessary, prepare a double or triple batch. It is normal for the seeds to make the blend a little gelatinous.

Substitutions

Try different sweeteners such as honey or stevia as desired.

Healthy Tidbit

Chia seeds have gained popularity in recent years as a super food, high in omega-3 fatty acids. They may also aid in digestion and hydration. The inspiring book *Born to Run*, about the Tarahumara, a tribe of superathletes in Mexico whose members sometimes run 50–100 miles in a day for enjoyment and recreation, reports that they have used chia seeds for centuries for quick and easy hydration.

Nutritional Analysis per Serving

Vitamin A	0.6 RE	Vitamin D	0.0 µg
Thiamin (B-1)	0.1 mg	Vitamin E	0.0 mg
Riboflavin (B-2)	0.0 mg	Calcium	74.5 mg
Niacin	0.9 mg	Iron	0.8 mg
Vitamin B-6	0.1 mg	Phosphorus	86.7 mg
Vitamin B-12	0.0 µg	Magnesium	37.5 mg
Folate (total)	5.4 µg	Zinc	0.5 mg
Vitamin C	4.5 mg	Potassium	50.3 mg

Aperitif

PER SERVING: 12.7 CALORIES ~ 0.0 G PROTEIN ~ 3.0 G CARBOHYDRATE ~ 0.0 G FIBER ~
0.0 G TOTAL FAT ~ 0.0 G SATURATED FAT ~ 0.0 MG CHOLESTEROL ~ 6.0 MG SODIUM

Serve before the meal to be sipped on while the meal is being prepared.

¾ cup water
2 teaspoons organic apple cider vinegar, with sediment
½ teaspoon honey

Combine all ingredients in a glass and stir well.
   Serves 1.

Substitutions
You may use a little stevia instead of the honey to eliminate the sugar, or you can just mix the vinegar and water together with no added sweetener. If you want to use this concoction for a cough or for immune-system stimulation, then add 1–2 cloves of minced garlic. It makes a delicious wellness drink when needed.

Healthy Tidbit
Apple cider vinegar stimulates digestion and increases pancreatic enzyme secretion for improved breakdown and absorption of nutrients from food. Apple cider vinegar has been used extensively for weight loss. The use of vinegar to fight infections and other acute conditions has historical roots all the way back to the father of medicine, Hippocrates, who recommended a vinegar preparation for cleaning ulcerations and for the treatment of sores. Oxymel, a popular ancient medicine composed of honey and vinegar, was prescribed for persistent coughs by Hippocrates and his contemporaries, and is still suggested by physicians today.

Nutritional Analysis per Serving

Vitamin A	0.0 RE	Vitamin D	0.0 µg
Thiamin (B-1)	0.0 mg	Vitamin E	0.0 mg
Riboflavin (B-2)	0.0 mg	Calcium	6.2 mg
Niacin	0.0 mg	Iron	0.0 mg
Vitamin B-6	0.0 mg	Phosphorus	0.9 mg
Vitamin B-12	0.0 µg	Magnesium	2.3 mg
Folate (total)	0.1 µg	Zinc	0.0 mg
Vitamin C	0.0 mg	Potassium	10.8 mg

Dairy-Free Eggnog

PER SERVING: 486.7 CALORIES ~ 12.1 G PROTEIN ~ 14.7 G CARBOHYDRATE ~ 4.1 G FIBER ~
44.6 G TOTAL FAT ~ 36.0 G SATURATED FAT ~ 248.0 MG CHOLESTEROL ~ 119.7 MG SODIUM

2 cups whole-fat coconut milk, or thick unsweetened almond milk

4 eggs

1 tablespoon pure maple syrup

½ teaspoon vanilla extract

1 teaspoon ground cinnamon

½ teaspoon ground nutmeg

¼ teaspoon ground cardamom

Ground nutmeg as garnish

Combine all ingredients in a blender and blend until smooth. Serve chilled, sprinkled with nutmeg.

Serves 3.

Substitutions

You can vary the ingredients to make your eggnog thinner or thicker. For thicker eggnog, use a little less milk and more eggs, or you can eliminate some of the egg whites. Using a higher ratio of egg yolks does increase the fat content quite a bit. If your blender is old or not very powerful, consider straining the eggnog before serving to ensure there are no stringy parts from the eggs left in the blend.

Healthy Tidbit

Raw eggs can be safe to consume. The risk of salmonella comes mostly from egg shells that haven't been washed well. Any time you add eggs to a dish that will not be cooked, wash the outside of the eggs very well before cracking them. There is a slight risk that salmonella can infect the egg through pores in the shell. Make sure your eggs are fresh and have been refrigerated before use. I have used organic, free-range eggs for years and have been giving my kids raw eggs since they were over the age of one. However, if you're worried about eating raw eggs and would like additional guidelines, be aware that the USDA notes that certain groups—including infants, young children, older adults, pregnant women, and people with weakened immune systems—can be more vulnerable to salmonella infections.

Nutritional Analysis per Serving

Vitamin A	108.3 RE	Vitamin D	1.3 µg
Thiamin (B-1)	0.1 mg	Vitamin E	0.7 mg
Riboflavin (B-2)	0.4 mg	Calcium	78.7 mg
Niacin	1.3 mg	Iron	3.9 mg
Vitamin B-6	0.2 mg	Phosphorus	293.7 mg
Vitamin B-12	0.6 µg	Magnesium	70.2 mg
Folate (total)	57.3 µg	Zinc	2.1 mg
Vitamin C	4.6 mg	Potassium	534.1 mg

Mintish Tea

PER SERVING: 0.9 CALORIES ~ 0.0 G PROTEIN ~ 0.2 G CARBOHYDRATE ~ 0.1 G FIBER ~
0.0 G TOTAL FAT ~ 0.0 G SATURATED FAT ~ 0.0 MG CHOLESTEROL ~ 8.4 MG SODIUM

This recipe, including the clever name, was created by Melody Frederic of Willamina, Oregon. She and her mother are so creative and inventive in the kitchen.

1 cup fresh nettle leaves*

4½ cups water

1 cup fresh mint or 2 tea bags peppermint tea

Stevia to taste

* If you can't find fresh stinging nettle, you can use ½ cup dried.

Combine nettle leaves and water in a large soup pot. Heat to boiling; reduce heat and simmer, covered, at least 30 minutes, or up to a few hours. Add mint tea, turn heat off, and allow to steep for 15 minutes. Strain through tea strainer or fine sieve. Add stevia to taste. Serve hot, or refrigerate and serve cold.

Yields 4 cups.

Kitchen Tip

Thirty minutes of simmering will produce a very mild-tasting tea that offers a mild anti-inflammatory benefit. If you would like to create a rich, thick tea with increased anti-inflammatory properties, transfer the brew to a crockpot and simmer for 12–18 hours. The resulting appearance may resemble pond water in August, but the stronger tea provides significant health benefits, including fighting off spring allergies. It can be served hot or cold, but is considered best hot.

Healthy Tidbit

This name of the beverage comes from the fact that stinging nettle, *Urtica dioica*, greatly resembles true nettle, which belongs to the mint family but is not itself a true mint. Nettles have been used over the years for various medicinal purposes. We mostly use nettles for their properties in fighting allergy symptoms and supporting the adrenals. The adrenal glands help support the stress response and control various other mechanisms in the body.

Nutritional Analysis per Serving

Vitamin A	5.4 RE	Vitamin D	0.0 µg
Thiamin (B-1)	0.0 mg	Vitamin E	0.0 mg
Riboflavin (B-2)	0.0 mg	Calcium	11.1 mg
Niacin	0.0 mg	Iron	0.1 mg
Vitamin B-6	0.0 mg	Phosphorus	0.9 mg
Vitamin B-12	0.0 µg	Magnesium	3.7 mg
Folate (total)	1.5 µg	Zinc	0.0 mg
Vitamin C	0.4 mg	Potassium	9.9 mg

Eggless Eggnog

PER SERVING: 104.0 CALORIES ~ 2.8 G PROTEIN ~ 10.7 G CARBOHYDRATE ~ 1.1 G FIBER ~
6.4 G TOTAL FAT ~ 1.2 G SATURATED FAT ~ 0.0 MG CHOLESTEROL ~ 54.1 MG SODIUM

3 cups water, divided

4 pitted dates

⅔ cup raw cashews

2 teaspoons honey

1 teaspoon vanilla extract

1 teaspoon ground cinnamon

¼ teaspoon ground nutmeg

¼ teaspoon ground allspice

Pinch ground cardamom

⅛ teaspoon salt

In a blender, blend 1 cup water, dates, and cashews until well blended. Add
remaining 2 cups water and remaining ingredients, and blend until smooth.
Serve cold, or heat and serve warm.

Serves 6.

Substitutions

To thin the eggnog, add more water. To thicken it, pour most of the mixture
into a separate container, add more raw cashews to the blender, blend until
smooth, add the reserved mixture back in, and blend again.

Healthy Tidbit

Holidays don't have to be filled with lots of foods that you later regret consuming. Make your choices carefully, and decide ahead of time what you think
you will be able to tolerate, such as a small piece of dessert. Or maybe you will
decide to double up on dinner proportions and enjoy the piece of bread you
usually avoid, but skip dessert. Whatever your strategy, make it realistic and
doable, and force yourself to follow it. Setting a goal and sticking to it will
reward you with good feelings after the fact. Try to give away leftovers or freeze
them for a later date to avoid
gorging again the second day.
Make smaller amounts of less
healthy items, such as desserts
and starches, so there are fewer
leftovers to tempt you.

Nutritional Analysis per Serving

Vitamin A	0.2 RE	Vitamin D	0.0 µg
Thiamin (B-1)	0.1 mg	Vitamin E	0.0 mg
Riboflavin (B-2)	0.0 mg	Calcium	15.5 mg
Niacin	0.2 mg	Iron	1.1 mg
Vitamin B-6	0.1 mg	Phosphorus	89.3 mg
Vitamin B-12	0.0 µg	Magnesium	46.1 mg
Folate (total)	4.7 µg	Zinc	0.9 mg
Vitamin C	0.2 mg	Potassium	132.7 mg

Chai

PER SERVING: 114.1 CALORIES ~ 4.7 G PROTEIN ~ 21.2 G CARBOHYDRATE ~ 2.5 G FIBER ~
2.3 G TOTAL FAT ~ 0.3 G SATURATED FAT ~ 0.0 MG CHOLESTEROL ~ 20.3 MG SODIUM

For the Spice Blend
2 tablespoons ground cardamom
1 tablespoon ground cloves
1 tablespoon ground cinnamon ·
1 tablespoon ground black pepper

For the Tea
1 cup almond milk
1 cup water
2 bags of organic black tea
2 tablespoons honey
1½ teaspoons grated gingerroot
1 teaspoon Spice Blend (recipe above)

To make the spice blend: Combine the ingredients. Store the mixture in a small glass jar.

Makes 5 tablespoons.

To make the tea: Combine all ingredients in a medium saucepan; heat to simmering. Stir well and remove from heat. Cover and allow to steep for about 10 minutes. Serve warm or cool, or refrigerate and serve cold.

Serves 2.

Substitutions
You can experiment with different spices, with the ratio of water and milk, or with a different type of milk.

Healthy Tidbit
Cloves are known for being the richest source of antioxidants in the spice world. Cloves are also high in a number of flavonoids, which supports their use for anti-inflammatory purposes. Clove oil has been used topically for pain relief, especially for dental and gum pain. Interestingly, based on the correlation often observed between

Nutritional Analysis per Serving

Vitamin A	0.2 RE	Vitamin D	0.0 µg
Thiamin (B-1)	0.0 mg	Vitamin E	0.0 mg
Riboflavin (B-2)	0.0 mg	Calcium	27.8 mg
Niacin	0.1 mg	Iron	1.2 mg
Vitamin B-6	0.0 mg	Phosphorus	3.9 mg
Vitamin B-12	0.0 µg	Magnesium	6.6 mg
Folate (total)	6.6 µg	Zinc	0.1 mg
Vitamin C	0.3 mg	Potassium	221.3 mg

gingivitis and inflammatory conditions, clove oil's effectiveness in treating dental pain may arise in part from its anti-inflammatory properties. Cloves are antiseptic in nature; use the essential oil in the home during the winter months to help cleanse the air. Lastly, cloves are very beneficial in supporting and aiding digestion.

Children's Chai

PER SERVING: 80.2 CALORIES ~ 4.6 G PROTEIN ~ 12.0 G CARBOHYDRATE ~ 2.4 G FIBER ~
2.3 G TOTAL FAT ~ 0.3 G SATURATED FAT ~ 0.0 MG CHOLESTEROL ~ 19.8 MG SODIUM

1 cup almond milk

1 cup water

½ teaspoon grated gingerroot

1 teaspoon Chai Tea Spice Blend (see page 165)

1 tablespoon honey

Combine all ingredients in medium saucepan; heat to simmering. Stir well and remove from heat. Cover and let stand for about 5 minutes. Remove cloves; serve warm.

Serves 2.

Substitutions
In addition to the cloves, you can add any whole spice such as allspice berries or cardamom pods. Make sure to strain out the whole spices before serving.

Healthy Tidbit
Involve your children in the kitchen and in your experiments. It will be fun to see what they come up with, because children's ideas flow a little more easily than adults? I have gotten some great ideas from my nine-year-old, who does experiments such as mixing coffee beans with honey, water, berries, and ice. That one, I have to admit, didn't turn out so well, but sometimes she comes up with a winning combination, like Sadie and Elisa's Mystery Chicken Noodle Soup (see recipe on page 228).

Nutritional Analysis per Serving

Vitamin A	0.2 RE	Vitamin D	0.0 µg
Thiamin (B-1)	0.0 mg	Vitamin E	0.0 mg
Riboflavin (B-2)	0.0 mg	Calcium	30.6 mg
Niacin	0.0 mg	Iron	1.1 mg
Vitamin B-6	0.0 mg	Phosphorus	2.0 mg
Vitamin B-12	0.0 µg	Magnesium	3.5 mg
Folate (total)	0.4 µg	Zinc	0.1 mg
Vitamin C	0.2 mg	Potassium	169.0 mg

Easy Almond Milk

PER SERVING: 91.4 CALORIES ~ 3.4 G PROTEIN ~ 3.4 G CARBOHYDRATE ~ 1.9 G FIBER ~
7.9 G TOTAL FAT ~ 0.6 G SATURATED FAT ~ 0.0 MG CHOLESTEROL ~ 3.3 MG SODIUM

1 cup organic whole almonds, blanched, skins removed (see below)

1 cup hot water

3 cups room-temperature water

Blend almonds with hot water in a blender until very smooth. Add remaining 3 cups water and process until very smooth. Strain through cheesecloth into a glass container. Refrigerate.

Yields 4½ cups (9 ½-cup servings).

Kitchen Tip

Blanch almonds by boiling them in water for 1–2 minutes. Then drain, cool, and pinch off the skins.

Substitutions

You can try this recipe with various seeds, soy beans, or other nuts. Nuts with skins, such as Brazil nuts and hazelnuts, should be blanched and skins removed. Cashews can be used with no blanching. Some recipes call for soaking the almonds overnight, but making almond milk on the fly is possible when you blanch them. So easy! You can add vanilla extract or a mild sweetener if desired.

Kitchen Tip

Making your own nut milks saves a lot of money. I don't always make my own, but I love knowing how to do so. I usually have nuts or seeds in my refrigerator that I can use in a pinch to make milk. For certain recipes, such as tapioca pudding, I prefer making the milk myself because I feel that fresh milk makes a much better tasting product. Same thing with flours: if a recipe calls for flour, I always have grains on hand that I can grind into a fine flour. You can do this easily in a coffee grinder or in a high-powdered blender or food processor.

Nutritional Analysis per Serving

Vitamin A	0.0 RE	Vitamin D	0.0 µg
Thiamin (B-1)	0.0 mg	Vitamin E	0.0 mg
Riboflavin (B-2)	0.2 mg	Calcium	45.1 mg
Niacin	0.5 mg	Iron	0.6 mg
Vitamin B-6	0.0 mg	Phosphorus	76.9 mg
Vitamin B-12	0.0 µg	Magnesium	43.6 mg
Folate (total)	7.9 µg	Zinc	0.5 mg
Vitamin C	0.0 mg	Potassium	113.1 mg

Nighty-Night Drink

PER SERVING: 62.4 CALORIES ~ 4.5 G PROTEIN ~ 2.7 G CARBOHYDRATE ~ 2.1 G FIBER ~
4.2 G TOTAL FAT ~ 1.5 G SATURATED FAT ~ 5.1 MG CHOLESTEROL ~ 31.9 MG SODIUM

This is a great drink to make for your kiddos before bed on special occasions. The warm milk and the butter help to increase acetylcholine, a neurotransmitter that stimulates the parasympathetic nervous system, which promotes sleep and decreases stress.

1½ cup unsweetened almond milk

1½ teaspoons butter

¼ teaspoon ground cinnamon

Heat all ingredients in a small saucepan over medium heat just until warm. Serves 3.

Substitutions

You can prepare this drink with hemp milk or other alternative milks (unsweetened). The butter isn't strictly necessary, but I think the fat is helpful before bedtime. Consuming a small amount of fat before bed can help stabilize the blood sugar and ensure better sleep. For a vegan version, try coconut oil instead of butter.

Healthy Tidbit

Sometimes children just need a little TLC. I started making this drink on special occasions when the children had stayed up past their bedtimes and seemed to need some help settling down. Making this treat is no longer really about the drink, but rather about our connection in the kitchen as we prepare it together or as I prepare it and the girls sit at the bar waiting for it to be served. Sometimes they don't even finish the drink. Still, I am happy to make it for them and happy to drink the rest of it after they have gone to bed. It tastes complete and comforting.

Nutritional Analysis per Serving

Vitamin A	17.8 RE	Vitamin D	0.0 µg
Thiamin (B-1)	0.0 mg	Vitamin E	0.1 mg
Riboflavin (B-2)	0.0 mg	Calcium	22.8 mg
Niacin	0.0 mg	Iron	0.9 mg
Vitamin B-6	0.0 mg	Phosphorus	0.7 mg
Vitamin B-12	0.0 µg	Magnesium	0.2 mg
Folate (total)	0.1 µg	Zinc	0.0 mg
Vitamin C	0.0 mg	Potassium	151.4 mg

Fermented Foods

Fermented foods are a significant source of beneficial bacteria and yeasts without the expense of a probiotic supplement. Fermenting foods takes some time, effort, and a little patience. It is easy to make mistakes during the fermentation process; sometimes it feels like you have a new baby to care for, depending on what you are fermenting. I think it is very fun, and my children love to see how the new things are growing.

Knowing that we always have a balance between friendly and unfriendly microorganisms in the body is helpful to our understanding of health. When we are healthy, the organisms maintain a pretty symbiotic balance. If we experience an infection, prolonged inflammation, or severe illness, the organisms become out of balance. How this happens is unknown. There is extensive research on probiotic balance as it relates to various illnesses, but scientists haven't yet determined which comes first: the illness or the imbalance in probiotics. At this point we are only able to note the relationship and attempt to improve the microflora balance in the body of someone who is ill. Various studies have proved probiotics to be beneficial at treating and preventing many illnesses, particularly those involving the gastrointestinal tract.[6]

Techniques for Fermenting Food

Using proper techniques during fermentation is very important. Here are a few rules to follow when you begin experimenting with fermenting your own foods:

+ Keep all of your equipment very clean. It may not need to be sterilized, but I often run my jars and containers through the dishwasher to at least sanitize them before use.

+ If your lacto-fermented goods are slimy, slippery, very mushy, smell funky in a bad sort of way, change color dramatically, or grow mold throughout, throw them out and start over.

+ Visit the following website, operated by the North Carolina Cooperative Extension Service, which offers a safety sheet describing normal and problematic fermentation results: http://www.ces.ncsu.edu/depts/food sci/ext/pubs/497-05.pdf.

+ If you are fermenting vegetables, keep them submerged completely, and err on the side of more salt.

Equipment for Fermenting Food

+ wide-mouth jars, in sizes ranging from 2 quarts to 1 gallon

+ yogurt maker or crockpot

+ cheesecloth

Almost Lactose-Free Yogurt

PER SERVING: 106.4 CALORIES ~ 5.6 G PROTEIN ~ 8.3 G CARBOHYDRATE ~ 0.0 G FIBER ~
5.7 G TOTAL FAT ~ 3.3 G SATURATED FAT ~ 18.5 MG CHOLESTEROL ~ 76.1 MG SODIUM

1 quart raw whole cow's milk or raw goat's milk*
1 cup whole milk yogurt

Heat the milk in a 2-quart saucepan until it reaches 185°F, measured with an instant-read cooking thermometer or a candy thermometer. Do not boil. When milk reaches this temperature, reduce heat and hold at 185°F for 2 minutes.

Remove from heat and pour into a clean glass bowl; cover with cloth, and let cool to 110°F. Mix in yogurt, whisking until smooth.

To ferment yogurt: If you have a yogurt maker, pour the milk mixture into sterile glass containers**, following manufacturer's directions. Ferment for 24 hours to ensure a yogurt with no lactose.

If you do not have a yogurt maker, use a slow cooker. Pour milk mixture into sterilized** 8-ounce glass jars. Place jars in slow cooker; add 1 inch warm water to slow cooker. Turn slow cooker to low and allow to stand, covered, 24 hours, monitoring closely to ensure a temperature between 110 and 120°F.

Serves 7.

Kitchen Tips

You can cool the yogurt faster by placing the glass bowl in a sink full of ice water to a level just below the rim of the bowl. You can test the temperature by dropping a bit on the inside of your wrist; it should be warmer than your skin but not scalding to the touch. Do not mix in the yogurt too soon (i.e., while the milk is still hot); doing so will kill the beneficial bacteria.

* If you cannot find raw milk, try to get organic whole milk with the least amount of processing, such as nonhomogenized.

** Sterilize the glass containers by pouring boiling water into them; drain and invert them before use. Or you can run them through the dishwasher on hot before use.

Kitchen Tip

Making yogurt is a learning process. Some people add milk powder for a thicker yogurt, but I think it is best to avoid the milk powder. Be patient with yourself while you practice!

Nutritional Analysis per Serving

Vitamin A	53.1 RE	Vitamin D	1.8 µg
Thiamin (B-1)	0.1 mg	Vitamin E	0.0 mg
Riboflavin (B-2)	0.3 mg	Calcium	200.0 mg
Niacin	0.2 mg	Iron	0.1 mg
Vitamin B-6	0.1 mg	Phosphorus	150.4 mg
Vitamin B-12	0.8 µg	Magnesium	18.1 mg
Folate (total)	9.4 µg	Zinc	0.7 mg
Vitamin C	0.2 mg	Potassium	238.3 mg

Cream Cheese "Curds and Whey"

PER SERVING: 34.6 CALORIES ~ 1.8 G PROTEIN ~ 2.7 G CARBOHYDRATE ~ 0.0 G FIBER ~
1.8 G TOTAL FAT ~ 1.1 G SATURATED FAT ~ 6.0 MG CHOLESTEROL ~ 24.7 MG SODIUM

2 cups Almost Lactose-Free Yogurt (see recipe on page 171)
Clean cloth napkin or cheesecloth
2-quart glass jar
Cotton string

Tie napkin or cheesecloth over the mouth of the jar so that napkin hangs into jar, forming a well. Spoon yogurt into napkin; flip edges of napkin over the top to cover. Let stand at room temperature for 6–8 hours. Place in refrigerator and let stand about 6 hours longer. Yogurt should drain at least 12 hours total, but can be left to drain up to 24 hours.

Open the napkin and spoon the cream cheese into a separate container; store in refrigerator.

Yields 1 cup cream cheese (8 2-tablespoon servings).

Kitchen Tip
Save the liquid, which is whey, to use in fermenting other foods, or add to baked goods in place of milk or water.

Nutritional Analysis per Serving

Vitamin A	17.3 RE	Vitamin D	0.6 µg
Thiamin (B-1)	0.0 mg	Vitamin E	0.0 mg
Riboflavin (B-2)	0.1 mg	Calcium	65.0 mg
Niacin	0.0 mg	Iron	0.0 mg
Vitamin B-6	0.0 mg	Phosphorus	48.9 mg
Vitamin B-12	0.2 µg	Magnesium	5.9 mg
Folate (total)	3.1 µg	Zinc	0.2 mg
Vitamin C	0.1 mg	Potassium	77.5 mg

Raw Milk Kefir

PER SERVING: 74.9 CALORIES ~ 3.9 G PROTEIN ~ 5.9 G CARBOHYDRATE ~ 0.0 G FIBER ~
4.0 G TOTAL FAT ~ 2.3 G SATURATED FAT ~ 12.3 MG CHOLESTEROL ~ 52.8 MG SODIUM

Production of kefir requires a "starter" of kefir grains, which are a culture of yeasts and bacteria. I prefer getting the grains from a friend or someone I know, but they are also available for sale on the Internet. You can try asking around your community for a source of kefir grains; check with a producer of raw milk.

2 tablespoons kefir grains

2 cups raw milk

2-quart glass jar

Pour the milk into the jar, and gently add the kefir grains. Cover with a clean towel or lid. Let stand at room temperature to ferment. Twelve hours of fermentation will produce a less-sour kefir; 24 hours will eliminate most of the lactose and create a probiotic-filled beverage. Carefully lift out the kefir grains and transfer them to a clean jar. Strain kefir through a clean cloth; refrigerate or allow to stand at room temperature for further fermentation. (Kefir can be kept at room temperature for up to 3 days).

Serves 4.

Nutritional Analysis per Serving

Vitamin A	37.3 RE	Vitamin D	1.6 µg
Thiamin (B-1)	0.1 mg	Vitamin E	0.0 mg
Riboflavin (B-2)	0.2 mg	Calcium	138.7 mg
Niacin	0.1 mg	Iron	0.0 mg
Vitamin B-6	0.0 mg	Phosphorus	103.1 mg
Vitamin B-12	0.6 µg	Magnesium	12.3 mg
Folate (total)	6.2 µg	Zinc	0.5 mg
Vitamin C	0.0 mg	Potassium	162.1 mg

Homemade Kombucha Scoby

Kombucha is a fermented beverage with great probiotic potential, offering a range of acidophilus and yeast strains beneficial to the gastrointestinal tract. Kombucha beverage is made by combining a kombucha culture, called a scoby (short for "symbiotic colony of bacteria and yeast"), with a caffeinated tea, either black or green, and sugar. The sugar feeds the culture. If left to ferment long enough, the beverage will no longer contain actual sugar content, only probiotics. Using inexpensive white sugar is fine because the culture utilizes all of it for making its own beneficial bacteria, yeasts, and acids.

2 cups water
⅓ cup sugar
2 bags black tea
2 16-ounce bottles raw kombucha, at room temperature

Heat water and sugar to boiling, stirring until sugar dissolves. Remove from heat. Add tea; let stand, covered, for 15 minutes. Remove the tea bags and pour mixture into a large glass jar. Allow tea to cool to room temperature. When tea has cooled, add kombucha. Cover with a cloth napkin or cheesecloth and secure with a rubber band. Allow to ferment in a warm, dark place for at least 3 weeks.

When fermentation is complete, carefully remove scoby from top of kombucha. Reserve the scoby to make more kombucha. Refrigerate in an airtight jar until ready to use again. An unused scoby will remain good for at least 3 months in the refrigerator.

Kitchen Tip
Share your scoby with your friends and neighbors so they can make their own batches.

Substitutions
You can try other types of teas, such as green tea or different varieties of black tea. Future batches of kombucha can be made from your homemade scoby rather than from commercially prepared kombucha (see following recipe). You won't have to purchase any raw kombucha again unless you kill your culture. Your culture is good as long as it is floating along the top and you don't see any mold growing on it. As I've stated, fermenting foods takes time and can involve a learning curve, so keep at it.

Kombucha from a Homemade Scoby

4 cups water
1 cup white sugar
4 bags black tea
1 batch Homemade Kombucha Scoby (see preceding recipe)
1 cup raw kombucha

Heat water and sugar to boiling in a medium saucepan, stirring until sugar dissolves. Turn off heat and add tea bags. Cover and let stand 15 minutes. Remove tea bags; cool to room temperature. Pour into large jar (half gallon or larger); add scoby and kombucha. Cover with a cloth napkin or cheesecloth; allow to ferment in a dark, warm place for 1–3 weeks, according to your preference. When fermentation is complete, carefully remove scoby and reserve. Refrigerate kombucha.

Substitutions
Experiment with fermenting for 1 week, 2 weeks, and 3 weeks to determine your taste preferences.

Healthy Tidbit
Kombucha is filled with beneficial organisms for your gastrointestinal tract. Drinking it is a very inexpensive way to make sure you and your family are getting probiotics in your diet daily. Make several batches, one week apart, so that you always have a mature batch to drink.

Water Kefir

Water kefir (that is, nondairy kefir) is easy to make, and the grains are easy to keep alive. You can use white sugar for this recipe because the culture in the grains consumes the sugar, producing acid and a nutritive fermented beverage full of beneficial yeasts and bacteria, the health-promoting probiotics.

2–4 tablespoons water kefir grains
4 cups filtered water
3 dried figs
½ to 1 lemon, sliced
¼ cup white sugar
1 2-quart glass jar
Clean cloth napkin
String or rubber band

Put all contents into jar; cover with cloth napkin, and tie cover in place with string or rubber band. Let stand at room temperature for 1–2 days. Remove lemon and figs and place in a clean 2-quart glass jar. Handling very gently, carefully pour the liquid through a fine nonmetallic strainer to remove the kefir grains. Add grains to the jar with lemon and figs to begin the process again. Enjoy the strained liquid as a beverage. It will be slightly fizzy and will be tart, due to the reduced sugar content.

Substitutions
The same lemon and fig can be used for at least 2 batches, and maybe 3 if your fermentation times are shorter. I have used a variety of different dried fruits to produce subtle new flavors.

Kitchen Tips
The difficulty of making water kefir is first acquiring the grains. I found mine by connecting with someone on the website mothering.com. You can go to the forums and find your geographical area. Then search under "water kefir," or start your own conversation on the forum asking if anyone in your area has water kefir grains they would be willing to share. If you want to purchase them commercially, it is possible to find both fresh and freeze-dried water kefir grains online. I have never purchased them this way, but many of the sources say they are organic and guaranteed to grow a culture.

Your grains will multiply rather quickly, so I encourage you to share them. If you want to store your grains, place them in a small jar with a couple teaspoons of sugar and store in the refrigerator. They should last this way for 2 weeks before you need to make a new batch.

Fermented Pink Sauerkraut

PER CUP: 43.1 CALORIES ~ 2.0 G PROTEIN ~ 10.1 G CARBOHYDRATE ~ 3.4 G FIBER ~
0.2 G TOTAL FAT ~ 0.0 G SATURATED FAT ~ 0.1 MG CHOLESTEROL ~ 618.8 MG SODIUM

1 medium green cabbage, grated

1 medium red cabbage, grated

½ cup whey (whey is a by-product of Cream Cheese "Curds and Whey";
see recipe on page 172)

2 tablespoons salt

1-gallon wide-mouthed jar

Combine cabbage, whey, and salt in a large nonmetallic bowl. Mix well, crushing cabbage with hands or heavy wooden spoon or mallet until juices are released, about 10 minutes. Spoon into 1-gallon glass jar or crock. Make sure all of the cabbage is below the liquid line; if not, add a small amount of water. Place gallon-sized plastic bag inside the jar and fill the bag with water; arrange it so the cabbage mixture is prevented from being exposed to any air. If needed, add a little more salt water to the cabbage to cover the vegetables completely. Cover the jar with a loose-fitting lid or towel, making sure to secure the towel with a large rubber band or string to keep bugs out and odors in. Some gas will need to escape during the process, so do not use a tight lid. Let jar sit at room temperature for at least seven days. Depending on the room's temperature, you may want to allow the sauerkraut to ferment a little longer to "sour" more. Once made, refrigerate the sauerkraut in the large jar, or divide into small jars.

Yields 12 cups.

Nutritional Analysis per Cup

Vitamin A	85.7 RE	Vitamin D	0.0 µg
Thiamin (B-1)	0.1 mg	Vitamin E	0.0 mg
Riboflavin (B-2)	0.1 mg	Calcium	73.0 mg
Niacin	0.5 mg	Iron	0.9 mg
Vitamin B-6	0.2 mg	Phosphorus	48.6 mg
Vitamin B-12	0.0 µg	Magnesium	21.3 mg
Folate (total)	45.3 µg	Zinc	0.3 mg
Vitamin C	67.6 mg	Potassium	313.3 mg

Fermented Garlic

PER SERVING: 45.9 CALORIES ~ 2.0 G PROTEIN ~ 10.2 G CARBOHYDRATE ~ 0.6 G FIBER ~
0.2 G TOTAL FAT ~ 0.0 G SATURATED FAT ~ 0.1 MG CHOLESTEROL ~ 395.4 MG SODIUM

10 large heads garlic

¼ cup whey (whey is a by-product of Cream Cheese "Curds and Whey";
see recipe on page 172)

½ cup filtered water

2 teaspoons salt

Preheat oven to 350°F.

To make it easy to peel the garlic, place whole heads of garlic on a baking sheet and roast in the oven for 10 minutes. Don't allow the garlic to cook. Remove from oven; separate and peel cloves of garlic. Allow to cool. (Alternatively, you could separate and peel the garlic cloves without first baking.) Place garlic in a 1-quart glass jar. Add remaining ingredients; add a bit more water, if necessary, to submerge garlic. Cover jar with a tight lid, and let stand at room temperature for 3 days. The garlic is ready to use immediately, or refrigerate up to 6 months.

Serves 12.

Nutritional Analysis per Serving

Vitamin A	0.4 RE	Vitamin D	0.0 µg
Thiamin (B-1)	0.1 mg	Vitamin E	0.0 mg
Riboflavin (B-2)	0.0 mg	Calcium	60.1 mg
Niacin	0.2 mg	Iron	0.5 mg
Vitamin B-6	0.4 mg	Phosphorus	49.9 mg
Vitamin B-12	0.0 µg	Magnesium	8.1 mg
Folate (total)	1.0 µg	Zinc	0.4 mg
Vitamin C	9.4 mg	Potassium	127.8 mg

Fermented Vegetables

PER SERVING: 30.8 CALORIES ~ 1.0 G PROTEIN ~ 6.5 G CARBOHYDRATE ~ 1.9 G FIBER ~
0.1 G TOTAL FAT ~ 0.0 G SATURATED FAT ~ 0.0 MG CHOLESTEROL ~ 142.5 MG SODIUM

This can be made with one vegetable or a combination of several, according to your tastes.

1 cup peeled and sliced carrots

1 cup asparagus, chopped into 1-inch pieces

1 cup pearl onions, sliced in halves

2 jalapeños, sliced (optional)

¼ cup whey (whey is a by-product of Cream Cheese "Curds and Whey";
see recipe on page 172)

½ cup filtered water

2 teaspoons salt

Place vegetables in 1-quart glass jar. Add remaining ingredients; add a bit more water, if necessary, to submerge vegetables. Cover jar with a tight lid and let stand at room temperature for 3 days. Use immediately, or refrigerate up to 3 months.

Yields 3 cups (4 ¾-cup servings).

Substitutions
Other vegetable ideas: beets, green beans, turnips, peeled gingerroot. Use 3 cups total.

Nutritional Analysis per Serving

Vitamin A	535.1 RE	Vitamin D	0.0 µg
Thiamin (B-1)	0.1 mg	Vitamin E	0.0 mg
Riboflavin (B-2)	0.1 mg	Calcium	19.8 mg
Niacin	0.6 mg	Iron	0.8 mg
Vitamin B-6	0.1 mg	Phosphorus	29.2 mg
Vitamin B-12	0.0 µg	Magnesium	8.5 mg
Folate (total)	23.2 µg	Zinc	0.3 mg
Vitamin C	3.7 mg	Potassium	167.2 mg

Fermented Pancakes

PER SERVING: 393.8 CALORIES ~ 11.4 G PROTEIN ~ 69.7 G CARBOHYDRATE ~ 5.8 G FIBER ~
8.3 G TOTAL FAT ~ 3.7 G SATURATED FAT ~ 140.4 MG CHOLESTEROL ~ 666.2 MG SODIUM

2 cups Gluten-Free Pancake and Baking Mix (see recipe on page 124)

½ cup whey (whey is a by-product of Cream Cheese "Curds and Whey";
see recipe on page 172)

½ cup water

1 ripe banana, mashed

3 eggs

2 teaspoons cinnamon

2 teaspoons coconut oil

1 teaspoon baking powder

At least one night before, whisk together Baking Mix, whey, and water in a
medium nonmetallic bowl until smooth. Cover with clean towel; place in a
warm spot overnight, or up to 2 days.

Combine remaining ingredients in a medium bowl, mixing until smooth;
stir into Baking Mix mixture.

Heat a pancake griddle or nonstick skillet over medium heat. Pour batter
onto skillet, using about ¼ cup per pancake. Cook until bubbles start to
appear, about 3 minutes; turn and cook until browned on other side, about 3
minutes.

Serves 4.

Nutritional Analysis per Serving

Vitamin A	64.3 RE	Vitamin D	0.8 µg
Thiamin (B-1)	0.3 mg	Vitamin E	0.4 mg
Riboflavin (B-2)	0.6 mg	Calcium	279.9 mg
Niacin	2.9 mg	Iron	2.5 mg
Vitamin B-6	0.6 mg	Phosphorus	480.8 mg
Vitamin B-12	0.7 µg	Magnesium	84.8 mg
Folate (total)	31.7 µg	Zinc	1.8 mg
Vitamin C	2.8 mg	Potassium	632.2 mg

Entrées

Recipes with this symbol are not strictly anti-inflammatory, therefore we suggest avoiding these recipes until you are feeling well and are ready to introduce a little variety to see how you do.

Spiced Lentil and Bean Burgers

PER SERVING: 70.5 CALORIES ~ 4.1 G PROTEIN ~ 10.4 G CARBOHYDRATE ~ 2.5 G FIBER ~
1.5 G TOTAL FAT ~ 0.4 G SATURATED FAT ~ 46.5 MG CHOLESTEROL ~ 310.3 MG SODIUM

½ cup lentils, cooked (see page 221)

½ cup short grain brown rice, cooked (see page 218)

½ cup black beans, cooked (see page 221)

2 eggs

1 teaspoon garlic powder

1 teaspoon onion powder

1 teaspoon cumin

½ cup unsweetened apple sauce

1 teaspoon salt

1 teaspoon ground black pepper

Preheat oven to 375°F.

Combine all ingredients in a large mixing bowl; stir until well mixed. Process half the mixture in a food processor until almost smooth. Mix with remaining mixture in bowl, and shape into 8 patties. Bake on a greased baking sheet for 30 minutes or until patties are crisp on the outside. You can broil both sides for a couple of minutes if you want them crisper.

Serves 8.

Substitutions

This recipe is easiest when you have leftover cooked legumes and rice. Just mash them together with spices and eggs, and turn your leftovers into a new meal. Don't hesitate to try various seasonings.

Healthy Tidbit

When legumes and grains are consumed together, they provide the body with complete protein. Proteins are made of amino acids. Grains have some amino acids and legumes have others, and when combined they contain all of the amino acids needed to complete a protein. This is an important concept to understand if you are a vegetarian or vegan. Protein is an important building block in every cell and tissue in the body, including bone, muscle, cartilage, skin, blood, hair, and nails. Your body uses proteins to make enzymes,

Nutritional Analysis per Serving

Vitamin A	21.2 RE	Vitamin D	0.3 µg
Thiamin (B-1)	0.1 mg	Vitamin E	0.1 mg
Riboflavin (B-2)	0.1 mg	Calcium	19.2 mg
Niacin	0.4 mg	Iron	1.0 mg
Vitamin B-6	0.1 mg	Phosphorus	74.9 mg
Vitamin B-12	0.1 µg	Magnesium	20.3 mg
Folate (total)	45.6 µg	Zinc	0.5 mg
Vitamin C	0.4 mg	Potassium	137.8 mg

hormones, and other chemicals needed for metabolism. Consuming complete proteins also helps to balance your blood sugar.

Macaro-No Cheese

PER SERVING: 266.1 CALORIES ~ 10.0 G PROTEIN ~ 33.8 G CARBOHYDRATE ~ 2.4 G FIBER ~ 10.6 G TOTAL FAT ~ 2.5 G SATURATED FAT ~ 6.1 MG CHOLESTEROL ~ 32.7 MG SODIUM

1 10-ounce package soft silken tofu, drained
1 cup unsweetened almond or hemp milk
½ cup tahini (sesame seed paste)
3 tablespoons nutritional yeast
1 teaspoon turmeric (optional)
1 teaspoon apple cider vinegar
Salt to taste
14 ounces uncooked elbow macaroni
4 cups boiling water
2 tablespoons butter, cut into 6–8 pieces

Preheat oven to 350°F.

Blend tofu and almond milk in a blender or food processor until smooth. Add tahini, nutritional yeast, turmeric, and vinegar, and blend until smooth. Season to taste with salt.

Boil macaroni in water for 3–4 minutes; drain, and rinse in cold water. Combine macaroni and tofu mixture in a large bowl. Spoon mixture into a lightly greased casserole dish. Top with butter; bake until golden and bubbly, about 20 minutes.

Serves 10.

Substitutions

If you're short on time, you do not absolutely need to bake this dish. If not baking it, you will need to cook the macaroni a few minutes longer: 8–10 minutes, or until tender but not mushy.

If the flavor isn't "cheesy" enough, then add more salt. Cheese is salty, and when I first made this dish I skimped on the salt and the flavor wasn't quite right.

The turmeric gives the dish the orange color of real mac and cheese, but it changes the

Nutritional Analysis per Serving

Vitamin A	22.1 RE	Vitamin D	0.0 µg
Thiamin (B-1)	1.0 mg	Vitamin E	0.1 mg
Riboflavin (B-2)	0.0 mg	Calcium	39.5 mg
Niacin	1.4 mg	Iron	1.5 mg
Vitamin B-6	0.1 mg	Phosphorus	170.5 mg
Vitamin B-12	0.6 µg	Magnesium	33.5 mg
Folate (total)	19.0 µg	Zinc	1.1 mg
Vitamin C	0.5 mg	Potassium	175.6 mg

flavor. For those who don't mind a white mac and cheese I would recommend leaving the turmeric out. The end product will look different, but it will taste better.

Healthy Tidbit

Nutritional yeast is very convenient to keep on hand. With its naturally salty character it can be added to many dishes in place of cheese. It even works well on popcorn and other snacks. My infant used to enjoy eating it plain. Nutritional yeast is high in proteins and the B vitamins. It is popular among vegans and vegetarians because it offers another complex source of amino acids.

You could use brewer's yeast instead of nutritional yeast. Brewer's yeast contains the mineral chromium whereas nutritional yeast does not. It is easier to find nutritional yeast. Finding a good-quality brewer's yeast can sometimes be a challenge.

A very small percentage of individuals seem to react adversely to nutritional yeast with itching or gastrointestinal upset. I suggest taking a tablespoon of nutritional yeast a few nights before you plan on preparing this recipe to make sure you can tolerate it.

Frittata Pizza

PER SERVING: 330.5 CALORIES ~ 18.5 G PROTEIN ~ 16.5 G CARBOHYDRATE ~ 3.4 G FIBER ~ 21.1 G TOTAL FAT ~ 5.0 G SATURATED FAT ~ 373.9 MG CHOLESTEROL ~ 666.3 MG SODIUM

3 cloves garlic, minced

2 tablespoons olive oil

1 cup diced broccoli

1 cup fresh, chopped spinach

8 eggs

2 tablespoons almond milk

Salt to taste (optional)

1½ cups spaghetti sauce

½ teaspoon freshly ground black pepper

½ cup grated vegan mozzarella cheese substitute (such as Vegan Rella Natural Cheese Alternative—Mozzarella Style)

Preheat oven to 400°F.

Sauté the garlic in oil in a large cast iron skillet until tender, about 2 minutes; add broccoli and sauté for 3–4 minutes. Stir in spinach. Whisk together eggs, almond milk, salt, and pepper in a medium bowl; add to skillet. Do not stir. Reduce heat to low, cover, and cook 5–10 minutes, or until eggs are firm and fork inserted in center comes out nearly clean.

Top frittata with spaghetti sauce and sprinkle with cheese. Broil until cheese is browned and sauce is warmed, about 3 minutes.

Serves 4.

Substitutions

Instead of the premade spaghetti sauce, you could use one of the sauces from the Dips and Spreads section for a very distinct flavor variation. The more you experiment in the kitchen, the more you will understand which combinations work well together and which don't. Here's one suggestion: brown some sausage in the same skillet in which you will make the frittata (leaving some of the resulting oil in the skillet for added flavor), add the cooked sausage to the frittata, then top the frittata with Mushroom Gravy (see recipe on page 113). As always, the cheese or cheese substitute is optional. If you tolerate some dairy, then perhaps try real cheese.

Healthy Tidbit

Tomatoes, though they are inflammatory for some individuals, contain an important anticancer nutrient called lycopene. Lycopene has been studied as having a chemo-preventive effect against prostate cancer and may reduce cancer-related symptoms such as pain and urinary tract symptoms.[7] If you are able to tolerate tomatoes without an adverse reaction, then enjoy tomatoes and know that you're getting the health benefits of lycopene.

Nutritional Analysis per Serving

Vitamin A	246.6 RE	Vitamin D	2.0 µg
Thiamin (B-1)	0.1 mg	Vitamin E	1.1 mg
Riboflavin (B-2)	0.6 mg	Calcium	101.3 mg
Niacin	4.0 mg	Iron	3.0 mg
Vitamin B-6	0.4 mg	Phosphorus	254.3 mg
Vitamin B-12	0.9 µg	Magnesium	43.4 mg
Folate (total)	88.2 µg	Zinc	2.0 mg
Vitamin C	25.0 mg	Potassium	570.0 mg

Veggie Noodle Stir-Fry

PER SERVING: 330.2 CALORIES ~ 4.3 G PROTEIN ~ 61.0 G CARBOHYDRATE ~ 2.7 G FIBER ~
8.4 G TOTAL FAT ~ 1.2 G SATURATED FAT ~ 0.0 MG CHOLESTEROL ~ 515.8 MG SODIUM

½ cup onion, chopped	½ cup water
3 cloves garlic, minced	2 tablespoons gluten-free tamari sauce
2 tablespoons olive oil	
2 large carrots, sliced diagonally	1 teaspoon sesame oil
2 cups sliced mushrooms	1 teaspoon honey
2 cups chopped kale	1 package (8 ounces) rice noodles

Sauté onion and garlic in olive oil in a large skillet or wok until translucent, about 5 minutes. Add carrots and sauté 3 minutes. Add mushrooms and kale and sauté 2–3 minutes, until kale is slightly wilted. Add water, tamari, sesame oil, honey, and noodles. Heat to simmering; cook until noodles are tender but not mushy, about 5–8 minutes.

Serves 4.

Substitutions

Any type of mushroom can be used in this recipe. Try all of your favorite vegetables. Collard or dark greens offer lots of nutrition, so make sure to include one of those when choosing your vegetables.

Healthy Tidbit

Avoid watching TV while eating, especially the news or anything with suspenseful drama. Watching upsetting or suspenseful programming keeps your nervous system in a stressed state, which inhibits your ability to digest food. Eat in a calm atmosphere. If you live alone, then plan to eat at least one dinner per week, preferably more, with other people. Living alone may increase heart disease risk; therefore, it is important to maintain regular contact with other people. Intimacy in all forms, either romantic, from friendship, or from volunteering, can help to fulfill your relationship needs. In the book *The General Theory of Love*, the authors explain how we thrive based on physical contact and attention, and the importance to our health of social connection within our peer group.

Nutritional Analysis per Serving

Vitamin A	1024.7 RE	Vitamin D	0.1 µg
Thiamin (B-1)	0.2 mg	Vitamin E	0.0 mg
Riboflavin (B-2)	0.3 mg	Calcium	80.6 mg
Niacin	2.5 mg	Iron	2.6 mg
Vitamin B-6	0.3 mg	Phosphorus	98.2 mg
Vitamin B-12	0.0 µg	Magnesium	24.0 mg
Folate (total)	28.7 µg	Zinc	0.8 mg
Vitamin C	45.2 mg	Potassium	445.2 mg

Chia Vegetable Stir-Fry

PER SERVING: 195.7 CALORIES ~ 5.8 G PROTEIN ~ 35.4 G CARBOHYDRATE ~ 4.4 G FIBER ~
3.9 G TOTAL FAT ~ 0.6 G SATURATED FAT ~ 0.0 MG CHOLESTEROL ~ 380.4 MG SODIUM

½ medium onion, sliced

1½ tablespoons peeled and minced gingerroot

4 garlic cloves, finely chopped

1 tablespoon olive oil

2 cups coarsely chopped kale

2 carrots, thinly sliced

½ bell pepper, thinly sliced

1 cup halved or sliced mushrooms

2 tomatoes, chopped

¾ cup water

3 tablespoons gluten-free tamari sauce

2 tablespoons chia seeds

1–2 tablespoons rice wine vinegar (optional)

½ teaspoon toasted sesame oil

5 cups cooked brown, or brown basmati, rice

In a wok or large skillet, heat olive oil over medium heat until it's hot but not smoking. Stir-fry onion, garlic, and ginger until softened, about 3 minutes. Add vegetables and stir-fry 4–5 minutes, or until kale is wilted. Stir in water, tamari, chia seeds, vinegar (optional), and sesame oil.

Cook, covered, until vegetables are crisp-tender, about 10 minutes. Serve over rice.

Serves 8.

Substitutions

Of course, this recipe can be prepared using all sorts of vegetables. The chia seeds offer a somewhat new and different taste and texture; they also add fiber and essential fatty acids.

Healthy Tidbit

Ginger is one of my favorite anti-inflammatory spices. It is warming and helps to stimulate digestion and appetite. Ginger has traditionally been used to treat nausea and vomiting. In our clinic, we have used ginger extensively for years as an effective treatment for arthritis symptoms. For therapeutic use, ginger needs to be given at a much higher dosage than can be achieved through diet, but including ginger in the diet is a good first step to attaining therapeutic effects and can help aid digestion immensely.

Nutritional Analysis per Serving

Vitamin A	540.8 RE	Vitamin D	0.0 µg
Thiamin (B-1)	0.2 mg	Vitamin E	0.0 mg
Riboflavin (B-2)	0.1 mg	Calcium	61.0 mg
Niacin	3.0 mg	Iron	1.5 mg
Vitamin B-6	0.3 mg	Phosphorus	155.9 mg
Vitamin B-12	0.0 µg	Magnesium	73.2 mg
Folate (total)	22.4 µg	Zinc	1.1 mg
Vitamin C	32.5 mg	Potassium	328.7 mg

Rich Veggie Stir-Fry

PER SERVING: 230.9 CALORIES ~ 4.3 G PROTEIN ~ 16.4 G CARBOHYDRATE ~ 4.6 G FIBER ~
11.0 G TOTAL FAT ~ 1.6 G SATURATED FAT ~ 0.0 MG CHOLESTEROL ~ 58.4 MG SODIUM

5 garlic cloves, minced

3 tablespoons olive oil or coconut oil

2 small zucchini, chopped

2 small yellow squash, chopped

2 cups chopped broccoli

1 cup coarsely chopped cauliflower

2 carrots, coarsely chopped

2 teaspoons dried thyme leaves

1 teaspoon dried rosemary leaves

1½ cups dry white wine, divided

Salt and freshly ground pepper to taste

Sauté garlic in oil in a large skillet until tender, about 2 minutes. Stir in vegetables and herbs and sauté 5 minutes. Add 1 cup wine and simmer until reduced by half, about 5 minutes. Add remaining ½ cup wine and simmer until vegetables are tender and sauce thickens, about 5 minutes. Season to taste with salt and pepper.

Serve over rice or with fish.

Serves 4.

Substitutions

Different vegetables can be used in this recipe. Any type of dry white wine, or a fortified wine such as dry marsala, can be used for the sauce. You can use the reducing process to make sauces for other foods as well. Practice on this recipe and you will begin to understand how to create tasty sauces.

Kitchen Tip

Reducing involves using wine or other liquids to thicken a sauce as you cook it. As you cook wine, the alcohol evaporates, leaving behind enough flavor to create a rich, savory sauce.

Nutritional Analysis per Serving

Vitamin A	572.9 RE	Vitamin D	0.0 µg
Thiamin (B-1)	0.2 mg	Vitamin E	0.0 mg
Riboflavin (B-2)	0.3 mg	Calcium	93.4 mg
Niacin	1.6 mg	Iron	2.4 mg
Vitamin B-6	0.6 mg	Phosphorus	134.7 mg
Vitamin B-12	0.0 µg	Magnesium	56.6 mg
Folate (total)	93.2 µg	Zinc	1.0 mg
Vitamin C	83.7 mg	Potassium	813.0 mg

Zucchini Mushroom Herb Casserole

PER SERVING: 237.5 CALORIES ~ 8.9 G PROTEIN ~ 31.3 G CARBOHYDRATE ~ 7.2 G FIBER ~
10.5 G TOTAL FAT ~ 5.7 G SATURATED FAT ~ 22.9 MG CHOLESTEROL ~ 825.8 MG SODIUM

⅓ cup uncooked long-grain brown rice

1 cup vegetable broth

1½ pounds cubed zucchini

1 pound chopped shiitake mushrooms

1 cup sliced green onions

4 cloves garlic, minced

3 tablespoons butter or olive oil

1 teaspoon garlic powder

1 teaspoon onion powder

1 teaspoon paprika

½ teaspoon dried basil leaves

½ teaspoon dried oregano leaves

1 teaspoon ground pepper

1 teaspoon salt

¼ cup nutritional yeast or brewer's yeast

Preheat oven to 350°F.

Combine the rice and chicken broth in a medium saucepan and heat to boiling. Reduce heat and simmer, covered, until rice is tender, about 20 minutes.

Sauté vegetables and garlic in butter in a large skillet until slightly softened, about 5 minutes. Stir in rice and remaining ingredients, except nutritional yeast. Spoon into a lightly greased medium casserole dish.

Bake uncovered for 20 minutes. Sprinkle with nutritional yeast before serving.

Serves 4.

Substitutions
Different vegetables work well with this dish. Try different grains as well. Sometimes I mix brown rice and buckwheat for a delicious flavor.

Healthy Tidbit
When baking at a temperature of 350°F or above, use coconut oil or organic, unsalted butter. For baking at lower temperatures, olive oil is fine. I stick to basic oils and avoid most processed oils. Oils that are refined for high heat may be fine to use every once in a while, but they are not my staple. I want to use oils that have undergone the least amount of processing and that are cold pressed and organic.

Nutritional Analysis per Serving

Vitamin A	168.7 RE	Vitamin D	0.6 µg
Thiamin (B-1)	2.6 mg	Vitamin E	0.3 mg
Riboflavin (B-2)	0.5 mg	Calcium	78.0 mg
Niacin	6.2 mg	Iron	2.5 mg
Vitamin B-6	0.8 mg	Phosphorus	349.8 mg
Vitamin B-12	2.0 µg	Magnesium	86.1 mg
Folate (total)	77.1 µg	Zinc	2.3 mg
Vitamin C	36.2 mg	Potassium	1009.2 mg

Gluten-Free Veggie Pasta

PER SERVING: 228.0 CALORIES ~ 7.8 G PROTEIN ~ 50.8 G CARBOHYDRATE ~ 3.9 G FIBER ~
9.0 G TOTAL FAT ~ 1.1 G SATURATED FAT ~ 0.0 MG CHOLESTEROL ~ 190.1 MG SODIUM

2 cloves garlic, minced

2 tablespoons olive oil

1 tablespoon miso paste

½ teaspoon dried oregano leaves

½ teaspoon dried basil leaves

1½ cups chopped zucchini

1½ cups chopped yellow summer squash

2 cups chopped broccoli

Salt and freshly ground pepper to taste

1 8-ounce package gluten-free penne pasta, cooked according
to package directions, warm

2 tablespoons nutritional yeast or brewer's yeast

Sauté garlic in oil in a large skillet over medium heat until tender, about 3 minutes; add miso paste and herbs, and sauté 1 minute. Stir in vegetables and sauté until tender and lightly browned, about 6 minutes. Season to taste with salt and pepper; toss with penne in a large serving bowl. Sprinkle with yeast.
    Serves 4.

Substitutions
You can use any vegetables with this recipe. I love the simplicity of the miso paste, brewer's yeast, and olive oil. It is a great combination.

Kitchen Tips
I like my cooked vegetables on the crunchy side, but I still aim for a little browning on the zucchini and squash. That means cooking them at a high-enough heat to sear the outside.

Nutritional Analysis per Serving

Vitamin A	47.7 RE	Vitamin D	0.0 µg
Thiamin (B-1)	1.3 mg	Vitamin E	0.0 mg
Riboflavin (B-2)	0.2 mg	Calcium	67.5 mg
Niacin	0.8 mg	Iron	1.3 mg
Vitamin B-6	0.3 mg	Phosphorus	72.2 mg
Vitamin B-12	1.0 µg	Magnesium	28.7 mg
Folate (total)	53.1 µg	Zinc	0.6 mg
Vitamin C	55.9 mg	Potassium	388.0 mg

Crunchy Burritos

PER SERVING: 911.6 CALORIES ~ 19.0 G PROTEIN ~ 128.1 G CARBOHYDRATE ~ 23.8 G FIBER ~
38.1 G TOTAL FAT ~ 5.0 G SATURATED FAT ~ 0.0 MG CHOLESTEROL ~ 844.2 MG SODIUM

4 teff tortillas, warm
1 cup cooked black beans, warm
1 cup green cabbage, finely chopped
1 cup barbecue-flavored rice chips, crushed into small pieces
1 avocado, cut into 8 slices
Kiwi Cucumber Salsa, as garnish (see recipe on page 79)

Place tortilla on a serving plate; top it with ¼ cup each of beans, cabbage, and rice chips, plus 2 slices avocado. Roll tortilla, tucking in ends.
   Serves 2.

Substitutions

Burritos are easy to make and can include a wide array of ingredients. This recipe is meant to be an easy dinner to throw together, but if you have a little more time you can sauté onions, garlic, and zucchini in a little olive oil to layer on top of the beans and before the green cabbage. The combo of zucchini, garlic, and onions cooks fast and are easy to prepare and clean up after. If you are making these burritos for children, especially children under the age of six, wrap the bottom part in aluminum foil. This helps little hands be able to hold the burritos together. My three-year-old daughter never ate her burritos until I started doing this for her. If it was served to her on a plate lying sideways, she would just pick it apart.

Healthy Tidbit

Let's discuss sodium intake. Excessive dietary sodium has been directly connected to elevated blood pressure and risk for stroke. Heart disease is the number-one killer in the United States. An easy, twofold strategy for reducing sodium in your diet is to stop eating from boxes and cans, and stop using the salt shaker at the table. In addition, when consuming foods like rice chips, keep them to a minimum and balance your sodium intake for the day by reducing in other areas. A recommended sodium intake for the average person is no more than 2,300 mg daily. If you have hypertension, diabetes, or kidney disease, then you should consume no more than 1,500 mg of sodium daily. If you are preparing these burritos and are on a low-sodium diet, skip the chips.

Nutritional Analysis per Serving

Vitamin A	42.7 RE	Vitamin D	0.0 µg
Thiamin (B-1)	0.3 mg	Vitamin E	0.0 mg
Riboflavin (B-2)	0.2 mg	Calcium	212.4 mg
Niacin	1.5 mg	Iron	4.4 mg
Vitamin B-6	0.2 mg	Phosphorus	190.3 mg
Vitamin B-12	0.0 µg	Magnesium	100.9 mg
Folate (total)	196.4 µg	Zinc	1.6 mg
Vitamin C	39.3 mg	Potassium	898.3 mg

Hummus Lettuce Wraps

PER SERVING: 249.4 CALORIES ~ 7.1 G PROTEIN ~ 30.7 G CARBOHYDRATE ~ 4.2 G FIBER ~
12.4 G TOTAL FAT ~ 0.1 G SATURATED FAT ~ 0.0 MG CHOLESTEROL ~ 655.0 MG SODIUM

These are a simple treat for lunch. Pack all of the fixings, and roll them up
fresh right before eating.

4 leaves of red or green leaf lettuce

1 cup prepared hummus

1 cucumber, cut into strips

¼ red onion, cut into very thin slices

1 cup sprouts

Top each lettuce leaf with ¼ cup hummus, slices of cucumber, onion, and
sprouts. Gently roll lettuce leaf, tucking in ends.
Serves 2.

Substitutions
Try loading your lettuce wraps with veggies, various dips or sauces, smoked
salmon, chicken, or baked tofu or tempeh.

Kitchen Tip
Lettuce leaves don't roll as tidily as tortillas; they may break or crack at the
spine. Don't worry about it. You'll figure out how to hold them together while
eating.

Healthy Tidbit
Wraps and burritos can offer most food groups. You can make warm wraps
with tortillas, veggies, rice, and beans, and you can make cold wraps with
lettuce, hummus, veggies, and a protein. Wraps can provide a satisfying meal
rather quickly, with plenty of options these days for making them gluten free
or grain free.

Nutritional Analysis per Serving

Vitamin A	271.6 RE	Vitamin D	0.0 µg
Thiamin (B-1)	0.1 mg	Vitamin E	0.0 mg
Riboflavin (B-2)	0.1 mg	Calcium	45.1 mg
Niacin	0.7 mg	Iron	1.3 mg
Vitamin B-6	0.2 mg	Phosphorus	77.4 mg
Vitamin B-12	0.0 µg	Magnesium	35.9 mg
Folate (total)	57.1 µg	Zinc	0.6 mg
Vitamin C	18.0 mg	Potassium	382.1 mg

Sweet Potato Corn Cakes

PER SERVING: 207.1 CALORIES ~ 5.1 G PROTEIN ~ 34.8 G CARBOHYDRATE ~ 5.1 G FIBER ~
5.8 G TOTAL FAT ~ 0.8 G SATURATED FAT ~ 0.0 MG CHOLESTEROL ~ 594.1 MG SODIUM

1 cup yellow corn meal

1 baked sweet potato, mashed

2 tablespoons chia seeds

2 cups vegetable broth

½ cup onion, diced

1 jalapeno pepper, minced

2 cloves garlic, minced

½ teaspoon chili powder

½ teaspoon salt

¼ teaspoon cumin

⅛ teaspoon cayenne pepper

1 tablespoon olive oil or coconut oil

Combine corn meal, potato, and chia seeds in a large bowl. Heat vegetable broth to boiling and pour over the mixture. Mix well, and set aside.

Sauté onion, pepper, garlic, and seasonings in oil in a medium skillet until tender, about 5 minutes.

Add the vegetables to the corn meal mixture and mix well. Shape into small hamburger-sized patties. Cook patties in a lightly greased nonstick skillet until browned on both sides, about 5 minutes per side.

Serves 4.

Healthy Tidbit

The salty-sweet combination is appealing to most people's taste buds. The sweet taste doesn't have to come from sweeteners but rather from naturally sweet foods. Polenta, or cornmeal, lends a richly satisfying sweetness to this recipe, and, of course, so do the sweet potatoes.

Nutritional Analysis per Serving

Vitamin A	575.9 RE	Vitamin D	0.0 µg
Thiamin (B-1)	0.2 mg	Vitamin E	0.0 mg
Riboflavin (B-2)	0.1 mg	Calcium	56.7 mg
Niacin	2.0 mg	Iron	1.9 mg
Vitamin B-6	0.3 mg	Phosphorus	296.5 mg
Vitamin B-12	0.0 µg	Magnesium	62.5 mg
Folate (total)	16.1 µg	Zinc	0.9 mg
Vitamin C	11.8 mg	Potassium	417.4 mg

Spaghetti Sauce with Gluten-Free Noodles

PER SERVING: 225.1 CALORIES ~ 6.4 G PROTEIN ~ 56.4 G CARBOHYDRATE ~ 4.0 G FIBER ~
6.2 G TOTAL FAT ~ 0.7 G SATURATED FAT ~ 0.0 MG CHOLESTEROL ~ 642.7 MG SODIUM

5 cloves garlic, minced

2 tablespoons olive oil

2 tablespoons dried basil leaves

1 tablespoon dried oregano leaves

1 tablespoon garlic powder

1 tablespoon onion powder

½ tablespoon chopped fresh rosemary, or ½ teaspoon
crumbled dried rosemary leaves

1 teaspoon salt

1 28-ounce can diced or stewed tomatoes

1 small sweet potato, steamed

1 12-ounce package gluten-free noodles, cooked, warm

Sauté garlic in oil in a large saucepan until translucent, about 2 minutes. Add seasonings and sauté 1 minute. Add tomatoes and heat to boiling; reduce heat and simmer, covered, 15–20 minutes. Purée half the sauce in a blender with the sweet potato; return to saucepan. Heat until hot. Serve over noodles.

Serves 6.

Kitchen Tip
If the sauce is too thick, add white wine or water and simmer a little longer to allow flavors to mingle. If you want a very smooth sauce, you can purée the entire batch.

Substitutions
Try adding steamed carrots or zucchini. If you are unable to tolerate tomatoes, you could use a roasted red pepper soup instead of the tomato sauce.

Healthy Tidbit
Purée steamed vegetables into sauces as a way to "sneak" more veggies into your kids' diets. Examples of vegetables that are easily disguised in purées are carrots, sweet potatoes, cauliflower, peas, or squash. Cooked legumes can also be puréed into sauces for added protein.

Nutritional Analysis per Serving

Vitamin A	404.6 RE	Vitamin D	0.0 µg
Thiamin (B-1)	0.0 mg	Vitamin E	0.0 mg
Riboflavin (B-2)	0.0 mg	Calcium	126.7 mg
Niacin	0.3 mg	Iron	2.9 mg
Vitamin B-6	0.1 mg	Phosphorus	28.5 mg
Vitamin B-12	0.0 µg	Magnesium	20.9 mg
Folate (total)	10.5 µg	Zinc	0.3 mg
Vitamin C	11.5 mg	Potassium	159.5 mg

Roasted Tempeh Melts

PER SERVING: 692.0 CALORIES ~ 27.7 G PROTEIN ~ 48.7 G CARBOHYDRATE ~ 5.0 G FIBER ~
43.5 G TOTAL FAT ~ 13.3 G SATURATED FAT ~ 62.0 MG CHOLESTEROL ~ 2414.0 MG SODIUM

½ cup mayonnaise

¼ cup ketchup

½ cup Zucchini Relish (see recipe on page 107) or sweet relish

4 slices gluten-free bread

2 servings Roasted Tempeh (see recipe on page 72), or
1 8-ounce package flavored tempeh, sliced

1 cup sauerkraut

8 slices Swiss cheese (omit if dairy intolerant)

Preheat oven to 400°F.

Combine mayonnaise, ketchup, and Zucchini Relish in a small bowl, mixing well.

Spread mayonnaise mixture on bread. Place bread on a baking pan; top with roasted tempeh, sauerkraut, and cheese. Bake until cheese melts, about 5 minutes.

Serves 4.

Substitutions

Another option would be to use the recipe for Faux Creamy Cheese Sauce (see recipe on page 111). You could also substitute turkey or sliced baked chicken for the tempeh.

Healthy Tidbit

Sauerkraut, especially if it's raw and contains live cultures, when consumed in moderation is a good way to get probiotics into your diet. Fermented foods haven't yet become a staple in most people's diets, but making an effort to include them will yield health benefits.

Nutritional Analysis per Serving

Vitamin A	187.7 RE	Vitamin D	0.3 µg
Thiamin (B-1)	0.2 mg	Vitamin E	0.0 mg
Riboflavin (B-2)	0.6 mg	Calcium	515.9 mg
Niacin	3.1 mg	Iron	3.5 mg
Vitamin B-6	0.4 mg	Phosphorus	478.8 mg
Vitamin B-12	2.0 µg	Magnesium	44.8 mg
Folate (total)	30.3 µg	Zinc	2.9 mg
Vitamin C	27.7 mg	Potassium	417.9 mg

Fish Patties

PER SERVING: 166.2 CALORIES ~ 18.8 G PROTEIN ~ 1.3 G CARBOHYDRATE ~ 0.4 G FIBER ~
9.2 G TOTAL FAT ~ 1.8 G SATURATED FAT ~ 133.3 MG CHOLESTEROL ~ 359.6 MG SODIUM

8 ounces cooked salmon, flaked

2 eggs

2 tablespoons minced parsley

1 tablespoon ground sunflower seeds

1 tablespoon ground pumpkin seeds

½ teaspoon salt

½ teaspoon garlic powder

⅛ teaspoon ground cayenne pepper

Preheat oven to 350°F.

Combine all ingredients until well mixed. Form into patties and place on lightly greased baking sheet. Bake until lightly browned and firm, about 15 minutes, turning halfway through cooking time.

Serves 4.

Substitutions

These are great to pack in a thermos for lunch. I usually prepare them when I have salmon left over from the night before. You can try other types of drier fish for this recipe. Fish that are more moist may need more of the ground seeds to help with the binding. You can use canned boneless, skinless salmon, but try to use fresh wild salmon.

Healthy Tidbit

Salmon is the super food of fish. It is an excellent source of omega-3 fatty acids, which support brain function and act to reduce inflammation in the body. Salmon doesn't concentrate heavy metals like some other types of fish; therefore, it is safer to consume regularly.

Nutritional Analysis per Serving

Vitamin A	66.5 RE	Vitamin D	0.5 µg
Thiamin (B-1)	0.2 mg	Vitamin E	0.2 mg
Riboflavin (B-2)	0.4 mg	Calcium	28.4 mg
Niacin	6.1 mg	Iron	1.5 mg
Vitamin B-6	0.6 mg	Phosphorus	238.8 mg
Vitamin B-12	2.0 µg	Magnesium	45.4 mg
Folate (total)	37.7 µg	Zinc	1.1 mg
Vitamin C	2.7 mg	Potassium	438.4 mg

Fish Tacos with Cilantro Yogurt Sauce

PER SERVING: 581.5 CALORIES ~ 29.7 G PROTEIN ~ 85.7 G CARBOHYDRATE ~ 9.5 G FIBER ~
13.2 G TOTAL FAT ~ 2.4 G SATURATED FAT ~ 60.2 MG CHOLESTEROL ~ 1309.2 MG SODIUM

1 pound tilapia fillets

1 teaspoon lemon juice

2 teaspoons dried dill weed

8 teff, or other wheat-free, tortillas

2 cups cabbage, finely chopped

2 carrots, shredded

1 cup minced onion

1 mango, peeled, seeded, cut into small pieces

¼ cup chopped cilantro

Cilantro Yogurt Sauce (recipe follows)

Preheat oven to 350°F.

Place tilapia on a lightly greased baking sheet or cast iron skillet; drizzle with lemon juice; sprinkle with salt and dill weed. Bake for 8–12 minutes, until fish is tender and flakes with a fork.

Meanwhile, wrap the tortillas in aluminum foil or in a clean kitchen towel, and place them in the oven to warm, about 8–10 minutes.

Place remaining ingredients in individual serving bowls. To make a taco, place a tortilla on the plate; top it with a fish fillet, additional ingredients as desired, and Cilantro Yogurt Sauce.

Serves 4.

Cilantro Yogurt Sauce

1 cup tomatillo salsa

1 bunch cilantro, finely chopped

½ cup Almost Lactose-Free Yogurt (see recipe on page 171)

Juice of 1 lime

¼ to ½ jalapeño, seeded, minced (optional)

¼ teaspoon salt

Combine all ingredients in a medium bowl, whisking until smooth.

Substitutions

You can use any kind of raw veggies for these tacos. Veggies are easier to include in a taco

Nutritional Analysis per Serving

Vitamin A	585.4 RE	Vitamin D	3.5 µg
Thiamin (B-1)	0.1 mg	Vitamin E	0.0 mg
Riboflavin (B-2)	0.2 mg	Calcium	258.6 mg
Niacin	5.3 mg	Iron	3.5 mg
Vitamin B-6	0.4 mg	Phosphorus	265.5 mg
Vitamin B-12	1.7 µg	Magnesium	54.9 mg
Folate (total)	79.9 µg	Zinc	0.8 mg
Vitamin C	49.1 mg	Potassium	728.3 mg

when they're chopped fine. In place of mango you could try pineapple or papaya.

For a dairy-free version of the sauce, just omit the yogurt. For a creamy dairy-free sauce, you can add ½ block of silken tofu.

Healthy Tidbit

Teff is an ancient gluten-free grain that enjoys a long history of use in traditional cooking. Purchase some from the bulk section of a health-food store and experiment. Use it to make cereals and add it to baked goods. There are also online sources for the grain and for teff tortillas. Teff is high in fiber, iron, and calcium, and provides eight amino acids. Because teff isn't used commonly, it hasn't undergone the extensive genetic modification that other, commonly used grains have been subject to.

Crusted Fish

PER SERVING: 278.2 CALORIES ~ 32.7 G PROTEIN ~ 12.5 G CARBOHYDRATE ~ 1.1 G FIBER ~ 10.6 G TOTAL FAT ~ 1.1 G SATURATED FAT ~ 72.6 MG CHOLESTEROL ~ 206.2 MG SODIUM

½ cup finely crushed barbeque-flavored rice chips

3 tablespoons sunflower seeds, ground in coffee grinder

1 pound sole or cod fillets

1 egg white, lightly beaten

Preheat oven to 375°F.

Combine chips and seeds on a large plate. Dip each fillet in egg white and then press it firmly into the rice chip mixture to coat on both sides. Place fillets on a lightly greased baking sheet or well-seasoned cast iron skillet. Bake for 10–14 minutes, until fish is tender and flakes with a fork.

Serves 3.

Substitutions

I have crushed many kinds of rice crackers, chips, seeds, and nuts to coat fish. It is very easy to experiment with different flavors. You don't need any special bread crumbs or any other gluten-containing product to add a tasty crunch to fish fillets.

Healthy Tidbit

Although seafood can offer a good source of fatty acids and protein, the mercury content in fish is a concern nowadays. Especially for infants, children, and women who are or who can become pregnant, fish containing high amounts of mercury should be avoided. Shark, king mackerel, swordfish, golden bass, sea bass, tilefish, Gulf Coast oysters, marlin, halibut, pike, lobster, and tomalley are high in mercury and should be avoided. If you want more information on mercury content in fish and other environmental dangers, visit ewg.org or epa.gov.

Nutritional Analysis per Serving

Vitamin A	6.3 RE	Vitamin D	1.7 µg
Thiamin (B-1)	0.3 mg	Vitamin E	0.0 mg
Riboflavin (B-2)	0.2 mg	Calcium	35.0 mg
Niacin	5.2 mg	Iron	1.0 mg
Vitamin B-6	0.4 mg	Phosphorus	339.3 mg
Vitamin B-12	2.3 µg	Magnesium	77.3 mg
Folate (total)	33.0 µg	Zinc	1.1 mg
Vitamin C	2.7 mg	Potassium	621.8 mg

Easy Teriyaki Salmon

PER SERVING: 379.1 CALORIES ~ 31.8 G PROTEIN ~ 8.2 G CARBOHYDRATE ~ 0.7 G FIBER ~ 23.7 G TOTAL FAT ~ 4.9 G SATURATED FAT ~ 82.2 MG CHOLESTEROL ~ 119.4 MG SODIUM

½ cup Teriyaki Sauce (see recipe on page 110)
1 pound salmon steaks or fillets

Preheat oven to 350°F.

Pour Teriyaki Sauce into a large baking dish. Place salmon skin side up in sauce. Bake for 12–18 minutes, or until salmon is tender and flakes with a fork. Be careful not to overcook the fish, or it will be too dry. Cook it until it flakes but is still bright pink; after you remove it from the oven, it will continue to bake a little longer.

Serves 3.

Substitutions

You can use this recipe as a basic baked salmon recipe, with or without any sauce. For a simpler taste, top the salmon with your favorite seasoning, such as lemon, capers, thyme, garlic, and a little bit of salt, and wrap it in aluminum foil to bake.

Healthy Tidbit

Exercise regularly every week. Although there is no stopping the aging process, research has shown that regular exercise improves physical condition and psychological wellness in people of all ages. In elderly patients, regular exercise can minimize the physiological effects of an otherwise sedentary lifestyle, help to improve memory and general well-being, and even increase active life expectancy. Exercise does this by limiting the development and progression of chronic disease and disabling conditions. Exercise can be started at any age and should be started as soon as you read this tidbit if you don't already have a regular practice. If you don't know where to start, hire a trainer at a gym for a few sessions. If your condition is physically limiting, but you would still like to start an exercise program, seek out a physical therapist to help you understand your options.

Nutritional Analysis per Serving

Vitamin A	23.8 RE	Vitamin D	0.0 µg
Thiamin (B-1)	0.3 mg	Vitamin E	0.0 mg
Riboflavin (B-2)	0.2 mg	Calcium	48.0 mg
Niacin	13.3 mg	Iron	1.1 mg
Vitamin B-6	0.9 mg	Phosphorus	383.7 mg
Vitamin B-12	3.7 µg	Magnesium	52.3 mg
Folate (total)	42.7 µg	Zinc	0.8 mg
Vitamin C	4.9 mg	Potassium	574.6 mg

Tangy Crusted Salmon

PER SERVING: 353.8 CALORIES ~ 30.8 G PROTEIN ~ 26.7 G CARBOHYDRATE ~ 2.8 G FIBER ~
13.5 G TOTAL FAT ~ 1.8 G SATURATED FAT ~ 82.7 MG CHOLESTEROL ~ 596.3 MG SODIUM

1 pound salmon

½ cup gluten-free bread crumbs, finely ground

2 tablespoons honey

2 tablespoons lemon juice

½ teaspoon lemon zest

1 clove garlic, minced

¼ teaspoon horseradish

½ teaspoon salt

Preheat oven to 425°F.

Place salmon, skin side down, on a lightly greased baking dish.

Combine remaining ingredients in a small bowl; spread topping over salmon.

Bake for 15 minutes, or until fish is tender and flakes with a fork.

Serves 3.

Substitutions

You can try other varieties of fish as well as other types of breadcrumbs. You could finely crush some rice crackers or rice chips that you have around. Flavored rice chips can make a good addition.

Healthy Tidbit

Spend time each week in a meditative state or doing some sort of reflection. This is the perfect recipe to give you a little extra time for doing so. Clean as you go so that while the salmon is baking you can sit and meditate for 10 minutes. If you don't have time for 10 minutes, try 5. Set the timer, and let family members know not to disturb you during this time, or have them meditate also. You don't need to know how. Just sit with good posture on a chair, focus on your breathing, and calmly breathe as deeply as possible. Every time your mind wanders, which will be often, gently bring it back to focusing on the breath. You will feel more calm and relaxed prior to enjoying your meal. Learn to look for 5- to 10-minute breaks in your day to allow yourself some reflection time.

Nutritional Analysis per Serving

Vitamin A	16.4 RE	Vitamin D	0.0 µg
Thiamin (B-1)	0.4 mg	Vitamin E	0.0 mg
Riboflavin (B-2)	0.8 mg	Calcium	35.7 mg
Niacin	13.9 mg	Iron	2.3 mg
Vitamin B-6	1.1 mg	Phosphorus	305.4 mg
Vitamin B-12	3.6 µg	Magnesium	45.2 mg
Folate (total)	63.3 µg	Zinc	1.0 mg
Vitamin C	4.9 mg	Potassium	797.5 mg

Shredded Chicken

PER SERVING: 134.0 CALORIES ~ 25.1 G PROTEIN ~ 0.2 G CARBOHYDRATE ~ 0.0 G FIBER ~
2.9 G TOTAL FAT ~ 0.6 G SATURATED FAT ~ 75.4 MG CHOLESTEROL ~ 273.1 MG SODIUM

3 chicken breasts

3 cups water

1 vegetable bouillon cube

Salt to taste

Place chicken, water, and bouillon cube in a crock pot, and cook on low for 8–12 hours. Use a fork to lightly shred the chicken; it should come right apart. Salt to taste. Use the shredded chicken in soups, curries, tacos, and over salad.

Serves 6.

Kitchen Tip

You can start the crock pot at night before going to bed or in the morning before you leave for the day. Once the chicken is finished cooking, your meal will be almost done. Freeze the broth for making soup later.

Substitutions

You can make shredded beef the same way.

Healthy Tidbit

The most important part of a healthy diet is balance and moderation. Limit your intake of animal proteins, but have ways to enjoy lean, healthy meats. A good rule of thumb to follow is that half your plate should be filled with vegetables.

Nutritional Analysis per Serving

Vitamin A	5.6 RE	Vitamin D	0.1 µg
Thiamin (B-1)	0.1 mg	Vitamin E	0.0 mg
Riboflavin (B-2)	0.1 mg	Calcium	9.2 mg
Niacin	9.9 mg	Iron	0.4 mg
Vitamin B-6	0.7 mg	Phosphorus	198.2 mg
Vitamin B-12	0.2 µg	Magnesium	24.2 mg
Folate (total)	2.8 µg	Zinc	0.7 mg
Vitamin C	1.1 mg	Potassium	354.9 mg

Turkey Burgers

PER SERVING: 162.5 CALORIES ~ 29.6 G PROTEIN ~ 4.5 G CARBOHYDRATE ~ 0.7 G FIBER ~
2.6 G TOTAL FAT ~ 1.0 G SATURATED FAT ~ 101.5 MG CHOLESTEROL ~ 100.6 MG SODIUM

1 pound ground turkey

1 egg

¼ cup finely chopped parsley

2 cloves garlic, minced

½ teaspoon dried sage

½ teaspoon dried thyme

½ teaspoon dried marjoram

½ teaspoon dried rosemary, chopped fine

Salt and freshly ground pepper to taste

2 tablespoons quinoa flakes or gluten-free rolled oats

Preheat oven to 450°F.

Mix all ingredients, except quinoa flakes, in large bowl until well blended. Form into patties that are slightly thicker on the edges and thinner in the middle (this allows for more even cooking). Place on broiler pan. Broil at 450°F for 3 minutes on each side. Reduce heat to 350°F and bake for another 25 minutes.

Serves 4.

Substitutions
You could use any ground meat to make these burgers, such as buffalo or lamb.

Kitchen Tip
Serve these burgers with a big tasty salad. Think about what you can add to your diet more than what you need to eliminate. Concentrate on getting more servings of vegetables and fruits per day and consuming additional fish and good oils. The rest should fall into place.

Nutritional Analysis per Serving

Vitamin A	54.6 RE	Vitamin D	0.3 µg
Thiamin (B-1)	0.0 mg	Vitamin E	0.1 mg
Riboflavin (B-2)	0.1 mg	Calcium	25.5 mg
Niacin	0.2 mg	Iron	1.8 mg
Vitamin B-6	0.1 mg	Phosphorus	54.3 mg
Vitamin B-12	0.1 µg	Magnesium	15.6 mg
Folate (total)	22.8 µg	Zinc	0.4 mg
Vitamin C	5.8 mg	Potassium	79.1 mg

Green Curry

PER SERVING: 519.0 CALORIES ~ 33.7 G PROTEIN ~ 28.4 G CARBOHYDRATE ~ 5.1 G FIBER ~
33.0 G TOTAL FAT ~ 26.4 G SATURATED FAT ~ 74.0 MG CHOLESTEROL ~ 1809.2 MG SODIUM

I have made this curry many times. Its long list of ingredients may seem daunting, but it is actually very quick and easy to prepare and very versatile; you
can change the veggies and protein source each time you make it. If you are
worried about having too much spice for the younger ones, omit the jalapeño
in the paste and add it to the spicy sauce, which is served on the side. You can
make double the paste and freeze it for an easy dinner in the future.

For the Green Curry Paste
1 stalk lemongrass

½ cup chopped cilantro

½ cup chopped fresh basil

¼ cup chopped purple onion

1 2-inch piece gingerroot, sliced

5 cloves garlic

½ jalapeño pepper, seeded

½ teaspoon ground coriander

½ teaspoon ground cumin

½ teaspoon ground white pepper

3 tablespoons fish sauce

1 teaspoon anchovy paste (or 2 anchovy fillets)

1 tablespoon lime juice

2 teaspoons pure maple syrup

¼ 14-ounce can whole coconut milk

For the Hot Sauce
¼ cup Green Curry Paste

1 jalapeño pepper, seeded

1 2-inch piece gingerroot, peeled and sliced

¼ cup chopped purple onion

2 cloves garlic

For the Green Curry
2 tablespoons coconut oil

Green Curry Paste

1 pound boneless, skinless chicken breast, sliced into ½-inch-thick strips

¾ 14-ounce can coconut milk

1 yellow pepper, julienned

3 small zucchinis, julienned

2 cups chopped broccoli florets
1 pint cherry tomatoes, halved
½ cup chicken broth (optional)
Fish sauce and fresh lime juice to taste (optional)
Hot Sauce (recipe included here)

To make the green curry paste: Remove tough outer leaves from lemongrass and cut off the end. Finely chop the stalk.

Combine lemongrass and remaining ingredients in a food processor or blender. Process until smooth, adding additional coconut milk and broth as needed to blend.

To make the hot sauce: Combine in a food processor or blender; process until smooth, adding a small amount of water if needed to blend.

To make the green curry: Heat coconut oil in a wok or large skillet over medium-high heat until hot; stir in Green Curry Paste. Stir-fry until fragrant, 1–2 minutes. Add chicken and coconut milk; heat to boiling. Reduce heat and simmer 5 minutes. Add vegetables and simmer until chicken is cooked and vegetables are tender but remain crunchy, about 10 minutes. If more liquid is needed or you want more sauce, add chicken broth, a couple of tablespoons at a time. Adjust flavors by adding more fish sauce or lime juice, and serve with Hot Sauce.

Serves 4.

Substitutions

Omit cherry tomatoes for individuals with arthritis or who are sensitive to tomatoes. Most fish sauces are gluten free, but make sure to check the label for thickeners.

Experiment with other vegetables of your choice—green beans, bamboo shoots, yellow squash, carrots, cabbage.

Healthy Tidbit

Various studies have shown that hot spices such as pepper, garlic, cayenne, and ginger have positive effects on digestion, nutrient absorption, fat breakdown, appetite control, and possibly LDL cholesterol levels (the "bad" cholesterol).

Nutritional Analysis per Serving

Vitamin A	170.3 RE	Vitamin D	0.1 µg
Thiamin (B-1)	0.3 mg	Vitamin E	0.4 mg
Riboflavin (B-2)	0.4 mg	Calcium	146.4 mg
Niacin	12.3 mg	Iron	5.9 mg
Vitamin B-6	1.3 mg	Phosphorus	434.7 mg
Vitamin B-12	0.2 µg	Magnesium	134.6 mg
Folate (total)	117.4 µg	Zinc	2.4 mg
Vitamin C	176.7 mg	Potassium	1537.8 mg

Turmeric Lentils with Chard

PER SERVING: 466.3 CALORIES ~ 26.8 G PROTEIN ~ 64.3 G CARBOHYDRATE ~ 31.0 G FIBER ~
11.9 G TOTAL FAT ~ 3.0 G SATURATED FAT ~ 7.8 MG CHOLESTEROL ~ 127.7 MG SODIUM

This is one of my favorite meals to make when I haven't gone grocery shopping. I always keep lentils on hand and usually have some form of green. I have experimented with this recipe in various ways, and they all turn out well. My current favorite modification is to add a little seasoned chicken sausage. It's easy to make this dish vegetarian, though, by eliminating the sausage.

2 cups red lentils

4 cups water

1 salt-free vegetable bouillon cube

2 tablespoons olive oil

1 tablespoon butter

1 tablespoon mustard seeds

1 onion, chopped

2 cloves garlic, minced

2 teaspoons turmeric

1 teaspoon ground coriander

½ teaspoon cumin

1 bunch Swiss chard, chopped

1 pound Italian chicken sausage, cooked (optional)

Salt to taste

Combine lentils, water, and bouillon in a medium saucepan; heat to boiling. Reduce heat and simmer, covered, until water is absorbed, about 30 minutes.

Heat oil and butter in a large saucepan over medium-low heat until hot but not smoking; add mustard seeds, cover, and cook for about 1 minute. Add onion, garlic, and spices, and sauté until onion is tender, about 5 minutes. Stir in chard and sausage (if using). Cook, stirring occasionally, until chard is wilted, about 2 minutes. Add lentils and cook about 5 minutes, until flavors are mingled. Season to taste with salt.

Serves 4.

Substitutions

Experiment with using any variety of cooking greens or sausage, or omit the sausage altogether. You can add different spices or use different types

Nutritional Analysis per Serving

Vitamin A	252.7 RE	Vitamin D	0.1 µg
Thiamin (B-1)	0.9 mg	Vitamin E	0.1 mg
Riboflavin (B-2)	0.3 mg	Calcium	103.8 mg
Niacin	2.9 mg	Iron	8.8 mg
Vitamin B-6	0.6 mg	Phosphorus	486.3 mg
Vitamin B-12	0.0 µg	Magnesium	164.7 mg
Folate (total)	475.3 µg	Zinc	5.0 mg
Vitamin C	18.8 mg	Potassium	1163.7 mg

of lentils. Try using a homemade stock in place of the bouillon; it increases the flavor dramatically.

Healthy Tidbit

Lentils are my favorite legume. They don't have to be soaked, so they are easy to prepare quickly. Even if my cupboards are relatively empty, I can usually make something tasty with lentils and chicken broth or vegetable broth in a very short amount of time. You can dilute the broth to half strength with water; this will help the liquid absorb into the lentils more easily. Lentils are high in iron, amino acids, and B vitamins. They help to stabilize blood sugar and have been shown to improve cholesterol levels.

Chicken Wraps

PER SERVING: 230.9 CALORIES ~ 29.1 G PROTEIN ~ 15.5 G CARBOHYDRATE ~ 2.5 G FIBER ~ 5.9 G TOTAL FAT ~ 1.3 G SATURATED FAT ~ 72.4 MG CHOLESTEROL ~ 844.7 MG SODIUM

For the Faux Peanut Sauce
2 tablespoons Sun Butter (see page 121)
2 tablespoons garlic black bean sauce
2 tablespoons minced gingerroot
2 cloves garlic
1 tablespoon gluten-free tamari sauce
4 tablespoons water

For the Chicken Wraps
1 pound boneless, skinless chicken breast
Juice of 1 lime
1 tablespoon gluten-free tamari
1 large carrot
1 head butter or Boston lettuce, separated into leaves
1½ cups bean sprouts
1 cup Cucumber Salad (see recipe on page 83)
Faux Peanut Sauce (recipe included here)

To make the Faux Peanut Sauce: Combine all ingredients in a blender; blend until smooth.

Yields ¾ cup sauce (4 servings).

To make the Chicken Wraps: Preheat oven to 350°F.

Place chicken breast in a lightly greased baking dish; top with lime juice and tamari. Bake until cooked, about 25–30 minutes.

With a vegetable peeler, shave the carrot into long strips. Arrange carrot, lettuce, sprouts, and Cucumber Salad on a serving platter. When chicken is cooked, cut into slices and arrange on the platter.

To assemble: Place chicken on lettuce leaf; top with desired ingredients and Faux Peanut Sauce. Roll into wraps.

Serves 4.

Substitutions

Instead of the Faux Peanut Sauce, you could use simple tamari, Bragg Liquid Aminos, Honey Mustard (see recipe on page 114), or Vegan Cashew Sauce (see recipe on page 117). You could use a variety of fillings, including shredded cabbage, pickled onions, green onions, scrambled eggs, and more.

Healthy Tidbit

Don't give up on eating out. You can always order a salad and tell them to hold the cheese. I get some of my best ideas from going out. This recipe is a perfect example. I love ordering lettuce wraps. I like them because I can control what I put in the wrap, so if I go back to that restaurant I will ask, "Can you just give me double the shredded carrots and omit the gluten noodles, please?" It is so helpful to be able to eat out. You just have to learn the art of ordering and the art of self-control. Simply decide ahead of time that you won't be ordering the fettuccini alfredo!

Nutritional Analysis per Serving

Vitamin A	400.9 RE	Vitamin D	0.1 µg
Thiamin (B-1)	0.1 mg	Vitamin E	0.0 mg
Riboflavin (B-2)	0.2 mg	Calcium	47.8 mg
Niacin	10.2 mg	Iron	2.1 mg
Vitamin B-6	0.8 mg	Phosphorus	245.9 mg
Vitamin B-12	0.1 µg	Magnesium	45.8 mg
Folate (total)	64.5 µg	Zinc	1.1 mg
Vitamin C	15.3 mg	Potassium	638.7 mg

Spiced Chicken

PER SERVING: 530.5 CALORIES ~ 28.3 G PROTEIN ~ 2.7 G CARBOHYDRATE ~ 0.6 G FIBER ~
45.4 G TOTAL FAT ~ 24.8 G SATURATED FAT ~ 118.3 MG CHOLESTEROL ~ 90.7 MG SODIUM

¾ cup coconut oil

⅔ cup lemon juice

2 tablespoons dried thyme leaves

2 teaspoons garlic powder

1 teaspoon ground cumin

½ teaspoon ground turmeric

4 pounds chicken, cut into pieces

Salt (optional)

Combine all ingredients except chicken in a small bowl, mixing well. Place chicken in a large zipper-lock bag or glass bowl; pour marinade over the top, tossing to coat well. Refrigerate for several hours or overnight.

Preheat oven to 350°F.

Arrange chicken in a single layer on a broiler-proof baking dish. Bake for 1 hour and then sprinkle with salt (optional), if desired.

Preheat broiler. Place chicken under broiler and broil 3–5 minutes or until golden brown. Chicken should be cooked to meat thermometer reading of 170°F.

Serves 8.

Substitutions
If you want more spice, add freshly ground black or white pepper. Cayenne makes a wonderful addition to this dish as well. Most of the time, because I have children, I don't make it too spicy, but my husband and I add spice prior to eating it, if needed.

Kitchen Tip
Water follows salt. This is an important chemistry tip to remember when cooking meats. It is best to undersalt until the meat is fully cooked. If you salt prior to cooking and the meat is resting in salt, the moisture will leave the meat. So if you want your meat to remain moist, salt only modestly until the meal is prepared, and salt before serving if desired.

Nutritional Analysis per Serving

Vitamin A	52.5 RE	Vitamin D	0.0 µg
Thiamin (B-1)	0.1 mg	Vitamin E	0.0 mg
Riboflavin (B-2)	0.2 mg	Calcium	39.8 mg
Niacin	8.7 mg	Iron	2.9 mg
Vitamin B-6	0.4 mg	Phosphorus	223.7 mg
Vitamin B-12	0.3 µg	Magnesium	27.5 mg
Folate (total)	13.2 µg	Zinc	1.9 mg
Vitamin C	8.4 mg	Potassium	301.1 mg

Turkey Balls with Brown Rice

PER SERVING: 386.0 CALORIES ~ 23.4 G PROTEIN ~ 24.5 G CARBOHYDRATE ~ 2.1 G FIBER ~
21.8 G TOTAL FAT ~ 5.0 G SATURATED FAT ~ 91.5 MG CHOLESTEROL ~ 613.4 MG SODIUM

This recipe was contributed by Kimberly Carson from Oregon Health and
Science University.

2 cups loosely packed fresh spinach leaves, chopped fine

3 cloves garlic, minced

1 tablespoon olive oil

1 pound ground turkey

3 tablespoons goat cheese (optional)

2 tablespoons gluten-free tamari (or Bragg Liquid Aminos)

2 tablespoons goddess dressing (e.g., Annie's)

2 cups cooked brown rice, warm

Preheat oven to 375°F.

Sauté the spinach and garlic in oil in a large skillet until spinach is wilted,
about 3 minutes. Drain excess liquid. Combine spinach, turkey, goat cheese,
tamari, and salt in a large bowl; mix well. Using a teaspoon, shape into 24
small balls and place on a foil-lined cookie sheet. Drizzle with dressing and
bake 15–18 minutes, or until browned and cooked through. Serve over rice.

Serves 4.

Substitutions

You can easily omit the goat cheese from this recipe. If your diet is already low
in dairy but you can tolerate a little bit, then a treat once in a while is a great
thing!

Healthy Tidbit

Routine is one of the most important things you can do for your health.
Adopting regular habits around time spent sleeping, waking, eating, and
exercising can help to regulate your hormone secretions. Routine is therefore
especially important for those who have hormone-related complaints such as
thyroid irregularities, adrenal
issues, or menstrual problems.
Routine can also help reduce
anxiety, improve breathing
patterns, and decrease susceptibility to infections.

Nutritional Analysis per Serving

Vitamin A	175.7 RE	Vitamin D	0.5 µg
Thiamin (B-1)	0.2 mg	Vitamin E	0.1 mg
Riboflavin (B-2)	0.3 mg	Calcium	68.7 mg
Niacin	7.4 mg	Iron	2.8 mg
Vitamin B-6	0.8 mg	Phosphorus	297.0 mg
Vitamin B-12	1.5 µg	Magnesium	76.4 mg
Folate (total)	40.2 µg	Zinc	3.9 mg
Vitamin C	4.9 mg	Potassium	368.1 mg

Porcupines

PER SERVING: 302.7 CALORIES ~ 26.8 G PROTEIN ~ 23.0 G CARBOHYDRATE ~ 1.7 G FIBER ~
9.3 G TOTAL FAT ~ 1.6 G SATURATED FAT ~ 0.6 MG CHOLESTEROL ~ 955.0 MG SODIUM

Inspired by Alice Black, my mother-in-law. These meatballs were my husband's favorite when he was growing up, so I had to include a version of them. We made them one year for our New Year's Eve party and everyone loved them.

½ cup uncooked short-grain brown rice	½ teaspoon celery salt
¾ cup water	¼ teaspoon garlic powder
1 pound ground buffalo	¼ teaspoon freshly ground pepper
⅓ cup chopped onion	2 tablespoons olive oil
1 egg (optional)	½ cup dry white wine
2 teaspoons Worcestershire sauce	1 cup Lentil or Roasted Red Pepper Soup
1 teaspoon salt	(see recipes on pages 232 and 234)

Soak rice with ½ cup water in medium sauce pan for at least an hour (see page 219). After soaking, heat to boiling: simmer 5 minutes. Drain well. Combine rice, ¼ cup water, buffalo, onion, egg (if using), Worcestershire sauce, and seasonings until well blended. Form into 1½-inch balls. Cook meatballs in oil in large skillet, turning occasionally until meatballs are browned on all sides. Pour in the soup and wine. Heat to boiling, reduce heat, cover, and simmer for 45 minutes, or until rice is tender, turning the meatballs occasionally. Add additional water if sauce becomes too thick. Spoon sauce over meatballs to serve.
    Serves 4.

Substitutions
You could use grass-fed beef for these meatballs. Another cooking method is to brown the meatballs and transfer them to a small baking dish. Pour the soup and wine over the meatballs and bake, covered, at 350°F for 45 minutes; uncover and bake for an additional 15 minutes.

Healthy Tidbit
Make sure to have a conscious relationship with food. Don't eat mindlessly. We have all been caught eating in the car, at our desk, or gulping down a quick snack in between commitments. Your relationship with food drastically affects your ability to achieve satiety and maintain proper weight. Having a poor

Nutritional Analysis per Serving

Vitamin A	83.6 RE	Vitamin D	0.0 mg
Thiamin (B-1)	0.3 mg	Vitamin E	0.0 mg
Riboflavin (B-2)	0.4 mg	Calcium	24.3 mg
Niacin	9.2 mg	Iron	3.7 mg
Vitamin B-6	1.1 mg	Phosphorus	308.5 mg
Vitamin B-12	1.3 µg	Magnesium	67.6 mg
Folate (total)	20.7 µg	Zinc	4.0 mg
Vitamin C	35.2 mg	Potassium	583.1 mg

relationship with food and eating the wrong types of foods will most often leave you hungry and lead to weight gain. Remember to slow down, chew and admire your food, eat in a relaxed environment, and don't overeat.

Delicious Meatloaf

PER SERVING: 386.9 CALORIES ~ 32.9 G PROTEIN ~ 9.3 G CARBOHYDRATE ~ 1.3 G FIBER ~ 23.9 G TOTAL FAT ~ 7.8 G SATURATED FAT ~ 169.4 MG CHOLESTEROL ~ 571.6 MG SODIUM

For the Meatloaf Glaze
1 2-ounce jar pimentos, drained
1 tablespoon honey
1 teaspoon ground cumin
1 teaspoon Worcestershire sauce
½ teaspoon hot sauce

For the Meatloaf
½ onion, coarsely chopped
1 carrot, coarsely chopped
5 cloves garlic
¼ cup Organic 5-Grain Cereal Mix (see recipe on page 123)
1 teaspoon chili powder
1 teaspoon dried thyme
1½ teaspoons salt
½ teaspoon ground black pepper
½ teaspoon cayenne pepper
1½ pounds ground beef
1½ pounds ground turkey
2 eggs

To make the meatloaf glaze: Double this recipe if you are using 2 loaf pans. Combine all ingredients in a blender; blend until smooth.

To make the meatloaf: Preheat oven to 325°F.

Combine onion, carrot, garlic, cereal, and seasonings in a food processor; process until vegetables are finely chopped. Stir together vegetable mixture, meat, and eggs until thoroughly blended. Pack mixture into a 3-pound loaf pan, or divide between 2 smaller loaf pans. Bake for 30 minutes, or until

Nutritional Analysis per Serving

Vitamin A	207.6 RE	Vitamin D	0.7 µg
Thiamin (B-1)	0.1 mg	Vitamin E	0.2 mg
Riboflavin (B-2)	0.4 mg	Calcium	66.8 mg
Niacin	8.3 mg	Iron	3.8 mg
Vitamin B-6	0.7 mg	Phosphorus	355.9 mg
Vitamin B-12	2.6 µg	Magnesium	47.4 mg
Folate (total)	23.1 µg	Zinc	6.6 mg
Vitamin C	7.8 mg	Potassium	535.5 mg

top begins to brown; spoon Meatloaf Glaze onto meatloaf. Continue baking until the center of the meatloaf reaches 155°F on a meat thermometer, about 1–2 hours, depending on whether you use 1 or 2 pans.

Serves 8.

Substitutions

Try various types of meat for this recipe. For a version with less animal protein and the added benefit of legumes, reduce the meat by half and substitute 1½ cups of cooked, mashed lentils. Another great additive is grated zucchini. It will help the meatloaf maintain its moisture.

Kitchen Tips

When you insert the thermometer probe, make sure it does not touch the bottom of the pan. To make a meatloaf shape without having to cut the cooked product out of the pan, pack the mixture into a loaf pan, then carefully turn the meatloaf out onto the center of a baking sheet lined with parchment paper. Smooth the edges if needed. It will hold its shape while baking.

Healthy Tidbit

Garlic affords significant health benefits, including but not limited to blood-thinning, antiseptic, antibacterial, and anti-inflammatory properties. Cooked garlic offers less medicinal effect, but it still shows benefit for cardiovascular conditions. Raw crushed garlic is extremely antimicrobial. Use caution when consuming raw garlic, as it can be irritating or caustic if used regularly in sensitive individuals.

Garlic Buffalo Meatballs and Linguini

PER SERVING: 332.4 CALORIES ~ 21.5 G PROTEIN ~ 41.2 G CARBOHYDRATE ~ 3.8 G FIBER ~ 9.2 G TOTAL FAT ~ 1.7 G SATURATED FAT ~ 62.0 MG CHOLESTEROL ~ 518.7 MG SODIUM

2 tablespoons olive oil, divided

1 pound ground buffalo

½ cup gluten-free bread crumbs

2 eggs

2 tablespoons minced fresh garlic, divided

1 tablespoon dried basil leaves

1 tablespoon dried oregano leaves

1 tablespoon dried parsley flakes

1 tablespoon garlic powder

1 teaspoon dried, crushed rosemary leaves

1 teaspoon dried marjoram leaves

1 teaspoon salt, divided

1 8-ounce package gluten-free linguine, cooked al dente, warm

⅓ cup minced fresh parsley

Preheat oven to 350°F.

Grease a 13×9-inch baking dish with 1 tablespoon olive oil, and place it in the oven while the oven is heating. Combine buffalo, bread crumbs, eggs,

1 tablespoon minced garlic, herbs, and 2 teaspoons salt in a medium bowl; mix well with hands until thoroughly blended. Form into golf ball–sized meatballs. Place about 1 inch apart in the hot baking dish.

Bake for 15 minutes; then turn meatballs and continue baking for about 10 more minutes, or until browned.

Sauté remaining 1 tablespoon minced garlic in remaining 1 tablespoon oil in a small skillet until tender but not browned, about 2 minutes.

While meatballs are baking, cook linguine. Toss linguine in serving bowl with sautéed garlic, fresh parsley, and remaining 1 teaspoon salt. Top with meatballs.

Serves 6.

Healthy Tidbit

Eat fresh, locally grown food as much as possible. Joining a neighborhood farm or a CSA (community supported agriculture) farm can be a great way to obtain local ingredients while also supporting family farms and reducing the use of fossil fuels to ship produce from far away. CSAs supply a group of subscribers with a weekly allotment of veggies and root crops, as well as extras like flowers, eggs, maple syrup, vinegars, and other items that are in season. The cost is around $350 or $450 per year, depending on how large a share of vegetables the customer wants. Some CSAs even offer meat from humanely raised, free-range, grass-fed animals.

Joining a CSA may encourage you to try new foods that you never would have purchased at the supermarket. All in all, becoming a "locavore" by buying fresh and local is good for the gut and for the environment. Books such as *The Omnivore's Dilemma*, by Michael Pollan, are informative resources. You can even start a garden and grown your own fruits and vegetables. There is nothing better than cooking together as a family, going out to your garden to pick fresh lettuce in the summer, and making a salad while sipping some red wine.

Nutritional Analysis per Serving

Vitamin A	65.3 RE	Vitamin D	0.3 µg
Thiamin (B-1)	0.2 mg	Vitamin E	0.2 mg
Riboflavin (B-2)	0.4 mg	Calcium	67.1 mg
Niacin	6.4 mg	Iron	5.0 mg
Vitamin B-6	0.7 mg	Phosphorus	200.6 mg
Vitamin B-12	1.0 µg	Magnesium	30.9 mg
Folate (total)	32.5 µg	Zinc	2.7 mg
Vitamin C	5.8 mg	Potassium	392.3 mg

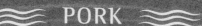

Pork and Chicken Patties

PER SERVING: 361.6 CALORIES ~ 30.5 G PROTEIN ~ 2.9 G CARBOHYDRATE ~ 0.7 G FIBER ~
24.7 G TOTAL FAT ~ 8.7 G SATURATED FAT ~ 156.9 MG CHOLESTEROL ~ 110.5 MG SODIUM

1½ pounds ground pork

1½ pounds ground chicken

1 egg

2 tablespoons red wine vinegar

1 teaspoon honey

1 tablespoon dried parsley

1 tablespoon garlic powder

1 tablespoon onion powder

1 tablespoon dried basil

2 teaspoons paprika

½ teaspoon ground fennel seed

¼ teaspoon dried oregano

Salt and freshly ground pepper to taste

Preheat oven to 450°F.

Mix all ingredients in large bowl until well blended. Form half the mixture into 8 patties that are slightly thicker on the edges, and thinner in the middle (this allows for more even cooking). Broil for 3 minutes on each side. Reduce heat to 350°F and bake for another 25 minutes. (Broiling first helps to keep moisture in while baking.)

Serves 8.

Substitutions

You are welcome to try a variety of meats for this recipe. Experiment with ground chicken, turkey, or buffalo. You can also vary the seasonings. These burgers are easy to make and easy to serve leftover the next day.

Healthy Tidbit

Pork has relatively high levels of saturated fats compared to some other meats, but lower levels of arachidonic acid (a chemical that triggers inflammation). Consume pork in moderation. In general, I suggest that my patients maintain a heavily plant-based diet with meats on the side. I included a few pork recipes in this book to offer variety.

Nutritional Analysis per Serving

Vitamin A	44.5 RE	Vitamin D	0.1 µg
Thiamin (B-1)	0.5 mg	Vitamin E	0.1 mg
Riboflavin (B-2)	0.4 mg	Calcium	41.3 mg
Niacin	8.4 mg	Iron	2.3 mg
Vitamin B-6	0.7 mg	Phosphorus	324.1 mg
Vitamin B-12	1.0 µg	Magnesium	42.4 mg
Folate (total)	10.0 µg	Zinc	3.3 mg
Vitamin C	0.9 mg	Potassium	750.5 mg

Polenta Lasagna

PER SERVING: 187.9 CALORIES ~ 9.2 G PROTEIN ~ 19.1 G CARBOHYDRATE ~ 2.0 G FIBER ~
8.0 G TOTAL FAT ~ 1.5 G SATURATED FAT ~ 31.1 MG CHOLESTEROL ~ 628.0 MG SODIUM

1 purple onion, chopped

1 cup mushrooms, chopped

5 cloves garlic, minced

¼ cup olive oil

1 pound chicken or pork Italian sausage

½ head cauliflower, chopped small

¼ cup dry white wine or water

1 teaspoon dried basil leaves

1 teaspoon dried oregano leaves

1 16-ounce jar spaghetti sauce

1 14.5-ounce can diced tomatoes

1 16-ounce package prepared polenta, cut lengthwise into thin slices

2 tablespoons pure maple syrup

1 cup Parmesan or Romano cheese (optional)

Preheat oven to 350°F.

Sauté onion, mushrooms, and garlic in oil in a large skillet until tender, about 5 minutes; add sausage and cauliflower. Sauté until sausage is cooked through and browned, about 10 minutes. Add wine and herbs, and simmer until wine is absorbed, about 3 minutes.

Combine spaghetti sauce and diced tomatoes in a medium bowl. Spoon a small amount of sauce into a lasagna pan or a 13 × 9-inch pan. Top with a layer of polenta; drizzle with maple syrup. Top with a thin layer of sauce; continue layering polenta, sauce, and maple syrup until all polenta is used, saving ⅓ of the sauce for the top. Spread sausage mixture over polenta and top with remaining sauce. Sprinkle with cheese, if desired. Bake 20–30 minutes.

Serves 12.

Substitutions

This simple, throw-together meal can tolerate lots of variations. You could use homemade polenta instead of store-bought. Just cook the polenta, chill it in a loaf pan, and slice it. I am a fan of how the cauliflower and

Nutritional Analysis per Serving			
Vitamin A	43.5 RE	Vitamin D	0.0 µg
Thiamin (B-1)	0.0 mg	Vitamin E	0.0 mg
Riboflavin (B-2)	0.1 mg	Calcium	36.0 mg
Niacin	0.5 mg	Iron	1.6 mg
Vitamin B-6	0.1 mg	Phosphorus	23.3 mg
Vitamin B-12	0.0 µg	Magnesium	8.0 mg
Folate (total)	17.6 µg	Zinc	0.2 mg
Vitamin C	18.0 mg	Potassium	130.7 mg

mushrooms complement each other, but you could experiment with other vegetables. The sausage adds flavor without much effort but is not needed if you are concerned about the seasonings in the sausage or if you are vegetarian. If you cannot tolerate tomatoes, you can easily substitute an organic puréed soup; for example, Roasted Red Pepper Soup (see recipe on page 234).

Healthy Tidbit
Mushrooms provide great immune support. Sautéed, they also offer a satisfying meatlike texture to vegetarian meals.

Grains

Grains are relatively easy to cook, and they make a hearty addition to many entrées, soups, and salads. Cooking them overnight in a crock pot brings out their natural sweetness and breaks them down for easier digestion.

To further enhance digestion, make it a goal to soak all of your grains before cooking. Soaking breaks down some of the hard-to-digest proteins. This step is especially important for a sensitive or ill person. Soaking the grain also helps the vitamins and minerals become easier to absorb. Soaking neutralizes phytic acid, which can interfere with proper absorption of the minerals calcium, magnesium, iron, zinc, and copper. Because grains are seeds, they contain an anti-enzyme that acts as protection, allowing them to withstand harsh winter conditions or long storage. Soaking helps to neutralize this substance.

Grains should be soaked for 12–24 hours. Cooking times for soaked grains are usually a little less than for dried grains; therefore, soaking can save you some time in the kitchen. After soaking grains overnight, you may notice little sprouts starting to form. You can prepare and eat the sprouted grain as you would an unsprouted grain.

Soaking is generally an optional step in rice cooking, but it will help people with sensitive digestion assimilate the rice more effectively. Fragrant basmati rice will hold its flavor better if soaked first. Because some of the water is absorbed during soaking, the cooking time is lessened, thus preserving flavor. The flavor of basmati rice is what suffers when it's not soaked, rather than the texture. Even soaking rice for 30 minutes before cooking will offer some benefit.

Grain Cooking Instructions

Grain (1 cup)	Cups water	Cook time (soaked)	Cook time (dry)	Cups yield
Amaranth	3	10–20 minutes	20–30 minutes	3
Basmati rice	1.5	10–20 minutes	15–25 minutes	2⅓–3
Brown rice, short and long grain	2	45 minutes	1 hour	3
Buckwheat (kasha)	2	10–20 minutes	20–30 minutes	2½
Millet	2	35–50 minutes	45–60 minutes	3
Oat berries	2½	20–30 minutes	45–60 minutes	3

Grain Cooking Instructions (cont'd.)

Grain (1 cup)	Cups water	Cook time (soaked)	Cook time (dry)	Cups yield
Oats, rolled	2	5–10 minutes	15 minutes	2
Oats, steelcut	3	15 minutes	25 minutes	3½
Quinoa	2	10–20 minutes	20–30 minutes	3
Teff	3	15 minutes	20–30 minutes	3½
Wild rice	3	45–60 minutes	60 minutes or more	4

Soaking Grains

1 cup grain (see table above for a list of some grains that are suitable for soaking)

1 tablespoon whey or apple cider vinegar

Warm water*

* Use the amount of water you would normally use to cook the grain, according to the table above.

Combine all ingredients in a medium saucepan or rice cooker; allow to soak overnight. The next day, cook according to the chart above, skimming off any scum that forms on the surface during cooking. You can use the same water you have soaked your grains in or discard it and use fresh water.

Legumes

Legumes and beans, a staple food in most cultures, can be a great source of affordable protein for those wanting to limit their animal consumption. Legumes are packed with vitamins and minerals and offer a cholesterol-smart choice. Choose dried beans over canned to avoid the chemicals and salt that may be added during the canning process. Soaking and cooking dried beans is extremely easy with a little advance planning.

Legumes offer an excellent dietary source of soluble fiber. Soluble fiber supports the body's regulation of cholesterol and has been shown to decrease LDL cholesterol, the "bad" cholesterol. In addition, it helps to regulate blood sugar levels—balancing the peaks and valleys—resulting in reduced diabetic tendency, better mood, and better weight control. Legumes also contain insoluble fiber, which helps improve constipation and other gastrointestinal problems.

Legumes are easy to store. I devote a section of my pantry to legumes and grains. If you have some legumes on hand, you can easily fix dinner in a pinch. If you are between paychecks and can't afford to go grocery shopping at the moment, a tasty dinner of rice and beans will satisfy the family while providing complete protein. Rice and beans is a favorite dish of mine to pack in school lunches. It is affordable, and I can warm it up in the morning to send in a thermos. My kids have grown to love rice and beans, the simple staple from around the world!

Most legumes should be soaked overnight before cooking. I soak them for at least eight hours, and sometimes longer depending on the legume. Unlike grains, the soaking water from legumes is best discarded in the morning. Cook them in fresh water. As beans soak, they release oligosaccharides into the water. Oligosaccharides, indigestible complex sugars, are the main reason why beans can produce gas. Soaking beans helps to minimize the gas-producing sugar as well as removing tannins and phytic acid, which can interfere with absorption of nutrients.

Another reason why legumes should be soaked is because they have not yet been washed. Depending on where they came from, they were picked, sorted, transferred, and have gone through many hands before they arrive in your home. Legumes can't be washed before packing because of the risk of developing mold. So make sure your beans are soaked and rinsed thoroughly. Some grains, such as split peas and lentils, don't need to be soaked; rinse them well in a strainer prior to use.

Legumes are high in a variety of nutrients including iron, calcium, and protein. When combined with whole grains like buckwheat, brown rice, millet, quinoa, and teff, legumes provide the full complement of essential amino acids needed by humans. We call this a complete protein. Most grains and legumes have a variety of amino acids but on their own don't provide a complete protein.

In a pinch, many legumes can be "flash soaked." Place beans in a medium to large saucepan (depending on the quantity of beans); add water to cover by 2 inches. Bring to a boil and continue boiling for at least 5 minutes. Remove from heat, and allow to soak for at least an hour. Beans that are listed in the table below as needing 8 hours or more soaking time won't do as well with the flash-soaking process. They have tougher shells and need more soaking time.

For extremely sensitive digestion, I suggest a triple-soak process. Soak the beans for 12 hours, pour off the water, rinse the beans, pick off anything that has floated to the top, and add new filtered water. Soak a second time for 12 hours and repeat the process above. Soak for a third 12-hour time period and then cook. This process continues the breakdown of the outer covering of the legume and promotes easier digestion.

Legume Soaking and Cooking Instructions

Legume (1 Cup Dry)	Cups Water	Soaking Time	Cooking Time	Cups Yield
Adzuki (aduki)	4	None	45–55 minutes	3
Anasazi	2½–3	5–8 hours	45–55 minutes	2¼
Black beans	4	5–8 hours	1–1½ hours	2¼
Black-eyed peas	3	None	1 hour	2
Cannellini (white kidney beans)	3	5–8 hours	45 minutes	2½
Cranberry bean	3	5–8 hours	40–45 minutes	3
Fava beans, skins removed	3	8 hours to overnight	40–50 minutes	1⅔
Garbanzos (chick peas)	4	8 hours to overnight	1–3 hours	2
Great Northern beans	3½	5–8 hours	1½ hours	2⅔
Green split peas	4	None	45 minutes	2
Green peas (freeze-dried), whole	6	5–8 hours	1–2 hours	2
Red kidney beans	3	5–8 hours	1 hour	2¼
Lentils, brown	2¼	None	45 minutes–1 hour	2¼

(cont'd.)

Legume Soaking and Cooking Instructions (cont'd.)

Legume (1 Cup Dry)	Cups Water	Soaking Time	Cooking Time	Cups Yield
Lentils, green	2	None	30–45 min	2
Lentils, red	3	None	20–30 minutes	2–2½
Lima beans, large	4	8 hours to overnight	45–1 hour	2½
Mung beans	2½	5–8 hours	1 hour	2
Navy beans	3	5–8 hours	45–60 minutes	2⅔
Pink chili beans	3	5–8 hours	50–60 minutes	2¾
Pinto beans	3	5–8 hours	1½ hours	2⅔
Small red beans (Mexican red bean)	4	5–8 hours	45–60 minutes	2
Soybeans	4	8 hours or overnight	3–4 hours	3
Yellow split peas	4	None	1–1½ hrs	2

Soaking Legumes

1 cup dried legumes
Water

Pick through the beans carefully, discarding any pebbles and any beans that look odd or rotten. Place beans in a medium saucepan or glass bowl, add water to cover by 2 inches, and soak overnight.

After soaking, discard any beans that have floated to the top; drain and rinse beans thoroughly. Prepare for cooking as described in the table above.

Sometimes legumes that have soaked overnight will sprout. Cook and use sprouted beans as normal.

Soups, Stocks, and Broths

Broths and stocks have been used for centuries to provide important nutrients. Including a small amount of apple cider vinegar in the cooking water helps leach minerals and other nutrients from the bones into the stock. The result is a stock rich in calcium, magnesium, phosphorus, and other trace minerals. Stocks also contain glucosamine, chondroitin, and gelatin, which can be helpful in preventing or diminishing the deleterious effects of arthritis or tendon and joint pain.

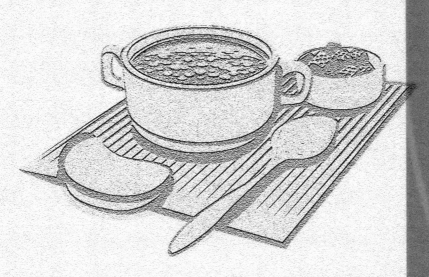

Wellness Broth

PER SERVING: 3.1 CALORIES ~ 0.2 G PROTEIN ~ 0.7 G CARBOHYDRATE ~ 0.2 G FIBER ~
0.0 G TOTAL FAT ~ 0.0 G SATURATED FAT ~ 0.0 MG CHOLESTEROL ~ 9.4 MG SODIUM

2 zucchinis, coarsely chopped	1–2 bunches of parsley, chopped large
3 stalks celery, coarsely chopped	1 tablespoon fresh grated gingerroot
1 onion, coarsely chopped	8 cups water
2 cups cut green beans	Salt (optional)
6 cloves garlic, chopped	

Combine all ingredients in a large saucepan; heat to boiling. Reduce heat and simmer until vegetables are very soft, about 40 minutes. Strain through a fine sieve, discarding vegetables.

Serve warm.

Yields about 2 quarts (8 8-ounce servings).

Substitutions

Include as much garlic and onion in this broth as possible. Mushrooms would also be a great addition, due to their immune-boosting properties.

Another, high-fiber version of this recipe calls for simmering the vegetables only until they are crisp-tender, about 8–10 minutes. Then place the mixture, including the cooking water, into a blender one pint at a time, and blend until smooth. (When hot liquids are whirled in a blender, the heat causes them to expand suddenly, so it's important to blend only small amounts of soup or other hot liquids at a time.)

Healthy Tidbit

This is my version of a Bieler's broth. Henry Bieler was a doctor who greatly believed in the healing power of fresh, whole foods. He developed a vegetable broth that he recommended as a detoxing remedy. We often suggest a "Bieler's broth fast" for our patients who have acute conditions such as urinary tract infection, upper respiratory tract infection, or other such ailments. The fast involves consuming only water and this broth for 3 days, in addition to taking certain herbal remedies. Most of the time patients who follow this regimen regain wellness quickly without having to take antibiotics.

Nutritional Analysis per Serving

Vitamin A	10.0 RE	Vitamin D	0.0 µg
Thiamin (B-1)	0.0 mg	Vitamin E	0.0 mg
Riboflavin (B-2)	0.0 mg	Calcium	11.3 mg
Niacin	0.1 mg	Iron	0.1 mg
Vitamin B-6	0.0 mg	Phosphorus	4.5 mg
Vitamin B-12	0.0 µg	Magnesium	4.7 mg
Folate (total)	4.1 µg	Zinc	0.0 mg
Vitamin C	2.5 mg	Potassium	32.3 mg

Chicken Broth

PER SERVING: 7.9 CALORIES ~ 1.0 G PROTEIN ~ 0.0 G CARBOHYDRATE ~ 0.0 G FIBER ~
0.3 G TOTAL FAT ~ 0.1 G SATURATED FAT ~ 4.0 MG CHOLESTEROL ~ 108.5 MG SODIUM

1 whole chicken (about 3½ pounds)
⅓ cup apple cider vinegar
1 bunch parsley

1 teaspoon salt
Water to cover (about 6 quarts)

Place the chicken, vinegar, parsley, and salt in a large slow cooker; add just enough water to cover chicken. Turn slow cooker to low and simmer for 12–15 hours. Strain through a fine sieve; chicken may be reserved for another use. Broth can be frozen in small containers for up to 6 months.

Yields about 6 quarts (24 8-ounce servings).

Substitutions

Any organic grass-fed meat would be fine for making stocks and broths.

Nutritional Analysis per Serving

Vitamin A	1.6 RE	Vitamin D	0.0 µg
Thiamin (B-1)	0.0 mg	Vitamin E	0.0 mg
Riboflavin (B-2)	0.0 mg	Calcium	9.0 mg
Niacin	0.2 mg	Iron	0.1 mg
Vitamin B-6	0.0 mg	Phosphorus	6.3 mg
Vitamin B-12	0.0 µg	Magnesium	3.4 mg
Folate (total)	0.4 µg	Zinc	0.1 mg
Vitamin C	0.3 mg	Potassium	14.1 mg

Fish Stock

PER SERVING: 56.1 CALORIES ~ 1.2 G PROTEIN ~ 2.1 G CARBOHYDRATE ~ 0.1 G FIBER ~
0.1 G TOTAL FAT ~ 0.0 G SATURATED FAT ~ 2.0 MG CHOLESTEROL ~ 13.8 MG SODIUM

1 whole snapper, including head, about 2 pounds
3 cloves garlic, minced
2 teaspoons lime juice
1 green onion, minced (white and green part)

1 teaspoon dried thyme leaves
About 4 cups water
1 onion, minced
1 cup wine
Bouquet Garni (see recipe on page 227)

Fillet the fish, removing any guts from the rib cage, and remove the gills. Set aside the fillets to cook for dinner, or freeze them for later use. Save the head and bones for making this stock. (If you prefer, ask the fishmonger to clean and fillet the fish for you, preserving the head and bones.)

Prepare the marinade by mixing together in a glass bowl the garlic, lime juice, green onion, and thyme. Break the fish bones in a few places to release the gelatin. Place the head and bones in the bowl with the marinade; toss thoroughly to coat. Add just enough water to cover the fish (too much water will dilute the flavors). Refrigerate for a couple of hours or overnight.

Combine fish mixture, onion, wine, and Bouquet Garni in a large saucepan; heat just to boiling. Immediately reduce heat, and simmer 20–25 minutes.
(Do not simmer longer.) Strain through a fine sieve, discarding bones and
vegetables.

Yields about 1 quart (4 8-ounce servings).

Substitutions

You can use any lean, nonoily fish such as flatfish, sea bass, or striped bass.
Experiment with other vegetables such as okra, plantain, pumpkin, or chives.
Chop vegetables into small pieces to ensure the most flavor.

For a full-bodied, brown fish stock, such as the type used for bouillabaisse,
before marinating, brown the bones and vegetables on a baking sheet in the
oven at 400°F for 15–20 minutes. Then proceed with the recipe as above. The
bones and vegetables will caramelize to give the stock an added depth and
richness.

For an even bolder stock, use salmon. Brown the head and bones in the
oven, and use red wine instead of white. You can add carrots to the salmon
stock for a hint of sweetness. (Carrots are not traditionally used in a white fish
broth.)

Kitchen Tips

Too much liquid will make the stock weak, so only use enough water to barely
cover the bones. When making a brown fish stock, you'll need slightly less
liquid, because the bones will have fallen apart and will take up less room.

Broths and stocks can be made very inexpensively. Use any leftover bones
from your meals, or befriend your local butcher and ask him or her to save
you the leftover bones from buffalo, lamb, or grass-fed beef. They will usually
give you soup bones for free or at a bargain price. I prefer using homemade
instead of store-bought broths and stocks because they have a deeper complexity of flavor and more nutrients. Store-bought broths, even organic ones, are
still more processed, are more watery, and offer significantly fewer nutrients.
Not to mention they are much more expensive! Keep homemade broths and
stocks on hand as bases for soups, to use as the liquid for cooking grains, and
to include in green drinks and
smoothies.

Nutritional Analysis per Serving

Vitamin A	2.3 RE	Vitamin D	0.6 µg
Thiamin (B-1)	0.0 mg	Vitamin E	0.0 mg
Riboflavin (B-2)	0.0 mg	Calcium	16.5 mg
Niacin	0.1 mg	Iron	0.2 mg
Vitamin B-6	0.1 mg	Phosphorus	23.1 mg
Vitamin B-12	0.2 µg	Magnesium	10.7 mg
Folate (total)	2.0 µg	Zinc	0.1 mg
Vitamin C	1.2 mg	Potassium	76.2 mg

Buffalo Stock

PER SERVING: 141.7 CALORIES ~ 2.6 G PROTEIN ~ 0.8 G CARBOHYDRATE ~ 0.1 G FIBER ~
13.8 G TOTAL FAT ~ 2.6 G SATURATED FAT ~ 18.1 MG CHOLESTEROL ~ 40.4 MG SODIUM

For the Bouquet Garni

3 sprigs fresh thyme	½ rib celery
3 sprigs fresh parsley	1 leek top (green part only)
1 bay leaf	6-inch length kitchen string

For the Buffalo Stock

2 pounds buffalo or beef bones (marrow bones and knuckle bones)	1 pound meaty buffalo rib bones or neck bones
1 calf's foot, cut into pieces (optional)	3 onions, coarsely chopped
½ cup apple cider vinegar	3 celery stalks, coarsely chopped
Water, to cover (about 6 quarts)	1 bunch parsley
	bouquet garni (recipe included here)

To make the bouquet garni: Arrange thyme, parsley, and bay leaf on top of celery rib; top with leek green. Tie tightly with kitchen string, making a neat package.

To make the stock: Place marrow bones, knuckle bones, and calf's foot in a large slow cooker and add vinegar and just enough water to cover. Let stand about 1 hour. Cook meaty bones in a lightly greased large skillet over medium-high heat until well browned on all sides, about 15 minutes, turning frequently. Add meaty bones and remaining ingredients to slow cooker. After the skillet has cooled slightly, add a small amount of cold water; heat to boiling, stirring with a wooden spoon to loosen coagulated juices. Pour into slow cooker or large stock pot. Add enough water to just cover bones, leaving at least an inch of room below the rim of the pot. Heat to boiling; reduce heat to low and barely simmer, covered, for at least 12 hours, or up to 24 hours. Add small amounts of water as necessary to cover. Strain stock through a fine sieve, discarding bones and vegetables. Use right away, or store in pint-size containers in the freezer for up to 6 months.

Yields about 6 quarts (24 8-ounce servings).

Substitutions

Other herbs can be used for the bouquet garni, such as tarragon, chives, marjoram, etc.

Nutritional Analysis per Serving

Vitamin A	217.1 RE	Vitamin D	0.0 µg
Thiamin (B-1)	0.0 mg	Vitamin E	0.0 mg
Riboflavin (B-2)	0.1 mg	Calcium	84.2 mg
Niacin	0.5 mg	Iron	3.2 mg
Vitamin B-6	0.2 mg	Phosphorus	35.3 mg
Vitamin B-12	0.0 µg	Magnesium	32.6 mg
Folate (total)	57.3 µg	Zinc	0.4 mg
Vitamin C	32.9 mg	Potassium	242.3 mg

Sadie and Elisa's Mystery Chicken Noodle Soup

PER SERVING: 101.6 CALORIES ~ 6.0 G PROTEIN ~ 18.5 G CARBOHYDRATE ~ 2.6 G FIBER ~ 3.1 G TOTAL FAT ~ 1.7 G SATURATED FAT ~ 7.9 MG CHOLESTEROL ~ 542.4 MG SODIUM

The spices in my kitchen are not marked, which makes it a little daunting for my nanny, Elisa, or my daughter Sadie to cook. But my daughter has really picked up a sense for what should go well together. The first time they made this recipe, my daughter selected all of the spices by smell. She put together a "mystery" seasoning blend that had never occurred to me: marjoram, chili powder, paprika, and cayenne. What a flavorful combination it makes!

1½ cups gluten-free spiral noodles, uncooked

1 onion, chopped

5 cloves garlic, minced

1 tablespoon coconut oil

3 tablespoons miso paste

2 tablespoons gluten-free tamari

2 large carrots, julienned

1 tablespoon dried marjoram leaves

1 tablespoon chili powder

1 tablespoon paprika

⅛ teaspoon cayenne pepper

1 cup Shredded Chicken (see recipe on page 202)

5 cups water

Salt and pepper to taste

1 bunch cilantro, stems removed, chopped

1 bunch green onions and tops, chopped fine

Cook noodles in a large pot of boiling water for half the time recommended on package; drain and reserve. Sauté onion and garlic in coconut oil in a large saucepan until softened, about 5 minutes. Add tamari, miso, carrots, and dried herbs and sauté 5 minutes. Add water, chicken, and reserved noodles; heat to boiling. Reduce heat and simmer for 10 minutes, or until noodles are cooked. Season to taste with salt and pepper; garnish with cilantro and green onions.

Serves 8.

Nutritional Analysis per Serving

Vitamin A	351.8 RE	Vitamin D	0.0 µg
Thiamin (B-1)	0.1 mg	Vitamin E	0.0 mg
Riboflavin (B-2)	0.1 mg	Calcium	51.4 mg
Niacin	1.6 mg	Iron	1.4 mg
Vitamin B-6	0.2 mg	Phosphorus	57.6 mg
Vitamin B-12	0.0 µg	Magnesium	19.0 mg
Folate (total)	22.8 µg	Zinc	0.5 mg
Vitamin C	7.0 mg	Potassium	231.4 mg

Healthy Tidbit

Make sure to get enough sleep. The amount needed varies from person to person, but getting adequate sleep is imperative to maintaining proper brain function and a positive mood. Regular exercise may help you get a good night's sleep, especially if you're older. In a small study published in the journal *Sleep Medicine*, researchers found that people age 55 years or more with chronic insomnia who started doing aerobic activities reported significantly better sleep, mood, and vitality after four months compared to those who did nonexercise activities.[8]

Thyroid Support Soup

PER SERVING: 117.3 CALORIES ~ 3.1 G PROTEIN ~ 25.8 G CARBOHYDRATE ~ 2.3 G FIBER ~ 1.1 G TOTAL FAT ~ 0.2 G SATURATED FAT ~ 0.0 MG CHOLESTEROL ~ 548.2 MG SODIUM

This macrobiotic-style recipe was adapted from one given to me by Cathe Frederic, of Grand Ronde, Oregon. She pointed out that macrobiotic dishes were served after the bombing of Hiroshima and were proven to reduce radiation sickness and to chelate heavy metals and radiation from the body.

4 cups water

1 ounce dried kelp, precut into thin strips or crumbled

1 cup cooked brown rice

1 onion, chopped

1 bunch cilantro, chopped

½ bunch parsley, chopped

4 cloves garlic, minced

Juice of 1 lemon

2 tablespoons miso paste

Salt to taste

1 avocado, diced, as garnish

Chopped parsley, as garnish

Kelp powder, as garnish

Heat water to boiling in a medium saucepan; add seaweed and simmer 4–5 minutes.

Add remaining ingredients, except miso paste, salt, and garnishes, and simmer until onion is tender, about 10 minutes. Stir

Nutritional Analysis per Serving

Vitamin A	64.9 RE	Vitamin D	0.0 µg
Thiamin (B-1)	0.1 mg	Vitamin E	0.0 mg
Riboflavin (B-2)	0.1 mg	Calcium	181.6 mg
Niacin	1.0 mg	Iron	2.4 mg
Vitamin B-6	0.2 mg	Phosphorus	72.3 mg
Vitamin B-12	0.0 µg	Magnesium	87.6 mg
Folate (total)	23.5 µg	Zinc	0.7 mg
Vitamin C	19.0 mg	Potassium	939.1 mg

in miso paste; season to taste with salt. Ladle soup into bowls and sprinkle with garnishes.

Serves 4.

Substitutions

As always, different vegetables can be used in this recipe, but aim to include cilantro, parsley, and some type of seaweed. Experiment with different types of seaweed: deep green kombu, dried black hijiki, chewy red dulse, emerald wakame, bright, leafy sea lettuce, or dark, toasted nori. These can be found in the ethnic section of most grocery stores.

Healthy Tidbit

If you don't consume animal protein, know that most seaweeds are a good source of amino acids. They are also high in vitamins A and C, as well as in potassium, iron, calcium, and magnesium (minerals that are concentrated in seawater). Seaweeds are one of the few vegetable sources of vitamin B-12, other benefit they provide to a vegetarian diet. Finally, seaweeds are high in another important mineral, iodine, which is vital to proper thyroid function. Due to the potential negative effects of radiation on thyroid function, seaweeds are good to consume following any radiation exposure, for example, from medical X rays or security screenings. The small amount of radiation delivered by these sources is well shy of a dangerous dose, but why not give your thyroid an added boost?

Chicken Dumpling Soup

PER SERVING: 159.7 CALORIES ~ 4.8 G PROTEIN ~ 29.7 G CARBOHYDRATE ~ 2.6 G FIBER ~
2.8 G TOTAL FAT ~ 0.6 G SATURATED FAT ~51.5 MG CHOLESTEROL ~ 1057.9 MG SODIUM

Here's another one created by Cathe Frederic, who hosts the very popular
Choctaw Medicine Women Group on Facebook.

½ cup unsweetened applesauce

1 egg

Salt to taste

1–1½ cups Gluten-Free Pancake and Baking Mix (see recipe on page 124)

4 cups Chicken Broth (see recipe on page 225)

Mix applesauce, egg, and salt in a medium bowl until well blended. Using a
wooden spoon, stir in 1 cup of flour; if needed, add additional flour until the
mixture is medium dough consistency. (The dough should be firm enough
to drop easily off a spoon in clumps.) Heat broth to boiling; reduce heat to
simmering. Using a wet teaspoon, gently form dough into balls, each slightly
smaller than a walnut; drop dumplings gently into broth, and simmer until
dumplings are cooked through, about 25 minutes.

Serves 4.

Substitutions
You can use all sorts of flour to make these little dumplings. Experiment with
seasoning them using different spices. The amount of flour will vary depending on the liquid consistency of your applesauce.

Healthy Tidbit
Envision great things. Imagine "infinite possibilities" whenever you want to
create change for the better. Believing is half the effort of attaining. Those who
show willingness to create, to change, to try, and to grow should inspire us all.
Always know that your mind has much power if you are willing to believe in
the possibilities!

Nutritional Analysis per Serving

Vitamin A	21.1 RE	Vitamin D	0.3 µg
Thiamin (B-1)	0.1 mg	Vitamin E	0.1 mg
Riboflavin (B-2)	0.1 mg	Calcium	28.7 mg
Niacin	1.3 mg	Iron	1.0 mg
Vitamin B-6	0.2 mg	Phosphorus	99.0 mg
Vitamin B-12	0.1 µg	Magnesium	24.7 mg
Folate (total)	10.0 µg	Zinc	0.7 mg
Vitamin C	0.3 mg	Potassium	173.6 mg

Lentil Soup

PER SERVING: 308.6 CALORIES ~ 15.6 G PROTEIN ~ 42.7 G CARBOHYDRATE ~ 16.9 G FIBER ~
5.2 G TOTAL FAT ~ 0.7 G SATURATED FAT ~ 0.0 MG CHOLESTEROL ~ 788.6 MG SODIUM

2 large onions, cubed

2 garlic cloves, diced

2 tablespoons olive oil

2 carrots, diced

1 small sweet potato, diced

2 stalks celery, diced

½ teaspoon paprika

1½ cups dry lentils

½ teaspoon salt

½ teaspoon ground black pepper

1 cup white wine

6 cups vegetable broth

2 bay leaves

¼ cup fresh parsley, chopped

Sauté onions and garlic in olive oil in a large saucepan until softened, about 5 minutes. Add sweet potato, carrots, celery, and paprika and sauté 10 minutes. Stir in remaining ingredients, except parsley. Heat to boiling; reduce heat and simmer, covered, until lentils are tender, about 45 minutes. Remove bay leaves. Ladle into bowls; sprinkle with parsley.

Serves 6.

Substitutions

You can use chicken broth instead of vegetable broth. You can also omit the wine and use more broth instead.

Kitchen Tip

Soups are welcome on cold days. They are an excellent option when you don't have many groceries left and nothing seems to go together to create an entrée. Soups can take on many flavors depending on what you start with and what you add. Lentils are a great addition to any soup because they go well with many flavors. Experiment with making soups from scratch using vegetable or chicken broth, garlic and onions, and other vegetables.

Nutritional Analysis per Serving

Vitamin A	685.8 RE	Vitamin D	0.0 µg
Thiamin (B-1)	0.5 mg	Vitamin E	0.0 mg
Riboflavin (B-2)	0.2 mg	Calcium	84.2 mg
Niacin	1.8 mg	Iron	4.6 mg
Vitamin B-6	0.4 mg	Phosphorus	589.1 mg
Vitamin B-12	0.0 µg	Magnesium	77.6 mg
Folate (total)	252.4 µg	Zinc	2.6 mg
Vitamin C	10.7 mg	Potassium	987.3 mg

Lentil Apricot Soup

PER SERVING: 289.3 CALORIES ~ 15.3 G PROTEIN ~ 41.0 G CARBOHYDRATE ~ 16.6 G FIBER ~
7.5 G TOTAL FAT ~ 1.0 G SATURATED FAT ~ 0.0 MG CHOLESTEROL ~ 466.7 MG SODIUM

This soup was introduced to me by my good friend Desiree LeFave, a licensed midwife who has a birth center near Salem, Oregon.

1 onion, chopped

2 cloves garlic, minced

⅓ cup dried apricots, minced

3 tablespoons olive oil

1½ cups red lentils

5 cups vegetable broth

½ teaspoon ground cumin

½ teaspoon dried thyme leaves

3 plum tomatoes, peeled, seeded, chopped

2 tablespoons fresh lemon juice

Salt and pepper to taste

Sauté onion, garlic, and apricots in olive oil in a large saucepan until tender, about 8 minutes. Add lentils, broth, and herbs. Heat to boiling; reduce heat and simmer, covered, 30 minutes, or until lentils are tender. Add tomatoes and simmer 10 minutes longer. Stir in lemon juice. Working in small batches, purée half the soup in a blender until smooth; return puréed soup to saucepan. Season to taste with salt and pepper.

Serves 6.

Substitutions

If you are diabetic, or for a slightly fresher taste, instead of using dried apricots, use 2 fresh apricots. Remove the pits, chop them into small pieces, then follow directions as above. If you don't have fresh tomatoes on hand, substitute 1 15-ounce can of tomatoes. If you cannot tolerate tomatoes, leave them out. If you don't have chicken broth, you can use chicken bouillon, prepared according to package directions. For a vegetarian option, use vegetable broth.

Healthy Tidbit

Chinese medicine holds that many diseases and many chronic pain conditions are triggered by a state of cold or dampness inside the body. For

Nutritional Analysis per Serving			
Vitamin A	138.2 RE	Vitamin D	0.0 µg
Thiamin (B-1)	0.5 mg	Vitamin E	0.0 mg
Riboflavin (B-2)	0.1 mg	Calcium	64.0 mg
Niacin	1.9 mg	Iron	4.8 mg
Vitamin B-6	0.4 mg	Phosphorus	524.6 mg
Vitamin B-12	0.0 µg	Magnesium	72.2 mg
Folate (total)	244.3 µg	Zinc	2.5 mg
Vitamin C	14.9 mg	Potassium	976.5 mg

pain patients, keeping the body warm can be an important part of treatment and recovery. Using warm compresses, drinking warm beverages, and avoiding the use of ice and iced drinks can help immensely with chronic pain of all sorts. Keeping warm by avoiding cold environments and cold beverages and foods may also help many other problems, such as weakened digestion, circulation issues, and thyroid complaints.

Roasted Red Pepper Soup

PER SERVING: 63.7 CALORIES ~ 2.0 G PROTEIN ~ 9.9 G CARBOHYDRATE ~ 2.9 G FIBER ~
1.8 G TOTAL FAT ~ 0.2 G SATURATED FAT ~ 2.5 MG CHOLESTEROL ~ 581.5 MG SODIUM

8 large red bell peppers (about 2¾ pounds), roasted,
peeled, and cut into 2-inch pieces

1 large onion, diced

5 large garlic cloves, minced

¼ jalapeño, seeded, minced

2 teaspoons olive oil

4 cups Chicken Broth (see recipe on page 225)

3 tablespoons white wine vinegar

½ teaspoon salt

½ teaspoon freshly ground black pepper

1 sprig fresh thyme

1 sprig fresh rosemary

1 bay leaf

2 tablespoons fresh chives, minced

To roast peppers:

Method 1—Using tongs or a long-handled fork, hold the pepper directly over a stovetop burner, turning frequently until all sides are black. Place peppers in a brown paper bag, and roll down top to seal. Let stand 15 minutes. Peel peppers by rubbing off blackened skin. Cut into halves; remove seeds.

Method 2—Preheat broiler to 400°F. Cut peppers in half lengthwise and discard the seeds and membranes. Place pepper halves, skin sides up, on foil-lined baking sheet, and press to flatten slightly. Broil for 15 minutes or until blackened. Place peppers in a brown paper

Nutritional Analysis per Serving

Vitamin A	379.0 RE	Vitamin D	0.0 µg
Thiamin (B-1)	0.1 mg	Vitamin E	0.0 mg
Riboflavin (B-2)	0.1 mg	Calcium	19.4 mg
Niacin	1.2 mg	Iron	0.7 mg
Vitamin B-6	0.4 mg	Phosphorus	39.7 mg
Vitamin B-12	0.0 µg	Magnesium	17.5 mg
Folate (total)	58.9 µg	Zinc	0.4 mg
Vitamin C	155.1 mg	Potassium	292.3 mg

bag and roll down top to seal. Let stand 15 minutes. Peel peppers by rubbing off blackened skin.

Sauté onion, garlic, and jalapeño in oil in a large saucepan until lightly browned, about 15 minutes. Add roasted peppers and remaining ingredients, except chives. Heat to boiling; reduce heat and simmer, covered, until vegetables are tender, about 20 minutes. Remove thyme and rosemary sprigs and the bay leaf.

Working in small batches, purée half the soup in a blender until smooth. Return puréed soup to saucepan. Ladle into bowls; garnish with chives.

Serves 8.

Substitutions

If your palate can handle a little spice, this soup does well with a bit of chili powder and/or cayenne pepper.

Healthy Tidbit

Red peppers fit into the *Solanaceae* (nightshade) family of vegetables, so they may increase inflammation in some individuals. For those who are not sensitive to red peppers, this is an easy, tasty recipe. I have also prepared a time-saving version of this recipe by using unroasted red peppers.

Sweet Things

Everyone at some time will crave something sweet. Sweet treats are okay in moderation. If you find yourself incessantly craving sweets, most likely there is a reason why, either a medical one or because of an imbalanced diet or excess stress. For the times when you want something sweet, please don't rush out and purchase a candy bar, ice cream, or cake. You can prepare a treat that will satisfy your sweet craving without having to fall off the wagon! For diabetics, most sweets should be eliminated, including all dried fruit. Keep some of the basics in your kitchen at all times so that you can make sweets when you desire them.

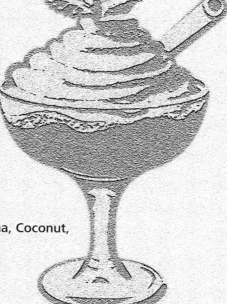

Ginger Candy and Ginger Syrup

PER SERVING: 70.2 CALORIES ~ 0.2 G PROTEIN ~ 18.7 G CARBOHYDRATE ~ 0.2 G FIBER ~
0.1 G TOTAL FAT ~ 0.0 G SATURATED FAT ~ 0.0 MG CHOLESTEROL ~ 1.9 MG SODIUM

This is a spicy-sweet treat to use as a garnish or to consume when sick. My
children have gotten used to the spiciness and love eating a few pieces when
they have a sore throat.

2 cups unpeeled gingerroot, very thinly sliced (about 2 large pieces)

1½ cups raw honey

Place ginger in a glass jar; pour honey over ginger to cover completely. If
needed, use a fork to push the ginger below the honey, or add more honey to
cover. For quicker crystallizing, it is best to use honey that is beginning to crys-
tallize, or make sure the honey is raw. In this case, heat the honey to a liquid
consistency before pouring over the ginger. Cover jar with a tight-fitting lid.
Let stand in a cool, dark place for 2–3 weeks before using.

The ginger slices and the ginger honey can be eaten plain, or added to
recipes.

Yields 1 cup ginger syrup (about 8 1-ounce servings) plus 2 cups crystallized
ginger (about 16 servings).

Substitutions
For added nutritional and antimicrobial value, you could add some cinnamon
sticks and whole cloves.

Healthy Tidbit
Consuming raw, local honey can have beneficial effects on seasonal allergies.
Though no scientific research yet supports its use for treating allergies, I have
had numerous patients stop needing their allergy medications after adopting a
habit of consuming raw, local honey daily during spring and fall, or whenever
they are likely to experience allergy symptoms. Honey, which shows significant antimicrobial properties, has been used traditionally for wound healing, a
benefit that is being rediscovered in modern medicine. Honey is very soothing
and can be used daily to help
ease ulcer symptoms.

Nutritional Analysis per Serving

Vitamin A	0.0 RE	Vitamin D	0.0 µg
Thiamin (B-1)	0.0 mg	Vitamin E	0.0 mg
Riboflavin (B-2)	0.0 mg	Calcium	2.5 mg
Niacin	0.1 mg	Iron	0.1 mg
Vitamin B-6	0.0 mg	Phosphorus	3.6 mg
Vitamin B-12	0.0 µg	Magnesium	3.9 mg
Folate (total)	1.3 µg	Zinc	0.1 mg
Vitamin C	0.5 mg	Potassium	44.1 mg

Tapioca Pudding

PER SERVING: 206.1 CALORIES ~ 4.8 G PROTEIN ~ 25.4 G CARBOHYDRATE ~ 1.3 G FIBER ~
10.2 G TOTAL FAT ~ 2.4 G SATURATED FAT ~ 62.0 MG CHOLESTEROL ~ 128.6 MG SODIUM

4 cups hot water, divided	2 teaspoons vanilla extract
1 cup blanched almonds	¼ teaspoon salt
⅓ cup honey	2 eggs, separated
⅓ cup tapioca	Ground nutmeg, as garnish
1 tablespoon coconut butter	

To blanch almonds: Pour boiling water over raw almonds in a small bowl; let stand 1 minute. Drain, rinse with cold water. Pinch off skins.

Process almonds and 1 cup hot water in the blender until almost smooth; add remaining 3 cups water and process until very smooth. Strain through cheesecloth into a medium saucepan. Stir in honey, tapioca, coconut butter, vanilla, salt, and egg yolks; heat to boiling, stirring constantly. Reduce heat and cook until tapioca turns clear, stirring frequently, about 10 minutes. Beat egg whites in a medium bowl with a hand mixer, or whisk until soft peaks form. Gently fold half the tapioca mixture into the egg whites. Transfer mixture back to saucepan. Turn off heat and beat mixture until smooth, 1–3 minutes. Spoon mixture into dessert dishes; sprinkle with nutmeg and chill.

Serves 6.

Substitutions

You can omit the egg from this recipe and it still turns out delicious, just a little denser. It would then serve 8 instead of 10. I don't suggest using almond milk in place of the puréed blanched almonds because freshly processed almonds add a rich flavor. You could use coconut extract instead of coconut butter if you are unable to find coconut butter. Of course, you can flavor the pudding with any additional seasonings you like.

Healthy Tidbit

Tapioca is a starch extracted from a root plant. For baking, it offers the binding power lacking from many gluten-free flours. It's a good substance to use in grain-free recipes, and as a thickener in place of cornstarch, which is often made from corn that has been genetically modified. Tapioca is free of cholesterol, low in unhealthy fats, and a good source of iron.

Nutritional Analysis per Serving

Vitamin A	27.1 RE	Vitamin D	0.3 µg
Thiamin (B-1)	0.0 mg	Vitamin E	0.2 mg
Riboflavin (B-2)	0.2 mg	Calcium	45.6 mg
Niacin	0.5 mg	Iron	0.9 mg
Vitamin B-6	0.1 mg	Phosphorus	92.5 mg
Vitamin B-12	0.2 µg	Magnesium	36.6 mg
Folate (total)	14.5 µg	Zinc	0.6 mg
Vitamin C	0.1 mg	Potassium	116.9 mg

Oat Cookies

PER COOKIE: 92.4 CALORIES ~ 2.1 G PROTEIN ~ 13.0 G CARBOHYDRATE ~ 1.3 G FIBER ~
4.1 G TOTAL FAT ~ 1.9 G SATURATED FAT ~ 12.0 MG CHOLESTEROL ~ 75.6 MG SODIUM

½ cup softened butter or coconut oil

½ cup honey

1 egg

1 teaspoon vanilla

¼ cup water

1 cup Gluten-Free Pancake and Baking Mix (see recipe on page 124)

½ cup almond meal

1 teaspoon baking powder

¼ teaspoon baking soda

⅛ teaspoon salt

2 cups gluten-free rolled oats

1 cup nuts or chopped dried fruit (optional)

Preheat oven to 350°F.

Beat butter and honey with a wooden spoon in a large bowl until smooth; beat in egg, vanilla, and water until smooth. In a separate bowl, combine flour, baking powder, baking soda, and salt. Add to egg mixture, blending until smooth. Stir in oats and optional nuts or dried fruit. Drop mixture by rounded tablespoons onto lightly greased cookie sheets. Bake for 15–17 minutes until lightly browned on bottoms.

Makes 3 dozen.

Substitutions

This recipe affords lots of room for experimentation. You can use any kind of nut, or add unsweetened carob chips for a modified chocolate chip oatmeal cookie. For extra crunch, add millet. I love adding millet to my baked goods; the small grain tastes like a little piece of candy when baked into cookies, muffins, and breads.

Kitchen Tips

This recipe produces a rather hard cookie that is crispy on the edges. They key is to bake it long enough. Others may prefer a different consistency. Let's talk about how changing the ingredients will change the cookie.

Nutritional Analysis per Cookie

Vitamin A	25.9 RE	Vitamin D	0.1 µg
Thiamin (B-1)	0.0 mg	Vitamin E	0.5 mg
Riboflavin (B-2)	0.0 mg	Calcium	19.4 mg
Niacin	0.1 mg	Iron	0.6 mg
Vitamin B-6	0.0 mg	Phosphorus	14.6 mg
Vitamin B-12	0.0 µg	Magnesium	7.3 mg
Folate (total)	1.2 µg	Zinc	0.1 mg
Vitamin C	0.0 mg	Potassium	14.1 mg

1. More eggs will produce a cookie with a more cakelike texture.

2. More baking soda will cause the cookie to spread out a little more and will lend it a nice brownness. Be careful when adding extra baking soda to a gluten-free recipe; it increases the pH of the dough, which may break down the protein structure of the grain and eggs required to hold the cookie together. If you are baking at high altitudes, you may want to omit the baking soda altogether.

3. Baking powder contains acid, so it will not reduce the acidity in the dough, and the resulting cookies will be puffier and lighter in color.

4. Adding more oil will cause the cookie to spread more; conversely, reducing the amount of oil will reduce the amount of spread.

5. Adding grated zucchini will soften the cookie, making it more moist and chewy.

6. To get a crispy cookie, you should use less liquid and more oil. You also should use a crystallized sugar like honey powder or maple syrup crystals, rather than liquid honey.

7. Liquids other than eggs, such as water or milk, will create a flatter cookie.

When I am experimenting with a cookie recipe, I mix my dough and then bake one cookie. That gives me a chance to test the cookie for taste and texture and to make needed additions. This is especially important when using gluten-free ingredients, which can require a little more finesse to get the dough to hold together during baking. Jump in and have fun with your kitchen experiments. If your cookies don't turn out, you can crumble them up and use them as a topping for fresh fruit. Decide to turn it into a positive and you won't need to waste anything!

Rice Crispy Treats

PER SERVING: 145.2 CALORIES ~ 3.1 G PROTEIN ~ 21.1 G CARBOHYDRATE ~ 3.1 G FIBER ~
5.4 G TOTAL FAT ~ 0.8 G SATURATED FAT ~ 0.0 MG CHOLESTEROL ~ 47.0 MG SODIUM

These freeze well, so make a large batch. Every Sunday you can thaw enough for the upcoming week.

3 cups gluten-free puffed rice cereal
½ cup coconut flour
2 tablespoons flax seeds
2 tablespoons chia seeds
2 tablespoons salba seeds
2 tablespoons protein powder (optional)
1 teaspoon ground cinnamon
1 cup brown rice syrup
½ cup sunflower butter or almond butter

Combine dry ingredients in a large bowl.

Heat brown rice syrup and sunflower butter in a small saucepan over low heat until melted. Pour half the syrup mixture over the cereal mixture; stir thoroughly. Add remaining syrup mixture and mix well. Mixture should be firm enough to stay in clumps when pressed between fingers. Press mixture into an oiled 13×9-inch pan. Cover and refrigerate until firm.

Cut into squares and store in airtight container until use.

Serves 18.

Healthy Tidbit

Salba seeds are not as well known as chia seeds or flax seeds, but they will be soon because of their superior nutritional quality. Salba seeds are higher in essential fatty acids than flax or hemp and contain more magnesium than many vegetables. They are high in calcium and fiber, and have powerful antioxidant content. Salba, which has undergone intensive clinical testing by Dr. Vladimir Vuksan of the University of Toronto, was shown to decrease inflammation (C-reactive protein), to lower blood pressure, and to decrease blood coagulation (blood clotting).[9]

Nutritional Analysis per Serving

Vitamin A	50.2 RE	Vitamin D	0.1 µg
Thiamin (B-1)	0.1 mg	Vitamin E	0.7 mg
Riboflavin (B-2)	0.1 mg	Calcium	16.0 mg
Niacin	0.8 mg	Iron	1.6 mg
Vitamin B-6	0.1 mg	Phosphorus	19.2 mg
Vitamin B-12	0.2 µg	Magnesium	6.5 mg
Folate (total)	14.1 µg	Zinc	0.1 mg
Vitamin C	2.1 mg	Potassium	29.9 mg

Raspberry Peach Syrup

PER SERVING: 72.8 CALORIES ~ 0.3 G PROTEIN ~ 19.4 G CARBOHYDRATE ~ 0.7 G FIBER ~
0.1 G TOTAL FAT ~ 0.0 G SATURATED FAT ~ 0.0 MG CHOLESTEROL ~ 1.9 MG SODIUM

½ cup raspberries

½ cup sliced peaches

½ cup honey

½ cup water

2 tablespoons arrowroot powder

Combine all ingredients in a medium saucepan; heat to boiling. Reduce heat and simmer, stirring frequently, and crushing fruit with a wooden spoon or potato masher as it softens. Simmer until fruit is very soft, about 15 minutes. Strain through a fine strainer, pressing on fruit to release syrup.

Yields 1 cup syrup (8 2-tablespoon servings).

Substitutions

Any berries work well for this easy-to-make syrup. For a thicker syrup, process in a blender or food processor until smooth, and strain through a fine strainer or cheesecloth to remove seeds.

Healthy Tidbit

Arrowroot powder is an excellent gluten-free thickener. It can also be used as a diaper rash powder. Most commercial baby powders contain added scents and other unwanted ingredients, but plain arrowroot powder offers the same benefits without any potential irritants. It is also much less expensive than baby powder. You can put it in a container with small holes for dispensing, just like regular powder. Please share this trick with others. Cornstarch has also been used as a rash powder and works great as long as the diaper rash is not a yeast rash. Yeast rashes can sometimes feed off the cornstarch and get worse.

Nutritional Analysis per Serving

Vitamin A	3.4 RE	Vitamin D	0.0 µg
Thiamin (B-1)	0.0 mg	Vitamin E	0.1 mg
Riboflavin (B-2)	0.0 mg	Calcium	4.3 mg
Niacin	0.2 mg	Iron	0.2 mg
Vitamin B-6	0.0 mg	Phosphorus	6.8 mg
Vitamin B-12	0.0 µg	Magnesium	3.6 mg
Folate (total)	8.8 µg	Zinc	0.1 mg
Vitamin C	2.8 mg	Potassium	49.5 mg

Strawberry Peach Crisp

PER SERVING: 372.6 CALORIES ~ 6.8 G PROTEIN ~ 47.4 G CARBOHYDRATE ~ 6.1 G FIBER ~
20.1 G TOTAL FAT ~ 11.5 G SATURATED FAT ~ 45.8 MG CHOLESTEROL ~ 270.8 MG SODIUM

3 cups strawberries, halved or quartered

2 peaches, cut into chunks

¼ cup honey or honey powder, divided

1¾ cups oats (gluten-free, if desired)

½ cup Gluten-Free Pancake and Baking Mix (see recipe on page 124)

2 teaspoons cinnamon

½ teaspoon nutmeg

¼ teaspoon salt

¾ cup butter or coconut oil, melted

Juice of 1 lemon

Preheat oven to 375°F.

Place fruit in a lightly greased 9-inch pie pan or baking dish. Pour honey over fruit.

Combine dry ingredients in a medium bowl; stir in butter, mixing well. Spoon mixture over fruit, and spread to cover.

Bake, covered, for 20 minutes, or until fruit is soft. Uncover and bake 5 minutes more or until top begins to crisp. Remove from oven.

Serves 8.

Substitutions

You can make crisps from berries, apples, pears, or other fruits, but seasonal fruits are the best. One year during peach season, my father and I visited a U-pick farm near my home. The peaches were beautifully ripe, so we couldn't stop ourselves from picking way more fruit than we needed. The aroma that filled the car on the drive home was intoxicating. Once home, we got to work cleaning peaches, freezing them, and, my favorite task, making peach crisps.

Healthy Tidbit

One cup of unsweetened strawberries contains only 55 calories, making them a great low-calorie treat. Strawberries are high in vitamin C, folic acid, potassium, and fiber.

Nutritional Analysis per Serving

Vitamin A	172.8 RE	Vitamin D	0.3 µg
Thiamin (B-1)	0.1 mg	Vitamin E	0.5 mg
Riboflavin (B-2)	0.0 mg	Calcium	45.8 mg
Niacin	0.9 mg	Iron	2.2 mg
Vitamin B-6	0.1 mg	Phosphorus	45.5 mg
Vitamin B-12	0.0 µg	Magnesium	17.7 mg
Folate (total)	17.8 µg	Zinc	0.3 mg
Vitamin C	37.3 mg	Potassium	195.0 mg

Sweet Cherry Cobbler

PER SERVING: 249.6 CALORIES ~ 4.1 G PROTEIN ~ 44.7 G CARBOHYDRATE ~ 4.1 G FIBER ~
7.3 G TOTAL FAT ~ 3.9 G SATURATED FAT ~ 15.3 MG CHOLESTEROL ~ 213.7 MG SODIUM

For the Filling

2 teaspoons organic cornstarch or arrowroot powder

1 tablespoon cold water

3 cups frozen dark sweet cherries, unthawed (14-ounce package)

2 tablespoons honey

¼ teaspoon ground cinnamon

Pinch salt

For the Topping

¾ cup Gluten-Free Pancake and Baking Mix (see recipe on page 124) or gluten-free oat flour

½ cup gluten-free rolled oats

¼ teaspoon baking soda

¼ teaspoon baking powder

⅛ teaspoon salt

3 tablespoons cold unsalted butter, cut into small bits, or substitute coconut oil, chilled and flaked into small bits

¼ cup thick unsweetened almond milk

2 tablespoons honey, divided

To make the filling: Preheat oven to 425°F.

Stir cornstarch into cold water in a small bowl until dissolved. Combine remaining filling ingredients in a 2-quart heavy saucepan; heat over moderate heat, stirring occasionally, until boiling, about 3 minutes. Reduce heat to simmer, and slowly add cornstarch mixture. Spoon filling into a 9-inch ceramic or glass pie plate (1 inch deep).

To make the topping: Whisk together flour, oats, baking soda, baking powder, and sea salt in a medium bowl. Blend in butter with pastry blender or fingers until mixture resembles coarse meal. Combine almond milk and 1 tablespoon honey; stir into the pastry mix with a fork until just blended. Drop dough in mounds over hot filling.

Drizzle with remaining 1 tablespoon honey.

Bake until topping is golden brown and fruit is bubbling, about 25 minutes. Cool slightly and serve warm.

Serves 6.

Substitutions

Cobblers are fun to prepare, easy to make gluten free, and a delicious treat. Experiment with using different fruits and berries.

Nutritional Analysis per Serving

Vitamin A	62.7 RE	Vitamin D	0.1 µg
Thiamin (B-1)	0.1 mg	Vitamin E	0.0 mg
Riboflavin (B-2)	0.0 mg	Calcium	33.5 mg
Niacin	0.6 mg	Iron	1.3 mg
Vitamin B-6	0.1 mg	Phosphorus	43.0 mg
Vitamin B-12	0.0 µg	Magnesium	11.7 mg
Folate (total)	2.1 µg	Zinc	0.3 mg
Vitamin C	0.6 mg	Potassium	61.4 mg

Healthy Tidbit

Cherries are very high in antioxidants. Concentrated cherry juice has been known to help with gout, a type of arthritis that causes pain in joints due to the buildup of a chemical called uric acid. Uric acid comes from the overconsumption of proteins or an inability to break them down effectively. Overconsumption of red meat can lead to gout. Cherries are remarkable at helping to ward off gout. Drinking unsweetened cherry juice at the initial onset of symptoms may lessen their severity and possibly prevent a full-blown attack.

Sadie's Peppermint Cake

PER SERVING: 444.8 CALORIES ~ 7.1 G PROTEIN ~ 67.1 G CARBOHYDRATE ~ 3.1 G FIBER ~ 18.4 G TOTAL FAT ~ 10.4 G SATURATED FAT ~ 102.7 MG CHOLESTEROL ~ 641.7 MG SODIUM

Adapted from the Vanilla Cake recipe in *Living with Crohn's and Colitis*. Adding the peppermint frosting was my daughter's inspiration. It makes a beautiful, delectable cake for the holidays.

For the Cake

3½ cups gluten-free Crêpe Flour Blend (see recipe on page 132)

1 tablespoon plus 1 teaspoon baking powder

1 teaspoon baking soda

1 teaspoon salt

1 cup butter or 1 cup coconut oil, melted

1¼ cup honey

4 large eggs

2 teaspoons vanilla extract

1½ cup almond milk

Honey Peppermint Frosting (recipe included here)

Fresh mint leaves, to decorate

For the Honey Peppermint Frosting

3 egg whites

⅔ cup honey

Pinch of salt

¼ teaspoon guar or xanthan gum

1 teaspoon peppermint extract

To make the cake: Preheat oven to 350°F.

Lightly oil two 8–9-inch round cake pans, and dust with gluten-free flour. Sift dry ingredients together into a medium bowl. Beat butter and honey in mixer on medium speed until light and fluffy,

Nutritional Analysis per Serving

Vitamin A	169.0 RE	Vitamin D	0.6 µg
Thiamin (B-1)	0.0 mg	Vitamin E	0.6 mg
Riboflavin (B-2)	0.1 mg	Calcium	128.3 mg
Niacin	0.2 mg	Iron	2.0 mg
Vitamin B-6	0.1 mg	Phosphorus	78.7 mg
Vitamin B-12	0.2 µg	Magnesium	5.9 mg
Folate (total)	24.0 µg	Zinc	0.4 mg
Vitamin C	0.3 mg	Potassium	142.6 mg

about 5 minutes. Add the eggs one at a time while beating on low speed. Add vanilla. Beat in half the flour mixture; beat on low speed until combined. Beat in almond milk; beat in remaining flour mixture until smooth. Divide batter between prepared pans. Bake 35–40 minutes, or until a fork inserted in the center comes out clean. Cool cake in pans for 20 minutes. Loosen cake from sides of pan with a sharp knife. Turn cake layers onto wire racks, using care when easing them out of pans. Cool completely before frosting.

Place 1 cake layer on a serving plate; frost with about ½ cup Honey Peppermint Frosting (recipe follows). Top with remaining cake layer and frost with remaining frosting. Decorate with mint leaves.

To make the frosting: Combine egg whites, honey, guar or xanthan gum, and salt in the top of a double boiler over hot water. While heating mixture, beat it with a handheld electric mixer on medium-high speed. Continue to beat for 7 minutes, or until the mixture forms soft mounds. Remove from heat, add peppermint extract, and continue beating until frosting forms stiff peaks, about 7–9 minutes.

Serves 12.

Substitutions

If you don't have guar gum, substitute ½ teaspoon of arrowroot powder. For a more festive appearance, purchase some mini peppermint candy canes, crush them into small pieces, and sprinkle them on the cake. Or leave them whole and use them to decorate the cake; that way, you and your guests can decide whether or not you want to eat them. This is a very fun holiday cake. Thank you, Sadie!

Healthy Tidbit

Emotions have physical effects. Have you ever noticed that when you hear bad news you can feel the shock travel down your entire body straight to your toes? Everyday stress has a similar, if less pronounced, impact on your body. Suppressing emotions—that is, ignoring unpleasant feelings or simply trying to push them out of your mind—is a coping strategy many people use, but it can be harmful. People who suppress an emotion after a distressing event may end up down the road reacting to similar situations with heightened anxiety. Learning to recognize, accept, and constructively express your feelings, and learning strategies for dealing with problems, can be very valuable in preventing the detrimental physical and mental effects of suppressed emotions.

Macaroons

PER SERVING: 238.0 CALORIES ~ 3.2 G PROTEIN ~ 16.7 G CARBOHYDRATE ~ 3.4 G FIBER ~
19.1 G TOTAL FAT ~ 12.2 G SATURATED FAT ~ 0.0 MG CHOLESTEROL ~ 68.9 MG SODIUM

3 cups shredded unsweetened coconut

1 cup almond flour/meal

½ cup pure maple syrup

¼ cup coconut butter

1 teaspoon vanilla extract

¼ teaspoon salt

Preheat oven to 350°F.

Combine all ingredients in a medium bowl and mix well. Form into balls about the size of a walnut and place on a greased baking sheet.

Bake for 10 minutes. Reduce oven to 250°F and bake for another 10 minutes. Remove from oven. Take one macaroon off the baking sheet, allow it to cool slightly, and then test. The outside should be hard, but the inside should be soft. For crisper macaroons, leave them on the baking sheets to cool. If they are perfect, then promptly remove them from the baking sheets and allow them to cool on racks.

Makes 20–25 small macaroons (10 servings).

Substitutions

For a chocolate (or "mock-chocolate") version, add 1 tablespoon cocoa or carob powder to the recipe.

Kitchen Tip

Coconut butter is naturally sweet and is a great source of healthy fat, especially for vegetarians or others who are trying to limit their animal consumption. Commercially prepared coconut butter is quite expensive. I make my own by simply grinding dried coconut in my Vitamix. I haven't tried this yet in a blender or food processor. If you don't have a Vitamix, I highly suggest purchasing one because you can use it to save a significant amount of money by making many items from scratch. I use mine to grind all my own flours, and to make sauces, dips, spreads, and drinks.

Nutritional Analysis per Serving

Vitamin A	0.0 RE	Vitamin D	0.0 µg
Thiamin (B-1)	0.0 mg	Vitamin E	2.8 mg
Riboflavin (B-2)	0.2 mg	Calcium	43.5 mg
Niacin	0.1 mg	Iron	1.0 mg
Vitamin B-6	0.0 mg	Phosphorus	27.5 mg
Vitamin B-12	0.0 µg	Magnesium	43.0 mg
Folate (total)	6.2 µg	Zinc	0.5 mg
Vitamin C	0.8 mg	Potassium	119.5 mg

Chia Pudding

PER SERVING: 366.2 CALORIES ~ 7.0 G PROTEIN ~ 20.9 G CARBOHYDRATE ~ 9.5 G FIBER ~
30.5 G TOTAL FAT ~ 20.9 G SATURATED FAT ~ 0.0 MG CHOLESTEROL ~ 23.4 MG SODIUM

1 15-ounce can coconut milk

⅔ cup chia seeds

½ cup almond milk

2 tablespoons pure maple syrup

1 teaspoon vanilla extract

Stevia to taste

Combine all ingredients, except stevia, in a large bowl. Refrigerate, covered, for at least 4 hours or overnight, until thickened. Add stevia to taste before serving.

Serves 4.

Substitutions
You can try other milks such as hemp milk or almond milk. You can add berries or fruit to make it a fruity flavored pudding. This recipe is very forgiving, quick, and easy.

Healthy Tidbit
When mixed with the liquid, the chia seeds will gel, creating a tapioca-like texture. It may take time to get used to this pudding, but once you learn to love the texture, you can enjoy the fact that this sweet treat is also extremely healthy and packed with beneficial fats.

Reducing carbs, such as baked goods and breads, and consuming healthy fats, such as coconut milk, can help you maintain an appropriate weight.

Nutritional Analysis per Serving

Vitamin A	1.0 RE	Vitamin D	0.0 µg
Thiamin (B-1)	0.2 mg	Vitamin E	0.0 mg
Riboflavin (B-2)	0.2 mg	Calcium	185.7 mg
Niacin	2.1 mg	Iron	6.1 mg
Vitamin B-6	0.2 mg	Phosphorus	329.5 mg
Vitamin B-12	0.0 µg	Magnesium	69.4 mg
Folate (total)	42.3 µg	Zinc	1.6 mg
Vitamin C	4.8 mg	Potassium	331.4 mg

Sun Butter Squares

PER SERVING: 180.6 CALORIES ~ 4.3 G PROTEIN ~ 21.5 G CARBOHYDRATE ~ 0.9 G FIBER ~
8.5 G TOTAL FAT ~ 2.2 G SATURATED FAT ~ 23.3 MG CHOLESTEROL ~ 369.7 MG SODIUM

2 cups Sun Butter (purchased or from recipe on page 121)

2 eggs

1 cup honey

1 teaspoon baking soda

Preheat oven to 350°F.

Combine all ingredients in a medium bowl, mixing until smooth. Pour into a lightly greased 8-inch square baking dish. Bake for 25–35 minutes, or until fork inserted in center comes out clean. Cool; cut into small squares.

Serves 16.

Healthy Tidbit

"Insulin resistance" is the term used to describe the body's inability to use insulin effectively to break down blood sugar (glucose) so it can easily pass through the cell membrane and enter the cell to be utilized as energy. When insulin isn't working properly, cells feel "hungry" for sugar; therefore, more insulin is released with the desired result of feeding sugar to the hungry cells. Over time, increased levels of insulin will overstimulate the receptors for insulin on cells, which can result in insulin resistance. This means that for each molecule of sugar needed to enter the cell, the body now needs more insulin to do the same job. Prolonged high levels of insulin will lead to weight gain and increased cholesterol. Help prevent insulin resistance with these four tips:

1. Consume fewer processed carbohydrates and less sugar. Consume slow-digesting carbohydrates, such as beans and legumes, and eat more vegetables.

2. Maintain a healthy body weight by exercising regularly, including a program of weight training.

3. Avoid liquid calories such as soda, juice, and alcohol.

4. Get plenty of sleep on a consistent schedule.

Nutritional Analysis per Serving

Vitamin A	10.1 RE	Vitamin D	0.1 µg
Thiamin (B-1)	0.0 mg	Vitamin E	0.1 mg
Riboflavin (B-2)	0.0 mg	Calcium	5.0 mg
Niacin	0.0 mg	Iron	0.2 mg
Vitamin B-6	0.0 mg	Phosphorus	13.3 mg
Vitamin B-12	0.1 µg	Magnesium	1.2 mg
Folate (total)	3.4 µg	Zinc	0.1 mg
Vitamin C	0.5 mg	Potassium	20.1 mg

Fruit Juice Jell-O

PER SERVING: 38.7 CALORIES ~ 1.7 G PROTEIN ~ 8.1 G CARBOHYDRATE ~ 0.1 G FIBER ~
0.1 G TOTAL FAT ~ 0.0 G SATURATED FAT ~ 0.0 MG CHOLESTEROL ~ 7.1 MG SODIUM

¼ cup cold water
1 envelope (1 tablespoon) unflavored gelatin
¾ cup boiling water
1 cup 100 percent fruit juice

Place cold water in a 1-quart bowl and sprinkle with gelatin; let stand until
gelatin is softened, about 2 minutes. Stir in boiling water, mixing until gelatin
dissolves.

Stir in fruit juice. Refrigerate until set, about 2 hours.

Serves 4.

Substitutions

This recipe can be chilled in a 5-inch gelatin mold. Any type of juice works.
To add fresh fruit, stir in ¼–½ cup berries or chopped fruit as the gelatin is
beginning to set. Refrigerate until set. For a more nutritious variation, try
adding shredded carrots or cabbage, a trick my husband's grandmother used
to employ.

Healthy Tidbit

Juice contains too much sugar to be consumed regularly as a beverage. I
recommend that the main beverage you drink be plain water. If you want to
drink green tea, herbal tea, or a cup of coffee, then it should be in addition to
the water you consume regularly. Juice should be reserved as a special treat.
This recipe dilutes juice with water to make a dessert. Children love Jell-O,
and with this recipe I can treat my kids without the processed sugars and dyes
contained in commercial Jell-O. I feel good about this special indulgence!

Nutritional Analysis per Serving

Vitamin A	1.4 RE	Vitamin D	0.0 µg
Thiamin (B-1)	0.0 mg	Vitamin E	0.0 mg
Riboflavin (B-2)	0.0 mg	Calcium	8.3 mg
Niacin	0.1 mg	Iron	0.2 mg
Vitamin B-6	0.0 mg	Phosphorus	6.3 mg
Vitamin B-12	0.0 µg	Magnesium	6.0 mg
Folate (total)	3.6 µg	Zinc	0.0 mg
Vitamin C	14.8 mg	Potassium	82.1 mg

Coconut Custard

PER SERVING: 222.6 CALORIES ~ 5.6 G PROTEIN ~ 13.8 G CARBOHYDRATE ~ 0.0 G FIBER ~
17.3 G TOTAL FAT ~ 13.5 G SATURATED FAT ~ 124.0 MG CHOLESTEROL ~ 56.5 MG SODIUM

1 14-ounce can coconut milk
¼ cup raw honey
¼ teaspoon ground nutmeg
1 teaspoon pure vanilla extract
4 eggs

Preheat oven to 325°F.

Whisk all ingredients together in a medium bowl until smooth and foamy, about 2 minutes. Place 6 8-ounce ramekins in a 13×9-inch baking pan; fill the baking pan with hot water to reach halfway up the side of the ramekins. Pour custard into ramekins. Bake for 25–30 minutes, or until set. To test, insert a knife into the center of one of the custards. It should come out clean.

Serves 6.

Substitutions
This recipe can also be baked in a 6-cup porcelain soufflé dish; bake for about 1 hour, or until set.

If a crystallized appearance is desired, sprinkle the custards with a small amount of maple sugar, honey crystals, or coconut palm sugar before baking.

You can also try other types of milk, such as a nice, thick hemp milk.

Healthy Tidbit
Coconut is a great source of protein and of medium-chain fatty acids. It comes in a variety of forms, such as ground, flaked, milk, flour, oil, or butter. I make use of all of these items for many different culinary purposes.

Nutritional Analysis per Serving

Vitamin A	54.0 RE	Vitamin D	0.7 µg
Thiamin (B-1)	0.0 mg	Vitamin E	0.4 mg
Riboflavin (B-2)	0.2 mg	Calcium	31.6 mg
Niacin	0.5 mg	Iron	2.8 mg
Vitamin B-6	0.1 mg	Phosphorus	130.1 mg
Vitamin B-12	0.3 µg	Magnesium	34.9 mg
Folate (total)	25.2 µg	Zinc	0.8 mg
Vitamin C	0.7 mg	Potassium	199.7 mg

Velvety Carob Pudding

PER SERVING: 192.7 CALORIES ~ 5.6 G PROTEIN ~ 25.4 G CARBOHYDRATE ~ 6.8 G FIBER ~
8.7 G TOTAL FAT ~ 0.7 G SATURATED FAT ~ 0.0 MG CHOLESTEROL ~ 84.4 MG SODIUM

Contributed by cooking instructor Robin Michelle Crout, of Tacoma, Washington.

1 cup cold almond or rice milk

4 tablespoons ground chia seeds

1 tablespoon finely ground flax seeds

2 tablespoons hazelnut butter or almond butter

2 tablespoons maple syrup

2 tablespoons honey

2 tablespoons raw or roasted carob powder

1 teaspoon vanilla extract

⅛ teaspoon salt

Blend all ingredients in a blender on high until smooth, scraping sides of blender with a rubber spatula if necessary. Pour into a serving bowl. Refrigerate for 1–2 hours, or until thickened.

Serves 4.

Suggested toppings: ground walnuts, sliced almonds, organic chocolate chips, shredded unsweetened coconut, a squeeze of orange, banana slices, or a sprig of fresh mint.

Substitutions

You could use organic unsweetened cocoa powder instead of the carob if you don't mind adding a little chocolate. In the summer, why not add a handful of pitted, sliced cherries to the ingredients and blend them in for a carob-cherry pudding? Alternately, you could add ½ teaspoon of organic peppermint extract or 1 tablespoon of strong coffee.

Healthy Tidbit

Carob, part of the legume family, is a popular alternative to chocolate or cocoa powder. It has a rich, deep flavor and offers a lot of nutrition. Carob is naturally sweet and is free of the caffeine and theobromine found in chocolate. It contains vitamins A, B-2, B-3, and D, and a small amount of protein. It is also high in calcium, phosphorus, potassium, and magnesium, and contains iron, manganese, barium, copper, and nickel.

Nutritional Analysis per Serving

Vitamin A	29.1 RE	Vitamin D	2.4 µg
Thiamin (B-1)	0.3 mg	Vitamin E	2.5 mg
Riboflavin (B-2)	0.4 mg	Calcium	92.3 mg
Niacin	4.1 mg	Iron	1.5 mg
Vitamin B-6	0.3 mg	Phosphorus	91.0 mg
Vitamin B-12	0.5 µg	Magnesium	39.4 mg
Folate (total)	68.4 µg	Zinc	0.8 mg
Vitamin C	22.7 mg	Potassium	165.0 mg

Berry Mango Sorbet

PER SERVING: 58.6 CALORIES ~ 0.9 G PROTEIN ~ 14.1 G CARBOHYDRATE ~ 1.2 G FIBER ~
0.4 G TOTAL FAT ~ 0.0 G SATURATED FAT ~ 0.0 MG CHOLESTEROL ~ 2.4 MG SODIUM

Another delicious creation from Robin Michelle Crout.

1 cup frozen strawberries or blackberries, partially thawed
1 cup frozen mango chunks, partially thawed
1 tablespoon honey
2 tablespoons almond milk
Juice and zest of one lemon (optional)

Combine all ingredients in a food processor or blender. Process, using the
pulse technique, until mixture is almost smooth but still partially frozen and
slushy. Serve immediately.
    Serves 4.

Substitutions
Raspberries work in this recipe, too, but some dislike their seed content. Blueberries do not work as well in this recipe.

Healthy Tidbit
Avoid getting into the habit of serving dessert after every dinner. Sweets
should be a surprise and a treat, not an expectation. I've noticed that children
in some families always expect a sweet after dinner. My children don't have
this expectation; therefore, when we do enjoy something sweet, it is fun and
festive. In addition, we never order desserts when we are eating out. I want
to prevent my daughters from becoming habituated to restaurant desserts;
that way the sweets we eat are usually healthier (except when we're at other
people's houses for dinner, when we relax the rules a little bit).

Nutritional Analysis per Serving

Vitamin A	0.0 RE	Vitamin D	0.0 µg
Thiamin (B-1)	0.0 mg	Vitamin E	0.1 mg
Riboflavin (B-2)	0.0 mg	Calcium	6.6 mg
Niacin	0.2 mg	Iron	0.4 mg
Vitamin B-6	0.0 mg	Phosphorus	4.8 mg
Vitamin B-12	0.0 µg	Magnesium	4.0 mg
Folate (total)	6.1 µg	Zinc	0.1 mg
Vitamin C	10.6 mg	Potassium	63.9 mg

Almond Cake with Banana, Coconut, and Pineapple Purée

PER SERVING: 361.9 CALORIES ~ 10.9 G PROTEIN ~ 36.7 G CARBOHYDRATE ~ 6.7 G FIBER ~ 22.4 G TOTAL FAT ~ 3.3 G SATURATED FAT ~ 46.5 MG CHOLESTEROL ~ 64.5 MG SODIUM

This recipe originally appeared in *Living with Crohn's and Colitis*.

For the Cake

2 eggs

¼ cup honey

3 very ripe bananas, mashed

2¾ cups almond flour/meal

½ teaspoon baking powder

Juice of ½ lemon

1 teaspoon vanilla extract

Tropical Fruit Topping (recipe follows)

Pineapple and banana slices, as garnish

For the Tropical Fruit Topping

(makes about 3 cups)

2 cups chopped pineapple

1 ripe banana

½ cup shredded coconut

To make the cake: Preheat oven to 350°F.

Beat eggs and honey with a mixer on medium speed until pale and fluffy, about 10 minutes; beat in bananas. Combine almond meal and baking powder; beat into egg mixture. Add lemon juice and vanilla, mixing until smooth. Pour into well-greased 9-inch round pan; bake for 45 minutes or until cake is golden brown and fork inserted in center comes out clean. Cool in pan on wire rack until completely cooled.

Loosen cake from edge of pan with a sharp knife. Invert onto a serving plate and ease cake out of pan. Pour Tropical Fruit Topping (recipe follows) over cake; decorate with sliced fruits.

To make the tropical fruit topping: While cake is cooling, place chopped pineapple, coconut, and banana in blender and blend until smooth.

Serves 8.

Healthy Tidbit

This is a great cake to serve at a child's first birthday party, before you've introduced dairy, gluten, sugar, or grains into their diet. We served this for my daughter's first birthday, and it was a hit with both the adults and children!

Nutritional Analysis per Serving

Vitamin A	26.3 RE	Vitamin D	0.3 µg
Thiamin (B-1)	0.1 mg	Vitamin E	9.8 mg
Riboflavin (B-2)	0.1 mg	Calcium	116.0 mg
Niacin	0.6 mg	Iron	2.2 mg
Vitamin B-6	0.3 mg	Phosphorus	53.5 mg
Vitamin B-12	0.1 µg	Magnesium	134.3 mg
Folate (total)	26.9 µg	Zinc	0.4 mg
Vitamin C	25.4 mg	Potassium	298.7 mg

Mini Pumpkin Pies

PER SERVING: 112.6 CALORIES ~ 3.4 G PROTEIN ~ 21.4 G CARBOHYDRATE ~ 1.7 G FIBER ~
2.4 G TOTAL FAT ~ 0.8 G SATURATED FAT ~ 62.8 MG CHOLESTEROL ~ 225.7 MG SODIUM

2 cups pumpkin purée, or 1 15-ounce can pumpkin

1 cup almond milk

¾ cup honey

4 eggs, lightly beaten

1 teaspoon butter, softened

1 teaspoon ground cinnamon

1 teaspoon salt

½ teaspoon ground ginger

Preheat oven to 375°F.

Whisk all ingredients together in a large bowl until smooth. Pour into 12 8-ounce ramekins. Place ramekins in two 13 × 9-inch baking pans; fill baking pans with hot water to reach halfway up the sides of the ramekins. Bake for 30–40 minutes, until a fork inserted in center of a ramekin comes out clean. Serve warm or cool.

Serves 12.

Substitutions

You can use most kinds of milk for this recipe. Fresh pumpkin, steamed and puréed, gives a better flavor than canned, but these little treats are still delicious—and very easy—even with canned pumpkin. I like this recipe for the holidays because it provides the familiar taste of a traditional favorite while omitting the crust, which is not missed at all.

Healthy Tidbit

Eating dinners together as a family on a regular basis has been shown to help teenagers ward off the temptations of drug experimentation. Creating a solid familial foundation reduces a teenager's feelings of isolation and creates a sense of worth and value. The more a person learns to value herself or himself and others, the less likely she or he will be to try illegal activities under peer pressure. Family dinners create a sense of belonging for all family members, including adults and younger children. If your toddler cannot sit at the table for the entire mealtime, have her sit as long

Nutritional Analysis per Serving

Vitamin A	665.5 RE	Vitamin D	0.3 µg
Thiamin (B-1)	0.0 mg	Vitamin E	0.2 mg
Riboflavin (B-2)	0.1 mg	Calcium	26.8 mg
Niacin	0.2 mg	Iron	1.1 mg
Vitamin B-6	0.1 mg	Phosphorus	48.5 mg
Vitamin B-12	0.2 µg	Magnesium	12.1 mg
Folate (total)	13.2 µg	Zinc	0.3 mg
Vitamin C	1.8 mg	Potassium	145.0 mg

as she can and then allow her to get up and move around while the rest of the family finishes the meal. As she gets older and continues to observe the tradition of family dinners, she will be able to sit at the table for longer periods without being forced.

Cinnamon Oranges

PER SERVING: 89.1 CALORIES ~ 1.4 G PROTEIN ~ 23.0 G CARBOHYDRATE ~ 3.2 G FIBER ~
0.3 G TOTAL FAT ~ 0.0 G SATURATED FAT ~ 0.0 MG CHOLESTEROL ~ 1.6 MG SODIUM

4 navel oranges, peeled and sliced into rounds

2 tablespoons orange juice

2 tablespoons lemon juice

1 tablespoon agave syrup

¼ teaspoon ground cinnamon

Arrange orange slices on a serving plate. Whisk orange juice, lemon juice, agave syrup, and cinnamon in a small bowl. Spoon over oranges; refrigerate and serve chilled.

Serves 4.

Substitutions

If you react to citrus, try this recipe with mangos, peaches, or pears.

Healthy Tidbit

A good laugh is worth more than you may know. Make sure to engage daily in activities that relieve stress and promote laughter, such as reading or watching something funny, or taking time to look at pictures from your past that remind you of happy memories. Laughter can increase your white blood cell count and is heart protective, so get your laugh on!

Nutritional Analysis per Serving

Vitamin A	36.2 RE	Vitamin D	0.0 µg
Thiamin (B-1)	0.1 mg	Vitamin E	0.0 mg
Riboflavin (B-2)	0.1 mg	Calcium	63.0 mg
Niacin	0.6 mg	Iron	0.2 mg
Vitamin B-6	0.1 mg	Phosphorus	34.2 mg
Vitamin B-12	0.0 µg	Magnesium	16.8 mg
Folate (total)	51.5 µg	Zinc	0.1 mg
Vitamin C	91.7 mg	Potassium	256.4 mg

Chocolate Syrup

PER SERVING: 156.9 CALORIES ~ 1.3 G PROTEIN ~ 25.7 G CARBOHYDRATE ~ 2.2 G FIBER ~
7.7 G TOTAL FAT ~ 6.4 G SATURATED FAT ~ 0.0 MG CHOLESTEROL ~ 26.0 MG SODIUM

1 cup cocoa powder

1 cup agave syrup

½ cup water

¼ cup plus 2 tablespoons coconut oil

2 teaspoons vanilla extract

½ teaspoon guar gum

⅛ teaspoon salt

Whisk all ingredients in a medium bowl until smooth. Store in a glass container in the refrigerator.

Yields 3 cups (12 servings).

Kitchen Tip

It is important to use a good-quality vanilla extract for this syrup. Because it contains coconut oil the syrup may harden in the refrigerator. Simply warm it slightly before use, as needed.

Healthy Tidbit

Dark chocolate and cocoa can help to reduce blood pressure and may improve the serum lipid profile. But can chocolate actually improve cardiometabolic outcomes? The current meta-analysis finds that higher levels of chocolate consumption are associated with a reduced risk of any cardiovascular disease and of stroke in particular. These findings may change physicians' dietary advice to patients.[10]

Nutritional Analysis per Serving

Vitamin A	0.0 RE	Vitamin D	0.0 µg
Thiamin (B-1)	0.0 mg	Vitamin E	0.0 mg
Riboflavin (B-2)	0.0 mg	Calcium	8.4 mg
Niacin	0.2 mg	Iron	1.1 mg
Vitamin B-6	0.0 mg	Phosphorus	52.5 mg
Vitamin B-12	0.0 µg	Magnesium	34.5 mg
Folate (total)	2.3 µg	Zinc	0.5 mg
Vitamin C	11.2 mg	Potassium	181.8 mg

Homemade Chocolate Spread

PER SERVING: 286.0 CALORIES ~ 1.2 G PROTEIN ~ 22.9 G CARBOHYDRATE ~ 1.2 G FIBER ~
22.4 G TOTAL FAT ~ 18.8 G SATURATED FAT ~ 0.0 MG CHOLESTEROL ~ 0.1 MG SODIUM

1 cup coconut butter

¾ cup cocoa powder

¾ cup agave syrup

2 teaspoons pure vanilla extract

Process all ingredients in a food processor or blender until smooth. If not using it right away, spoon into small storage containers and freeze for future use.

Yields 2½ cups (10 4-tablespoon servings).

Kitchen Tip

Commercially prepared coconut butter is quite expensive. I make my own by simply grinding dried coconut in my Vitamix.

Substitutions

You could substitute carob for the cocoa powder, and you could try adding a nut butter such as Sun Butter (see recipe on page 121). Adding finely ground hazelnuts would yield a spread similar to Nutella.

Nutritional Analysis per Serving

Vitamin A	0.0 RE	Vitamin D	0.0 µg
Thiamin (B-1)	0.0 mg	Vitamin E	0.0 mg
Riboflavin (B-2)	0.0 mg	Calcium	0.1 mg
Niacin	0.0 mg	Iron	2.2 mg
Vitamin B-6	0.0 mg	Phosphorus	0.1 mg
Vitamin B-12	0.0 µg	Magnesium	0.1 mg
Folate (total)	0.0 µg	Zinc	0.0 mg
Vitamin C	10.1 mg	Potassium	1.2 mg

Sandwiches

Sandwiches are convenient, offer a wide range of ingredient choices, and can be a good way to get vegetables into children. Using bread as the basis for a sandwich is the easiest and most obvious choice, but you can also consider other options, such as tortillas, flatbread, or the pancakes left over from breakfast. Because children's diets can perhaps be less restrictive, some of the ingredient ideas that I've listed here aren't strictly considered part of the anti-inflammation diet. For example, I've listed cheese or cream cheese as a possible sandwich filling. Cream Cheese "Curds and Whey" (see recipe on page 172) may be easier to digest than commercial cream cheese. Harder cheeses are a little easier to digest than soft cheeses, so if you or your child is somewhat dairy intolerant, stick to harder cheeses.

Besides sliced bread, consider using any of the following creative alternatives. Gluten-free versions of most of these can be made or purchased.

- bagels
- buns
- crackers
- crêpes
- English muffins
- flatbread
- matzo
- muffins
- naan
- pancakes
- rice cakes
- rolls
- tortillas

For fillings, start with a combination of colorful, nutrient-dense vegetables. Then add a tasty spread, or turn to last night's leftovers. Here are some ideas:

- avocado, cucumber, and sprouts
- shredded carrots, cucumbers, sunflower seeds, avocado, and cream cheese
- grilled vegetables (bell peppers, onions, mushrooms, eggplant, zucchini) with pesto sauce
- grilled vegetables with hummus
- sharp cheddar with apple slices
- brie cheese with mustard and sprouts
- cheese, tomato, sprouts or lettuce, and pesto sauce
- turkey loaf with tomato, and lettuce or sprouts
- sliced chicken or turkey, cranberry sauce, and lettuce

✦ sliced chicken or turkey, honey mustard, tomato, and lettuce or sprouts

✦ sliced beef with mayonnaise or horseradish, sliced tomato, and cucumbers

✦ chicken salad made from celery, lettuce, and tomato

✦ tuna/cucumber/green pepper salad with tomato

✦ cream cheese and strawberries

✦ cream cheese, cherry chutney, turkey, lettuce

✦ salmon salad with lettuce or sprouts

✦ cream cheese, smoked salmon, red onion, and capers

✦ chicken salad with relish and spinach

✦ egg salad with lettuce or spinach

✦ spinach, tomato, bacon, mayo

✦ "Sadie's special": turkey, grilled onions, sweet relish, mayo, mustard, lettuce

✦ Sun Butter or almond butter with jelly

✦ Sun Butter or almond butter with honey

✦ Sun Butter or almond butter with honey and banana

✦ nitrite-free and hormone-free turkey cold cuts with roasted red pepper sauce, lettuce, and sauerkraut

Lunch Ideas for Kids

Lunch is the meal that sets the stage for the afternoon. The food eaten for lunch will play a role in determining the quality of the rest of the day for you and your children. Preparing ahead of time to pack a healthy, high-quality lunch is integral to improving or maintaining health and productivity. Consuming a balanced meal at lunchtime will help adults stay sharper and more energized, and help children to perform well in school and be better behaved. Make sure the lunch you eat and the one you provide for your kids, whether prepared ahead of time at home or purchased at a restaurant or school cafeteria, meet anti-inflammatory guidelines.

- frozen fruit with agave syrup
- frozen peas
- sandwiches on gluten-free bread
- wraps on gluten-free tortillas
- bean and cheese burritos on gluten-free tortillas
- salmon salad with rice crackers
- chicken sausage, heated and packed in a thermos
- fish or chicken patties, heated and packed in a thermos, with dipping sauce
- French toast
- pancakes
- peanut butter and jelly sandwiches made with pancakes
- frozen edamame, served cold, or heated and packed in a thermos
- squash, heated and packed in a thermos
- sweet potatoes, heated and packed in a thermos
- rice and beans, heated and packed in a thermos
- soup, heated and packed in a thermos
- salad, with dressing on the side
- frozen grapes
- smoked salmon
- smoothies
- sushi balls
- fruit

- mini quiches
- homemade granola bars
- red pepper roll-ups: roasted red pepper rolled in slices of turkey
- pepperoni
- muffins
- custards
- gluten-free pasta salads
- hard boiled or poached egg
- fresh veggies with dip
- steamed veggies: carrots, zucchini, asparagus, green beans, yellow beets

Using Leftovers

- If you cook chicken breasts, steak, or turkey for dinner, prepare an extra serving and slice it for sandwiches the next day instead of purchasing lunch meat.
- If you're making a salad for dinner, slice some extra vegetables, such as cucumbers, carrots, bell peppers, and celery, to add to your child's lunch the next day. Make extra dressing and pour it into the dip container. Always pack salad dressing separately to keep the salad fresh and crisp until lunchtime.
- While you're making dinner, boil a few eggs. Pack the eggs whole, make deviled eggs, or use them in egg salad.
- Boil extra pasta, couscous, or quinoa. Use it to make a salad for lunch by cutting vegetables very small, tossing them with the grain or pasta, and adding salad dressing or a little lemon juice, oil, and salt.
- Use leftover rice to make burritos with beans and cheese.
- Use extra rice to make a stir-fried rice with vegetables; quickly reheat it and pack it in a thermos the next morning.
- Grill extra vegetables and use them in sandwiches or pack them alone in a thermos.

Conclusion

Thank you so much for caring for your health enough to purchase this book. If you adopt the changes I've suggested, prepare yourself for big improvements in your health and your overall well-being. Creating health feels wonderful and is contagious to those around you. Please share your knowledge with others, and give them the support they need to begin caring for themselves the way you have done. I am so proud of you for taking this step, and I am excited to hear about your progress. I invite you to e-mail me with your comments, suggestions, and testimonials. You can find a link to my e-mail address at either of my two websites: www.drjessicablack.com or www.afamilyhealingcenter.com.

Notes

Introduction

1. P. M. Barnes, B. Bloom, and R. L. Nahin, "Complementary and Alternative Medicine Use Among Adults and Children: United States, 2007," (2008), http://www.cdc.gov/nchs/data/nhsr/nhsr012.pdf (accessed 10 July 2012).

Chapter 1

1. S. Vasto et al., "Alzheimer's Disease and Genetics of Inflammation: A Pharmacogenomic Vision," *Pharmacogenomics* 8, no. 12(2007): 1735–45; C. Holmes, et al., "Systemic Inflammation and Disease Progression in Alzheimer Disease," *Neurology* 73, no. 10: 768–74.

2. T. T. Issac, H. Dokainish, N. M. Lakkis, "Role of Inflammation in Initiation and Perpetuation of Atrial Fibrillation: A Systematic Review of the Published Data," *Journal of the American College of Cardiology* 50, no. 21 (2007): 2021–28.

3. A. M. Iacopino, "Inflammation in Systemic Health and in Periodontal Disease." Medscape Dentistry and Oral Health, 2011, http://www.webmd .com (accessed March 14, 2012).

4. P. Kardos and J. Keenan, "Tackling COPD: A Multicomponent Disease Driven by Inflammation," *Medscape General Medicine* 8, no. 3 (2006): 54.

5. L. Barclay, "One-Hour Plasma Glucose Levels May Be a Marker for Cardiovascular Risk," *Diabetes Care*, 2009; D. Stocker, et al., "A Randomized Trial of the Effects of Rosiglitazone and Metformin on Inflammation and Subclinical Atherosclerosis in Patients with Type 2 Diabetes," *American Heart Journal* 153, no. 3 (2007): 445.e1–445.e6.

6. S. Vasto et al., "Inflammation and Prostate Cancer," *Future Oncology* 4, no. 5 (2008): 637–45; E. Siegel, et al., "The Effects of Obesity and Obesity-Related Conditions on Colorectal Cancer Prognosis" *Cancer Control* 17, no. 1 (2010): 52–57.

7. Centers for Disease Control, "National Vital Statistics Report," 51 (4). DHHS Publication number 2011-1120, http://www.cdc.gov/nchs/products /nvsr.htm (accessed September 10, 2012).

Chapter 2

1. J. O'Keefe, N. Gheewala, and J. O. O'Keefe, "Dietary Strategies for Improving Post-Prandial Glucose, Lipids, Inflammation, and Cardiovascular Health," *Journal of the American College of Cardiology* 51, no. 3 (2008): 249–55.

2. Janet Kim, "Expert Interview with David Katz, MD, MPH," February 15, 2011, http://www.medscape.com/viewarticle/737342 (accessed January 12, 2012).

3. V. Verallo-Rowell et al., "Novel Antibacterial and Emollient Effects of Coconut and Virgin Olive Oils in Adult Atopic Dermatitis," *Dermatitis* 19, no. 6 (2008): 308–15.

4. D. Iggman, "Role of Different Dietary Saturated Fatty Acids for Cardio-metabolic Risk," *Journal of Clinical Lipidology* 6, no. 2 (2011): 209–23.

5. Jessica Black and Dede Cummings, *Living with Crohn's and Colitis: A Comprehensive Naturopathic Guide to Complete Digestive Wellness* (Long Island City, NY: Hatherleigh Press, 2010), 59.

6. J. Rudant et al., "Household Exposure to Pesticides and Risk of Childhood Hematopoietic Malignancies: The ESCALE Study (SFCE)," *Environmental Health Perspectives* 115, no. 12 (2007): 1787–93.

7. J. R. Richardson et al., "Elevated Serum Pesticide Levels and Risk of Parkinson Disease," *Archives of Neurology* 66, no. 7 (2009): 870–75.

8. Black and Cummings, *Living with Crohn's and Colitis*, 59.

9. S. L. Kraeuter and R. Schwartz, "Blood and Mast Cell Histamine Levels in Magnesium-Deficient Rats," *The Journal of Nutrition* 110, no. 5 (1980): 851–58, http://www.ncbi.nlm.nih.gov/pubmed/6445415 (accessed August 10, 2012).

10. Black and Cummings, *Living with Crohn's and Colitis*, 24.

11. F. Jacka, "The Association Between Habitual Diet Quality and the Common Mental Disorders in Community-Dwelling Adults: The Hordaland Health Study," *Psychosomatic Medicine* 73 (2011): 483–90.

12. L. Pelsser et al., "Effects of a Restricted Elimination Diet on the Behaviour of Children with Attention-Deficit Hyperactivity Disorder (INCA Study): A Randomised Controlled Trial," *Lancet* 377, no. 9764 (2011): 446–48, 494–503.

13. Y. Jiang, S. K. Noh, and S. I. Koo, "Egg Phosphatidylcholine Decreases the Lymphatic Absorption of Cholesterol in Rats," *Journal of Nutrition* 131, no. 9 (2001): 2358–63.

14. Sandra Yin, "Low-Sugar Diet Can Reduce Irritable Bowel Symptoms," Presented October 31, 2011, http://www.medscape.com/viewarticle/752779 (accessed June 10, 2012).

15. D. Jenkins, "Nuts as a Replacement for Carbohydrates in the Diabetic Diet," *Diabetes Care* 2011, 34, no. 8 (2011): 1706–1711.

16. H. Ferdowsian, "Does Diet Really Affect Acne?" *Skin Therapy Letter* 15, no. 3 (2010): 1–2.

17. L. Azadbakht et al., "Effects of the Dietary Approaches to Stop Hypertension (DASH) Eating Plan on Cardiovascular Risks Among Type 2 Diabetic Patients: A Randomized Crossover Clinical Trial," *Diabetes Care* 34, no. 1 (2011): 55–57.

18. J. Ludvigsson, "Celiac Disease Confers a 1.6-Fold Increased Risk of Asthma: A Nationwide Population-Based Cohort Study," *Journal of Allergy and Clinical Immunology* 127, no. 4 (2011): 1071–73.

19. J. H. O'Keefe, N. Gheewala, and J. O. O'Keefe, "Dietary Strategies for Improving Post-Prandial Glucose, Lipids, Inflammation, and Cardiovascular Health," *Journal of the American College of Cardiology* 51, no. 3 (2008) 249–255.

20. Ibid.

21. S. Arora and S. McFarlane, "The Case for Low-Carbohydrate Diets in Diabetes Management," *Nutrition and Metabolism* 2 (2005): 16–24.

22. D. Kromhout et al., "N-3 Fatty Acids, Ventricular Arrhythmia-Related Events, and Fatal Myocardial Infarction in Postmyocardial Infarction Patients with Diabetes," *Diabetes Care* 34, no. 12 (2011): 2515–20.

23. M. Thorogood et al., "Risk of Death from Cancer and Ischaemic Heart Disease in Meat and Non-Meat Eaters," *British Medical Journal* 1994, 308, no. 6945 (1994): 1667–70; J. Chang-Claude, R. Frentzel-Beyme, and U. Eilber, "Mortality Patterns of German Vegetarians after 11 Years of Follow-Up," *Epidemiology* 3, no. 5 (1992): 395–401; J. Chang-Claude and R. Frentzel-Beyme, "Dietary and Lifestyle Determinants of Mortality among German Vegetarians," *International Journal of Epidemiology* 22, no. 2 (1993): 228–36.

24. The National Center on Addiction and Substance Abuse at Columbia University, "2011 Family Dinners Report from the National Center on Addiction and Substance Abuse at Columbia University," http://www .casacolumbia.org/templates/PressReleases.aspx?articleid=653&zoneid=87 (accessed June 5, 2012).

Chapter 3

1. A. Lund, "Markers of Chronic Inflammation with Short-Term Changes in Physical Activity," *Medicine and Science in Sports and Exercise* 43, no. 4 (2011): 578–83.

2. Ibid.

3. N. Ranjit et al., "Psychosocial Factors and Inflammation in the Multi-Ethnic Study of Atherosclerosis," *Archives of Internal Medicine* 167, no. 2 (2007): 174–81.

4. WebMD, "Get More Out of Each Day: Quick Tricks for Diet, Exercise, Stress," reviewed by Kathleen M. Zelman, MPH, RD, LD, http://www.web md.com/balance/diet-exercise-stress-10/slideshow-stress (accessed May 10, 2012).

5. Emma Hitt, "Large, Prospective Analysis Links Lack of Sleep to Weight Gain," (2006), http://www.medscape.com/viewarticle/536938 (accessed June 6, 2012).

6. M. Miller and F. Cappuccio, "Inflammation, Sleep, Obesity and Cardio-vascular Disease," *Current Vascular Pharmacology* 5, no. 2 (2007): 93–102.

7. J.-L. Pepin et al., "Comparison of Continuous Positive Airway Pressure and Valsartan in Hypertensive Sleep Apnea Patients," *American Journal of Respiratory and Critical Care Medicine* 2010, 182, no. 7 (2010): 954–60.

8. M. R. Irwin et al., "Sleep Loss Activates Cellular Inflammatory Signaling," *Biological Psychiatry* 2008, 64, no. 6 (2008), 538–40.

9. Caroline Cassels, "Lack of Sleep in Children Linked to ADHD Symptoms," (2009), 123: e857–e864, http://www.medscape.org/viewarticle /702399 (accessed June 6, 2012).

10. V. Seegers, "Short Sleep Duration and Body Mass Index: A Prospective Longitudinal Study in Preadolescence," *American Journal of Epidemiology* 173, no. 6 (2011): 621–29.

11. S. Boyles, "Air Pollution Linked to Risk of Diabetes," (2010), http://www .medscape.com/viewarticle/729946 (accessed February 14, 2012).

12. Z. J. Andersen et al., "Chronic Obstructive Pulmonary Disease and Long-Term Exposure to Traffic-Related Air Pollution: A Cohort Study" *American Journal of Respiratory and Critical Care Medicine* 183, no. 4 (2011): 455–61.

13. J. Hart et al., "Exposure to Traffic Pollution and Increased Risk of Rheumatoid Arthritis," *Environmental Health Perspectives* 117, no. 7 (2009): 1065–69.

14. A. C. Steinmann, "Fragranced Consumer Products and Undisclosed Ingredients," *Environmental Impact Assessment Review* 29 (2009): 32–38.

15. California Air Resources Board (CARB), "Report to the California Legislature: Indoor Air Pollution in California," Sacramento, CA: California Environmental Protection Agency, 2005.

16. W. W. Nazaroff and C. J. Weschler, "Cleaning Products and Air Fresheners: Exposure to Primary and Secondary Air Pollutants," *Atmospheric Environment* 38 (2004): 2841–65.

17. U.S. Environmental Protection Agency, "Fish Consumption Advisory," http://www.epa.gov/hg/advisories.htm (accessed May 2, 2012).

18. U.S. Environmental Protection Agency, "Background Report on Fertilizer Use, Contaminants, and Regulations," 1999, http://www.epa.gov/oppt /pubs/fertilizer.pdf (accessed July 17, 2012).

Chapter 4

1. A. Danese, "Elevated Inflammation Levels in Depressed Adults with a History of Childhood Maltreatment," *Archives of General Psychiatry* 65, no. 4 (2008): 409–16.
2. P. Carter et al., "Fruit and Vegetable Intake and Incidence of Type 2 Diabetes Mellitus: Systematic Review and Meta-Analysis," *British Medical Journal* 341 (2010): c4229.
3. A. Q. Pham et al., "Cinnamon Supplementation in Patients with Type 2 Diabetes Mellitus," *Pharmacotherapy* 27, no. 4 (2007): 595–99.
4. Environmental Working Group, "Sugar in Children's Cereals," 2011, http://breakingnews.ewg.org/report/sugar_in_childrens_cereals/more_sugar (accessed June 19, 2012).
5. A.S. Lillard and J. Peterson, "The Immediate Impact of Different Types of Television on Young Children's Executive Function," *Pediatrics* 2011, 128, no. 4 (2011): 644–49.
6. N. T. Williams, "Probiotics," *American Journal of Health-System Pharmacy* 67, no. 6 (2010): 449–58.
7. F. Haseen et al., "Is There a Benefit from Lycopene Supplementation in Men with Prostate Cancer? A Systematic Review," *Prostate Cancer and Prostatic Diseases* 12, no. 4 (2009): 316–24.
8. K. J. Reid et al., "Aerobic Exercise Improves Self-Reported Sleep and Quality of Life in Older Adults with Insomnia," *Sleep Medicine* 11, no. 9 (2010): 934–40.
9. V. Vuksan et al., "Supplementation of Conventional Therapy with the Novel Grain Salba (Salvia hispanica L.) Improves Major and Emerging Cardiovascular Risk Factors in Type 2 Diabetes: Results of a Randomized Controlled Trial," *Diabetes Care* 11 (2007): 2804–10, http://www.ncbi.nlm.nih.gov/pubmed/17686832 (accessed August 12, 2012)
10. A. Buitrago-Lopez et al., "Chocolate Consumption and Cardiometabolic Disorders: Systematic Review and Meta-Analysis," *British Medical Journal* 343 (2011): d4488.

Diet and Treatment Strategies for Common Ailments

When approaching illness, it is of utmost importance to consider what the body is trying to achieve by creating the illness and to help the body move through the illness, rather than merely suppressing the symptoms. Ibuprofen for pain and arthritis, for example, can only help for so long. Likewise, medications for blood pressure or ADD will only help for short amounts of time because they are working contrary to the body, not with the body. We want to accomplish wellness by supporting the body's natural healing processes and reversing the disease process.

The following are some common ailments, what types of dietary changes are most effective for treating them, and simple supplements to support the body in each case.

Arthritis Pain

- Remove all tomatoes, nightshade vegetables, and potatoes from the diet. Remove all gluten from the diet. Go strict on the anti-inflammation diet.

- Take hot-and-cold showers every day (see description on page 37).

- Begin light exercise, yoga, or movement every day to keep joints loose and less stiff.

- Consider the following herbal medicines: turmeric and ginger in capsule or tincture form.

- Consider the following nutraceutical medicines: adrenal support such as Strength by Herb Fusion (see Resources).

Asthma, ADD, ADHD, or Autism

- Stick to the anti-inflammation diet. Make sure to avoid *all* food dyes, sugars, artificial sugar substitutes, and gluten. Eliminate all food allergies if known.

- Add a probiotic supplement such as Restore by Herb Fusion, high-dosage fish oil, magnesium such as Tranquility by Herb Fusion (see Resources), and B vitamins to support the adrenals. Consider digestive enzymes before each meal.

- Follow a strict regular routine of eating, sleeping, and regular activities.

Body Odor

- Stick to the anti-inflammation diet, and consider doing an elimination and challenge diet. Avoid all dairy.
- Improve your digestion and make sure you are having regular bowel movements. For women, make sure hormones are balanced.
- Make sure to sweat regularly through strenuous exercise or saunas.
- Drink plenty of filtered water, at least half your body weight in ounces daily.
- Take a high-quality probiotic like Restore from Herb Fusion (see Resources) or zinc tablets daily.

Cancer

- Start a very strict anti-inflammation diet and eliminate most animal products. Eat mostly vegetables, fruits, and good fats such as those contained in salmon. Reduce grains and meats. Follow a strict anti-inflammation diet.
- Exercise strenuously to your tolerance every day. Exercise is your ticket to producing repair chemicals in your body. If you are physically fit, you should be exercising pretty hard. You can work your way into it or get a trainer. If you are not physically fit, get a trainer and do as much work as you can. If you are not fit enough to exercise, you still need to get outside and walk every day. Even if you can only walk a block, do so, and work up to more.
- Do some form of meditation or visualization daily that includes imagining yourself appearing and feeling healthy.
- Believe in something bigger than yourself. Pray daily and give thanks for what you have now and what you will have in the future. You have to be able to see yourself surviving.
- Watch funny movies, or find other ways to make sure you are laughing daily. Laughter boosts the immune response.
- Take additional antioxidant supplements.
- Take a high-potency probiotic supplement.
- Take high-dose fish oil, making sure you purchase a good quality one with no hidden heavy metals.

Chronic Ear Infections

- Avoid all dairy, including all fermented dairy products. If this doesn't help after two weeks, avoid all gluten and sugar as well. Drink more water. For babies, don't have them drink while lying down with a bottle. No side-lying breastfeeding, at least until the ear infections have cleared.

- Consider the following homeopathic medicines: chamomilia, belladonna, and pulsatilla.

- Use garlic mullein eardrops for acute treatment: three drops, warmed, in each ear three times per day for at least ten days in a row. Note: If anything is draining from the ear prior to the drops, or if rupture is suspected, do not use the ear drops.

Chronic Headache or Migraine

- Follow a strict anti-inflammation diet. Make sure to remove all migraine triggers from the diet such as wine, cheese, and chocolate.

- During a headache, you can try ice to the head and heat to the feet. Put yourself in a dark room for relaxation.

- Try acupressure to the following areas (you can look them up online): LI4, LV3, GB41.

- For women, treat stress or hormone imbalance.

- Take Strength for the adrenals and Tranquility for sleep and additional adrenal support (both from Herb Fusion, see Resources).

Chronic Sinus Infections

- Eliminate all dairy and sugar from the diet.

- Do a nasal lavage daily with sea salt and water or probiotics and water. You can purchase a neti pot online or in health-food stores or most drugstores. I personally don't like a neti pot and don't think you need one to get the job done. You can use a small dropper from a tincture bottle and save money by not purchasing a neti pot.

- Consider the following homeopathic medicines: kali bic (kali bichromicum), nat mur (natrum muriaticum).

- If you also have acid reflux or heartburn or are constantly clearing your throat or coughing in the morning, treat yourself for reflux. Chronic sinus conditions are often related to reflux.

- Chronic sinus infections are also related to chronic stress. Reduce stress by using a stress-moderating technique of your own, such as exercise or meditation.

- Take an adrenal-support supplement such as Strength from Herb Fusion (see Resources).

- If you don't sleep well, take a magnesium supplement like Tranquility, from Herb Fusion, nightly before bed.

Cough

- Remove all dairy, gluten, juice, and sugar from the diet. Increase mushrooms, herbal teas, and filtered water.
- Consider the following homeopathic medicines: drosera, spongia, ant tart (antimonium tartaricum), phos (phosphorous).
- Do some form of hydrotherapy such as hot and cold showers (see description on page 37) or constitutional hydrotherapy. Try warming socks.

Diarrhea

- Eat light and only to appetite. That is, if you don't have an appetite, don't make yourself eat, but *do* continue drinking water. Make sure to hydrate with a hydration drink and/or a nutritive broth, either a vegetable broth, a meat stock, or the Wellness Broth (see recipe on page 224). The BRAT diet may be helpful: bananas, rice, apples, and toast. I suggest a brown or wild rice and gluten-free toast.
- Consider the following homeopathic medicines: arsenicum, podophyllum.
- Consider the following nutraceuticals: saccharomyces, charcoal capsules.

Fever

- Eat light and only to appetite. That is, if you don't have an appetite, don't make yourself eat, but *do* continue drinking water. Hydrate with a hydration drink and nutritive broth, either a vegetable broth, a meat stock, or the Wellness Broth (see recipe on page 224). Absolutely no dairy, gluten, sugar, or juice.
- Do at least one constitutional hydrotherapy treatment daily, and up to three in a child with a high fever. (Instructions can be found at http://www.naturalopinion.com/nmp/nmp5/Conshydr.htm.) Make sure to get as much sleep as possible, and don't overdo activity during the day when the fever lessens a little. Often it will increase again at night.
- The Mayo clinic says not to treat a fever as long as it stays under 101°F.
- Consider the following homeopathic medicines: belladonna, ferrum phos (ferrum phosphoricum), chamomilia.

Gas, Bloating, or Regular Abdominal Discomfort

- Steam or cook most of your foods, including vegetables and fruits. It is okay to consume melons and avocado raw, but all other foods should be at least lightly steamed.
- Begin a strict anti-inflammation diet for at least one month and then begin introducing foods to see which foods may contribute to gas and bloating.

- Chew your food very well (try to chew at least 19–21 times before swallowing).
- Consider using the following homeopathic medicines: carb veg, lycopodium, colocynthis, mag phos.
- Consider the following teas: Peppermint, fennel, or anise.

Hashimoto's Disease (Thyroiditis) or Graves' Disease

- In addition to following the anti-inflammation diet, eliminate all grains until you can get the thyroid under control. Have your doctor check your TPO (thyroid peroxidase) levels before and after grain elimination so you can see the result improve. Avoid raw goitrogens, foods that suppress thyroid functioning, resulting in a goiter (enlarged thyroid).
- Exercise as much as you are able.
- Get proper sleep, and take your thyroid hormones at the same time each day if you currently have a prescription. Don't take your thyroid hormone with any other foods, especially calcium-containing foods.
- Consider taking selenium and other antioxidants.
- Treat the adrenal glands by taking Tranquility and Strength by Herb Fusion (see Resources).

Heart Disease or Diabetes

- Stick to the anti-inflammation diet strictly. Absolutely no fried foods and no fast foods. Avoid eating out as much as possible. Stick to the basics of a very clean diet. Don't consume sugars or any sugar substitutes.
- Exercise every day. Keep yourself moving. If you aren't physically fit, hire a trainer to come up with a program designed specifically for you.
- Take high-dose fish oil. For diabetes, add chromium picolinate, alpha-lipoic acid, and cinnamon supplements.

Heartburn

- Eliminate tomatoes, caffeine, chocolate, wine or other alcohol, and spicy foods.
- Do heel drops every day first thing in the morning. To do heel drops, drink 10 ounces of water on an empty stomach and rise onto heels; drop down with some force onto the heels. Repeat this sequence of rising onto toes and dropping back onto heels 10 times. Make sure you are not using enough force to cause any pain elsewhere in the body.
- Don't eat late at night.

- Take baking soda before bed at night: ¼ teaspoon in a little bit of water can reduce symptoms dramatically.
- Consider the following homeopathic medicines: nux vomica, carbo veg.

Inflammatory Bowel Disease

- Eliminate all grains from the diet. Be strict with elimination of gluten and dairy.
- It is also helpful to steam or cook all foods during any flare-ups.
- Exercise to build strength and muscle mass.
- Take probiotics such as Restore from Herb Fusion (see Resources).
- Include ginger and turmeric daily to decrease inflammation.
- Use digestive enzymes to aid digestion.

Muscle Spasm, Muscle Twitching, or Muscle Pains

- Begin anti-inflammation diet and do an elimination diet and a reintroduction diet to see if there are foods that specifically cause the pain. (See my previous book, *The Anti-Inflammation Diet and Recipe Book*, for more discussion on this subject.)
- Use magnesium either in topical form or in oral form daily. My favorite form that is digested and absorbed well is aspartate. Try Tranquility from Herb Fusion (see Resources).
- Try getting regular massages, being careful not to get massaged too deeply. You're looking for effleurage and movement of lymphatic vessels.
- Do dry skin brushing (see description on page 54) nightly before bed, and take hot and cold showers (see description on page 54) every morning.
- In a pinch, some of my patients have sworn by drinking pickle juice!
- Consider the following homeopathic medicine: mag phos (magnesia phosphorica).

Psoriasis and Eczema

- Stick to the anti-inflammation diet, and consider doing an elimination and challenge diet. Consider eliminating all eggs for four weeks and reintroducing them to see if they cause problems. Skin issues sometimes are related to egg intolerance.
- Make sure to sweat regularly through exercise or saunas.
- Drink plenty of filtered water, at least half your body weight in ounces daily.
- Take zinc and B vitamins and a good probiotic such as Advanced BM, from Herb Fusion (see Resources).

- For psoriasis, avoid all echinacea, vitamin C, and ginsengs.
- Take high-dosage, high-quality fish oil.

Vomiting

- Eat light and only to appetite. That is, if you don't have an appetite, don't make yourself eat, but *do* continue drinking water. Make sure to hydrate with a hydration drink and/or a nutritive broth, either a vegetable broth, a meat stock, or the Wellness Broth (see recipe on page 224).
- Consider the following homeopathic medicines: ipecac, nux vomica, colchicum.

Substitutions Chart

Use this chart to help you modify favorite recipes to meet the anti-inflammation diet (AI diet). Because some people may need or want to avoid eggs, egg substitutions are included even though eggs are generally allowed on the AI diet. Baking with gluten-free flours can sometimes present challenges in terms of creating satisfactory taste and texture. I find that blending different kinds of flour helps significantly with the taste. Utilizing flours that have natural binding capability, such as tapioca and arrowroot, has generally increased my success in gluten-free baking.

Eliminated Food	Substitution	Directions
Butter	Blend of organic butter and olive oil (use as a spread) Blend of organic butter and coconut oil (use for baking) Nonhydrogenated vegan spread	Substitute equal quantities
Chocolate	Carob powder is nutritionally superior to chocolate	Substitute 3 tablespoons for 1 ounce chocolate
	Unsweetened carob chips	Substitute equal quantities
Commercial eggs	Organic eggs are fine for some individuals. Or you can experiment with the following binders:	
	Flax seeds soaked overnight in water or boiled for 15 minutes	1–2 tablespoons seeds in ½–1 cup of water
	Soft tofu, for scrambles or baked goods	¼ cup in place of 1 egg
	Banana, to bind baked goods (adds a sweet taste)	½–1 banana in cookies or muffins
	Arrowroot powder (use as a binder for nongluten flours)	1 tablespoon for each cup of nongluten flour
	Guar gum (you need only a very small amount)	¼–½ teaspoon for muffins, breads, and other baked goods

Eliminated Food	Substitution	Directions
Commercial eggs	Xantham gum	1 teaspoon for each cup of nongluten flour
Cow's milk	Hemp milk, rice milk, sesame seed milk, almond milk (or other nut milk), oat milk, coconut milk	Substitute equal quantities
Peanuts, peanut butter	Almonds, almond butter, sunflower butter	Substitute equal quantities
Potatoes	Yucca root, taro root, Jerusalem artichokes (sunchokes)	Cook similar to potatoes
Sugar	Honey (twice as sweet as processed cane sugar)	1 teaspoon for each cup of nongluten flour
	Pure maple syrup	½ amount called for in recipe
	Brown rice syrup	½–¾ amount called for in recipe
	Stevia	Extremely small amount needed for adding sweetness
Wheat flour	When substituting these flours, you may want to add a little more baking powder or baking soda to help the baked goods rise. Use a blend of at least 2 different flours.	
	Almond meal	May need a binder (see above)
	Amaranth (can have a strong taste)	Needs a binder (see above) Use up to 25% in a blend
	Arrowroot powder	Acts as a binder Use up to 25% in a blend
	Buckwheat	Needs a binder
	Coconut flour	Needs a binder
	Garbanzo	Needs a binder Use up to 25% in a blend
	Millet	Needs a binder Use up to 50% in a blend
	Oat (made from gluten-free oats)	May need a binder
	Quinoa (can taste bitter; should be mixed with other flours)	Needs a binder Use up to 33% in a blend

(cont'd.)

Substitutions Chart (cont'd.)

Eliminated Food	Substitution	Directions
Wheat flour	Rice (can be grainy; mix with other flours)	Needs a binder Use up to 33% in a blend
	Sorghum	Needs a binder Use up to 25% in a blend
	Soy (can have a beany flavor)	Needs a binder Use up to 25% in a blend
	Tapioca flour	Should be mixed with other flours Acts as a binder Use up to 50% in a blend
	Teff	Needs a binder Use up to 75% in a blend

Solid Food Introduction Chart

To help ensure proper gastrointestinal health, timely food introduction is vital for babies and toddlers. Introducing foods too young can lead to allergies and other problems. Introduce foods slowly and carefully, and pay close attention to potential reactions. For example, if you introduce squash and your baby develops cradle cap within a couple of days, then most likely the baby isn't yet ready for squash. It is important to steam or cook most foods before introducing them. Acceptable raw foods are noted in the chart that spans the following two pages; if the food in question is not listed, steam and purée it before serving it to your baby. As children get older, they will be able tolerate more raw foods. Refer to Chapter 4 for more information regarding food choices for infants and children.

The chart on pages 280–281 is meant to be read across both pages; a single page version can be downloaded from hunterhouse.com on the page for this book.

	Vegetables	Fruits	Grains	Meat/Protein Foods
0–3 Months	None	None	None	None
3–6 Months	None	None	None	None
6 Months	Sweet potato, squash, peas, pumpkin—start with vegetables before fruits	Avocado, banana are okay raw. Apricot, nectarines, peaches, pears, plums	None	None
7 Months	Zucchini, yellow squash	Mango, pear, papaya are okay raw	None	None
8 Months	Asparagus, carrots, green beans	Nectarines, peaches, pears, plums are okay raw Apples	Rice cereal Homemade porridge—with rice, oat, quinoa, millet	None
9 Months	Broccoli, parsley, okra	Apricot, apple, cantaloupe, honeydew, kiwi, plums, watermelon, peeled and cut grapes are all okay raw	Barley added to porridge, oatmeal	Tahini, ground nuts/seeds, organic chicken and turkey Wild salmon
10 Months	Cauliflower, snow peas, spinach, brussels sprouts, kale, rutabaga, turnips, ground sprouts	Coconut milk is okay raw. Rhubarb		Beans: pinto, black, white, navy, split peas, lentils, tofu (watch for reaction)
11 Months	Artichokes, beets, corn, cucumbers, onions, green and sweet peppers	Dates, pineapple, prunes are okay raw	Brown rice and other whole grains	Organic lean lamb, buffalo, thinned nut butters—not peanut butter
12–18 Months	Eggplant, white potatoes—introduce slowly	Berries, cherries, citrus fruits, tomatoes are okay raw	Wheat—introduce and wait 4 days	Organic lean beef
18–24 Months			Continue whole-grain porridge	
2–3 Years				

Eggs and Dairy	Nutritional Enhancers	Fluids	Misc.
None—unless using dairy formula	None	Only breast milk (BM) or formula	Establish regular routine and provide tender loving care
None	None	BM or formula. Begin introducing water at 4 months	Routine and TLC
None	None	BM or formula and water. Let baby take small sips of water from your cup	Begin introduction with 1 food at a time; wait 4 days for reaction.
None	None	BM or formula. Let baby try to hold small cup of water	Continue to introduce, always doing so slowly
Hard- or soft-boiled egg yolk	None	BM or formula and water	Let baby practice feeding self with spoon and finger foods. Continue introducing foods one at a time
Hard- or soft-boiled egg yolk	Brewer's yeast, powdered kelp, spirulina—sooner if iron deficient	BM or formula and water	Consistency of foods should begin to be thicker with small chunks
Hard- or soft-boiled egg yolk		BM or formula and water	Continue self-spoon feeding practice
Organic yogurt, cottage cheese, hard cheeses		BM or formula and water	
Organic whole milk, egg whites—introduce and wait 4 days	Wheat germ, honey	BM or formula as needed and water	A 1-year-old can eat one thing at a time placed on their plate
		BM or formula as needed	A 2-year-old can eat 2 things at a time
		BM or formula as needed	A 3-year-old can eat 3 things at a time

Resources

Online Resources

Dr. Jessica Black—www.drjessicablack.com
The author's website offers health tips, cooking tips, and weekly menu planners that can be e-mailed directly to you. It also includes a blog dedicated to exploring ideas for following an anti-inflammation diet and lifestyle.

A Family Healing Center—www.afamilyhealingcenter.com
The website of Drs. Jason and Jessica Black's naturopathic medical clinic.

ABC Homeopathy—www.abchomeopathy.com
Visit this site to learn about homoeopathy. It also helps you choose medicines on your own.

American Association of Naturopathic Physicians—
www.naturopathic.org
The official site for the national organization of naturopathic physicians. It offers useful information about naturopathy and will help you find doctors in your area.

Azure Standard—www.azurestandard.com
At this website you can order many bulk and natural foods at lower prices than if you were to purchase them in stores. It requires a minimum order, but you can join others in your area to collectively place orders.

Bastyr University—www.bastyr.edu
Naturopathic medical school located in Seattle, Washington.

The Center for Food Safety: The True Food Network—
www.truefoodnow.org
A resource on current eating trends and how to embrace healthier dietary habits.

Centers for Disease Control and Prevention—www.cdc.gov
Offers information about diseases, disease prevalence, acute disease outbreaks, vaccinations, and much more.

The Chopra Center—www.chopra.com
A site for learning how to balance body, mind, and spirit.

Coconut Research Center—www.coconutresearchcenter.com
Information on coconut.

Eating with Purpose—www.eatingwithpurpose.com
Real-life solutions to eating real food.

Elana's Pantry—www.elanaspantry.com
Gluten-free recipes.

Environmental Protection Agency—www.epa.gov
Offers current advice relating to foods, environmental concerns, and much
more. The mission of this governmental agency is to protect human health
and the environment.

Environmental Working Group—www.ewg.org
Wonderful site on environmental toxins: how they are present in our surroundings, and what you can do to limit exposure.

Fly Lady—www.flylady.net
A site for helping women to stop procrastinating and create better lifestyle
habits.

GAPS Diet—www.gapsdiet.com
Information about the GAPS (Gut and Psychology Syndrome) diet. Includes
recipes.

Glycemic Index—www.glycemicindex.com
An easy way to look up the glycemic index of foods. This website can help you
choose foods with lower GIs that will make you feel more full and help you to
control your appetite better.

Herb Fusion, LLC—www.herb-fusion.com
Offers physician-designed herbal products for energy, sleep, stress, and general
health. Dr. Black and her husband have developed these products based on
their years of experience treating patients in their clinic.

Keeper of the Home—www.keeperofthehome.org
Great GAPS ideas and recipes.

Kelly Mom—www.kellymom.com
Great site offering tips on breastfeeding and parenting.

Know the Cause—www.knowthecause.com
Information on potential causes of health problems.

Livestrong—www.livestrong.org
This website will soon become a favorite. It provides reliable, up-to-date, re-searched health information on almost anything you have questions about.

Mayo Clinic—www.mayoclinic.com
A site to help you learn more about various conditions and the current allo-pathic approach to treating them. The site even supplies some information regarding natural treatments.

Mothering Magazine—www.mothering.com
This is a great site that helps people connect with similar interests when it comes to raising children. People share information and even kefir grains and kombucha scobies through this network.

National College of Naturopathic Medicine—www.ncnm.edu
Naturopathic medical school located in Portland, Oregon, and the school from which the author and her husband graduated.

National Library of Medicine—www.nlm.nih.gov
Operated by the federal government, this is the premier library of health information. Use it to access articles, journals, and other health resources for specific information.

North Carolina State University—
http://www.ces.ncsu.edu/depts/foodsci/ext/pubs/497-05.pdf
Food safety sheet on fermenting and pickling foods.

Nourishing Days—www.nourishingdays.com
Great recipes and some information on fermenting.

Oregon Association of Naturopathic Physicians—www.oanp.org
Oregon's state organization for naturopathic physicians. Can help you locate a physician in your area of the state.

Helpful Books

Black, Jessica. *The Anti-Inflammation Diet and Recipe Book: Protect Yourself and Your Family from Heart Disease, Arthritis, Diabetes, Allergies—and More.* Alameda, CA: Hunter House, 2005.

Black, Jessica, and Dede Cummings. *Living with Crohn's and Colitis: A Comprehensive Naturopathic Guide for Complete Digestive Wellness.* Long Island City, NY: Hatherleigh Press, 2010.

Brantley, Jeffrey. *Calming Your Anxious Mind: How Mindfulness and Compassion Can Free You from Anxiety, Fear, and Panic.* Oakland, CA: New Harbinger Publications, 2003. This book offers concrete suggestions on how to begin a meditation practice and break the habitual thinking that can lead to anxieties.

Eden, Donna. *Energy Medicine: Balancing Your Body's Energies for Optimal Health, Joy, and Vitality.* New York: Tarcher, 2008. An excellent book that offers many ideas on daily tapping routines to increase the flow of energy in the body and to help make healing possible.

Fallon, Sally. *Nourishing Traditions: The Cookbook That Challenges Politically Correct Nutrition and the Diet Dictocrats.* Warsaw, IN: New Trends Publishing, 1999. A great cookbook and an excellent resource for making fermented foods.

Gates, Donna, and Linda Schatz. *The Body Ecology Diet: Recovering Your Health and Rebuilding Your Immunity.* Carlsbad, CA: Body Ecology, 2006. Discusses increasing gastrointestinal resistance and overall health through the use of probiotics.

Gottschall, Elaine Gloria. *Breaking the Vicious Cycle: Intestinal Health Through Diet.* Baltimore, Ontario, Canada: Kirkton Press, 1994. Investigates the link between food and intestinal disorders such as Crohn's disease, ulcerative colitis, diverticulitis, celiac disease, cystic fibrosis, and chronic diarrhea.

Kamm, Laura Alden. *Intuitive Wellness: Using Your Body's Inner Wisdom to Heal.* New York: Atria Books/Beyond Words, 2006. A remarkable memoir about Kamm's health journey.

Kinderlehrer, Jane. *Confessions of a Sneaky Organic Cook, or How to Make Your Family Healthy When They're Not Looking!* New York: New American Library, 1972. Although older, this book contains many good ideas. You can probably find an inexpensive used copy online.

Lair, Cynthia. *Feeding the Whole Family: Cooking with Whole Foods.* Seattle, WA: Sasquatch Books, 2008. This fun book provides many ideas for quick family meals.

Lipton, Bruce H. *The Biology of Belief: Unleashing the Power of Consciousness, Matter and Miracles.* Carlsbad, CA: Hay House, 2008. A great book on how emotions and thoughts can control your destiny.

Remen, Rachel Naomi. *Kitchen Table Wisdom: Stories that Heal.* New York: Riverhead Trade Books, 1997. Remen is one of a growing number of physicians exploring the spiritual dimension of the healing arts.

Santorelli, Saki. *Heal Thy Self: Lessons on Mindfulness in Medicine.* New York: Three Rivers Press, 2000. Santorelli, director of the Stress Reduction Clinic at the University of Massachusetts Medical Center, offers a collection of inspirational essays and meditations he uses in his eight-week course on mindful awareness, available to both healing professionals and patients.

Index

Boldface page numbers refer to recipes.